Oxidative Stress and Inflammation: From Mechanisms to Therapeutic Approaches

Oxidative Stress and Inflammation: From Mechanisms to Therapeutic Approaches

Editor

Juan Gambini

MDPI • Basel • Beijing • Wuhan • Barcelona • Belgrade • Manchester • Tokyo • Cluj • Tianjin

MDPI

Editor
Juan Gambini
University of Valencia
Spain

Editorial Office
MDPI
St. Alban-Anlage 66
4052 Basel, Switzerland

This is a reprint of articles from the Special Issue published online in the open access journal *Biomedicines* (ISSN 2227-9059) (available at: https://www.mdpi.com/journal/biomedicines/special_issues/oxidative_stress_inflammation_mechanisms_therapeutic).

For citation purposes, cite each article independently as indicated on the article page online and as indicated below:

LastName, A.A.; LastName, B.B.; LastName, C.C. Article Title. *Journal Name* **Year**, *Volume Number*, Page Range.

ISBN 978-3-0365-6023-6 (Hbk)
ISBN 978-3-0365-6024-3 (PDF)

Contents

Juan Gambini and Kristine Stromsnes
Oxidative Stress and Inflammation: From Mechanisms to Therapeutic Approaches
Reprinted from: *Biomedicines* **2022**, *10*, 753, doi:10.3390/biomedicines10040753 1

Daniele La Russa, Alessandro Marrone, Maurizio Mandalà, Rachele Macirella and Daniela Pellegrino
Antioxidant/Anti-Inflammatory Effects of Caloric Restriction in an Aged and Obese Rat Model: The Role of Adiponectin
Reprinted from: *Biomedicines* **2020**, *8*, 532, doi:10.3390/biomedicines8120532 7

Heba Al Housseiny, Madhu Singh, Shaneeka Emile, Marvin Nicoleau, Randy L. Vander Wal and Patricia Silveyra
Identification of Toxicity Parameters Associated with Combustion Produced Soot Surface Chemistry and Particle Structure by In Vitro Assays
Reprinted from: *Biomedicines* **2020**, *8*, 345, doi:10.3390/biomedicines8090345 17

Dmitry V. Chistyakov, Olga S. Gancharova, Viktoriia E. Baksheeva, Veronika V. Tiulina, Sergei V. Goriainov, Nadezhda V. Azbukina, Marina S. Tsarkova, Andrey A. Zamyatnin Jr., Pavel P. Philippov, Marina G. Sergeeva, Ivan I. Senin and Evgeni Yu. Zernii
Inflammation in Dry Eye Syndrome: Identification and Targeting of Oxylipin-Mediated Mechanisms
Reprinted from: *Biomedicines* **2020**, *8*, 344, doi:10.3390/biomedicines8090344 35

Laura Bordoni, Donatella Fedeli, Marco Piangerelli, Iwona Pelikant-Malecka, Adrianna Radulska, Joanna J. Samulak, Angelika K. Sawicka, Lukasz Lewicki, Leszek Kalinowski, Robert A. Olek and Rosita Gabbianelli
Gender-Related Differences in Trimethylamine and Oxidative Blood Biomarkers in Cardiovascular Disease Patients
Reprinted from: *Biomedicines* **2020**, *8*, 238, doi:10.3390/biomedicines8080238 57

Sihui Ma, Takaki Tominaga, Kazue Kanda, Kaoru Sugama, Chiaki Omae, Shunsuke Hashimoto, Katsuhiko Aoyama, Yasunobu Yoshikai and Katsuhiko Suzuki
Effects of an 8-Week Protein Supplementation Regimen with Hyperimmunized Cow Milk on Exercise-Induced Organ Damage and Inflammation in Male Runners: A Randomized, Placebo Controlled, Cross-Over Study
Reprinted from: *Biomedicines* **2020**, *8*, 51, doi:10.3390/biomedicines8030051 71

Isabelle Guinobert, Claude Blondeau, Bruno Colicchio, Noufissa Oudrhiri, Alain Dieterlen, Eric Jeandidier, Georges Deschenes, Valérie Bardot, César Cotte, Isabelle Ripoche, Patrice Carde, Lucile Berthomier and Radhia M'Kacher
The Use of Natural Agents to Counteract Telomere Shortening: Effects of a Multi-Component Extract of *Astragalus mongholicus* Bunge and Danazol
Reprinted from: *Biomedicines* **2020**, *8*, 31, doi:10.3390/biomedicines8020031 89

Adnan Shahidullah, Ji-Young Lee, Young-Jin Kim, Syed Muhammad Ashhad Halimi, Abdur Rauf, Hyun-Ju Kim, Bong-Youn Kim and Wansu Park
Anti-Inflammatory Effects of Diospyrin on Lipopolysaccharide-Induced Inflammation Using RAW 264.7 Mouse Macrophages
Reprinted from: *Biomedicines* **2020**, *8*, 11, doi:10.3390/biomedicines8010011 103

Taurean Brown, DeLawrence Sykes and Antiño R. Allen
Implications of Breast Cancer Chemotherapy-Induced Inflammation on the Gut, Liver, and Central Nervous System
Reprinted from: *Biomedicines* **2021**, *9*, 189, doi:10.3390/biomedicines9020189 . . . . **113**

Spyridon Methenitis, Ioanna Stergiou, Smaragdi Antonopoulou and Tzortzis Nomikos
Can Exercise-Induced Muscle Damage Be a Good Model for the Investigation of the Anti-Inflammatory Properties of Diet in Humans?
Reprinted from: *Biomedicines* **2021**, *9*, 36, doi:10.3390/biomedicines9010036 . . . . **129**

Tamotsu Tsukahara, Hisao Haniu, Takeshi Uemura and Yoshikazu Matsuda
Therapeutic Potential of Porcine Liver Decomposition Product: New Insights and Perspectives for Microglia-Mediated Neuroinflammation in Neurodegenerative Diseases
Reprinted from: *Biomedicines* **2020**, *8*, 446, doi:10.3390/biomedicines8110446 . . . . **149**

Francesca Oppedisano, Roberta Macrì, Micaela Gliozzi, Vincenzo Musolino, Cristina Carresi, Jessica Maiuolo, Francesca Bosco, Saverio Nucera, Maria Caterina Zito, Lorenza Guarnieri, Federica Scarano, Caterina Nicita, Anna Rita Coppoletta, Stefano Ruga, Miriam Scicchitano, Rocco Mollace, Ernesto Palma and Vincenzo Mollace
The Anti-Inflammatory and Antioxidant Properties of n-3 PUFAs: Their Role in Cardiovascular Protection
Reprinted from: *Biomedicines* **2020**, *8*, 306, doi:10.3390/biomedicines8090306 . . . . **163**

Elisa Sanchez-Morate, Lucia Gimeno-Mallench, Kristine Stromsnes, Jorge Sanz-Ros, Aurora Román-Domínguez, Sergi Parejo-Pedrajas, Marta Inglés, Gloria Olaso, Juan Gambini and Cristina Mas-Bargues
Relationship between Diet, Microbiota, and Healthy Aging
Reprinted from: *Biomedicines* **2020**, *8*, 287, doi:10.3390/biomedicines8080287 . . . . **181**

Chuan-Mu Chen, Hsiao-Ching Lu, Yu-Tang Tung and Wei Chen
Antiplatelet Therapy for Acute Respiratory Distress Syndrome
Reprinted from: *Biomedicines* **2020**, *8*, 230, doi:10.3390/biomedicines8070230 . . . . **195**

Keiichiro Matoba, Yusuke Takeda, Yosuke Nagai, Tamotsu Yokota, Kazunori Utsunomiya and Rimei Nishimura
Targeting Redox Imbalance as an Approach for Diabetic Kidney Disease
Reprinted from: *Biomedicines* **2020**, *8*, 40, doi:10.3390/biomedicines8020040 . . . . **213**

biomedicines

MDPI

Editorial

Oxidative Stress and Inflammation: From Mechanisms to Therapeutic Approaches

Juan Gambini * and Kristine Stromsnes

Freshage Research Group, Department of Physiology, Faculty of Medicine, Insitute of Health Research-INCLIVA, University of Valencia and CIBERFES, Avda. Blasco Ibañez, 15, 46010 Valencia, Spain; kristine.stromsnes@uv.es
* Correspondence: juan.gambini@uv.es

Oxidative stress and inflammation are two phenomena that are directly involved in practically all pathologies and especially in aging. Oxidative stress, which is associated with the redox state, constitutes an important mechanism in many physiological processes, such as adaptations to physical exercise, cell signaling, and hypothalamic appetite regulation. Inflammatory mediators are known to be essential in mechanisms such as the generation of gastric mucus for the protection of the stomach and for the repair of tissues via the mobilization of stem cells. However, when these two phenomena are deregulated, their actions are harmful. In this Special Issue, we ask ourselves several questions: How and when should we allow or block oxidative stress and inflammation? What is the advisable dose of antioxidant or anti-inflammatory therapy associated with aging? Are diet, physical exercise, and decreased psychological stress the best therapies for oxidative stress and inflammation control? In this Special Issue, we have published 14 articles: 7 original research articles and 7 reviews. They describe everything from the inflammatory and oxidative processes involved in different diseases to functional foods containing molecules that counteract these phenomena.

In order to reflect upon the comments made in this Special Issue in a coherent way, the publications have been divided into two sections that we will comment on below.

Environmental pollution has become a major public health risk in recent decades, causing millions of deaths worldwide. Among pollutants, we find harmful or harmful components that can be both physical, chemical, and biological. Identifying these compounds is the starting point to combat them.

In their original research article, Heba Al Housseiny et al. [1] have identified and reflected how the exposure of a product called PM2.5, which is derived from the combustion of matter, is associated with a decrease in lung function, impaired immunity, and exacerbations in lung disease. Their results show how these particles are capable of reducing cell viability and increasing the inflammatory parameters and oxidative stress in lung epithelial cells. These data suggest that effective mitigation strategies are necessary to address not only the identification of polluting particles but also their possible neutralization and treatments that avoid their toxicity [1].

Acute respiratory distress syndrome is one of the pathologies of the respiratory system. This condition presents with the acute onset of respiratory failure that leads to bilateral pulmonary infiltrates seen on chest radiographs, hypoxemia, etc., and that can result in direct lung lesions, pneumonia, sepsis, and even death. Globally, it has an incidence of around 15 to 80/100,000 inhabitants per year, and so far, no beneficial drug therapy has been developed; however, it has been found that platelets play a fundamental role in this disease. Therefore, Chuan-Mu Chen et al. [2] describe studies that show the possible benefits of antiplatelet therapy for prevention and treatment via the control of platelet activity and describe the mechanisms of action that are involved.

Dry eye syndrome affects approximately 40% of the adult population. It manifests as hyperemia, glare, fatigue, and eye irritation. The most critical consequences of this

Citation: Gambini, J.; Stromsnes, K. Oxidative Stress and Inflammation: From Mechanisms to Therapeutic Approaches. *Biomedicines* **2022**, *10*, 753. https://doi.org/10.3390/biomedicines10040753

Received: 22 February 2022
Accepted: 11 March 2022
Published: 23 March 2022

desiccant stress are inflammation and damage to the ocular surface, which, in severe cases, can lead to blindness, scarring, opacification or ulceration of the cornea, and blurred vision. Treatments for this condition include lubricating drops, anti-inflammatory therapy, or immunosuppressants such as cyclosporine. However, all of these treatments can cause adverse effects that limit their use. For this reason, in their original article, Dmitry V. Chistyakov et al. [3] have tested a therapy with a new ophthalmic formulation containing a zileuton solution based on dimethylsulfoxide. Their results showed the high efficacy of the proposed therapy. On the one hand, DMSO decreased the activity of pro-inflammatory protagladins, and on the other hand, zileuton decreased the cytokine levels released by T cells. In this way, the two compounds presented synergistic activity that opens the door to more effective anti-inflammatory therapies against said pathology [3].

Gender differences in cardiovascular diseases (CVD) as well as the identification of biomarkers for disease detection are challenges that are of great importance today. In the original study by Laura Bordoni et al. [4], they recruited 547 individuals comprising both men and women with or without cardiovascular disease to identify useful biomarkers to characterize gender differences in CVD. The study evaluated blood parameters such as plasma membrane fluidity, erythrocyte lipid hydroperoxides, and trimethylamine (TMA). Lower plasmatic TMA was observed in male CVD patients compared to in the healthy male controls, while higher levels of TMA were measured in female CVD patients with respect to the female controls. Diphenyl−1-pyrenylphosphine (DPPP) was significantly lower in male CVD patients compared to in the healthy controls, while no significant changes were measured in females with or without CVD. The results obtained allowed Laura Bordoni et al. to conclude that TMA could be an effective marker for the detection and prevention of CVD and that the DPPP value could be predictive biomarker of CVD in men [4].

Breast cancer remains as one of the most common cancers today. As advances in diagnostic and treatment methods continue to become more effective, the survival rate continues to increase. However, the chemotherapy that is administered, although effective, still presents important adverse reactions, such as difficulty concentrating and remembering or alterations in processing speed. Patients may also experience symptoms of gastrointestinal (GI) issues, such as diarrhea and vomiting as well as long-term hepatotoxicity or liver damage. In their review, Taurean Brown et al. [5] describe how the series of symptoms experienced by cancer patients are interconnected and mediated by inflammatory responses. Therefore, new therapeutic approaches could help improve the quality of life in breast cancer patients after treatment [5].

Protecting the kidneys is essential in the management of diabetes-derived problems. There is good evidence to illustrate the causal link between oxidative stress and the progression of diabetes-related kidney disease (DKD). Currently, the only therapeutic options that are for DKD are limited to systemic interventions for the metabolic changes related to diabetes, such as dyslipidemia, hypertension, and hyperglycemia. Given the important role that oxidative stress plays in various aspects of kidney injury, the redox imbalance could be considered to be potential therapeutic target for renal failure in diabetic patients. This review article written by Keiichiro Matoba et al. [6] shows recent therapeutic approaches to prevent DKD by targeting the antioxidant effects of newly developed antihyperglycemic agents.

In their review, Spyridon Methenitis et al. [7] discuss the possibility of exercise-induced muscle damage being a suitable model of inflammation for the evaluation of nutraceutical anti-inflammatory properties. Low-grade, subclinical inflammation is one of the main pathophysiological mechanisms underlying most chronic and non-communicable diseases. In this sense, the use of functional foods, those with bioactive compounds and, in this case, with an anti-inflammatory capacity, could be a model to take into consideration in humans. The capacity of these compounds could be highly valued since it is known that bioavailability is a key point in their effectiveness [7].

Compounds with pharmacological activities with the possibility of having great therapeutic power have been found in nature.

Telomere shortening and oxidative stress have been linked to aging and patients with cancer and inflammatory diseases. In 2016, the *New England Journal of Medicine* published an article showing how danazol, a synthetic androgen, promotes telomere lengthening in circulating human leukocytes, comparing its effects to a hydroethanolic root extract that is known to stimulate telomerase activity. These findings open the door for treatments for associated diseases, telomeres, or aging. In this Special Issue, Isabelle Guinobert et al. [8] show how danazol, similar to extracts from the Astragalus mongholicus plant, has positive effects on telomerase-dependent telomere lengthening in human lymphocytes in their review. These findings create possibilities for new treatments for diseases that are associated with aging [8].

Diospirin is a medicinal compound derived from the Diospyros lotus, which has anticancer, antituberculous, and antileishmanial activities against Leishmania donovani. Adnan Shahidullah et al. [9] describe a modulatory role in the inflammatory response induced by lipopolysaccharides (LPS) in mouse macrophages through the inhibition of nitric oxide and several cytokines via the ER-stressed calcium-p38 MAPK/CHOP/Fas pathway. These effects have not been shown previously and could have important therapeutic uses [9].

Prolonged strenuous exercise can induce unfavorable biological changes and symptoms, including inflammatory responses that can lead to intestinal barrier dysfunction. Many athletes use non-steroidal anti-inflammatory drugs to treat inflammation-induced algesthesia. Sihui Ma et al. [10] have verified how hyperimmunized milk supplementation, obtained after immunizing cows against specific antigens, protects intestinal function, exerts anti-inflammatory effects, and promotes the development of immunity against various pathogens. This could be a viable nutritional approach for preventing intense exercise-induced symptoms.

Caloric restriction has been shown to be a powerful intervention to extend both lifespan and health span in various animal models, from yeast to primates. Furthermore, in humans, caloric restriction has been found to induce cardiometabolic adaptations that are associated with better health. Daniele La Russa et al. [11] studied the long-term effects of caloric restrictions on the inflammatory and redox balance in aged, obese rats. They found that caloric restriction not only induces weight loss but also positively modulates both the anti-inflammatory and antioxidant pathways while also improving the circulating adiponectin levels in obese old rats. Along with achieving normal weight, these adaptations, which are induced by caloric restriction, suggest that the redox and inflammatory imbalance in obese aged rats appears to be caused by obesity rather than by aging [11].

Microglia play an important role in the development of neurodegenerative diseases, but the mechanisms of action have yet to be specified. When activated, they can express pro-inflammatory cytokines that act on the surrounding brain and spinal cord, something that can have a detrimental effect on nerve cells when they acquire a chronic inflammatory function and promote neuropathologies. In their bibliographic review, Tamotsu Tsukahara et al. [12] set out to clarify the mechanism of action by which the porcine liver decomposition product, which is rich in phospholipids, exerts beneficial effects on cognitive functions in healthy humans. The authors propose that this food is function due to its possibility of enhancing visual memory and delay recall as well as to improve Hasegawa's Dementia Scale-Revised scores and the Wechsler Memory Scale in healthy adults and discuss whether it would be convenient to use it in patients with neurodegenerative diseases. Additionally, they reinforce their hypothesis by outlining other recent findings showing the bidirectional interactions between lysophospholipids, microglia, and age-related neurodegenerative diseases [12].

Fatty acids (n-3 PUFA) are long chain polyunsaturated fatty acids that contain 18, 20 or 22 carbon atoms and that exert a multitude of benefits on human health. Specifically, eicosapentaenoic acid (EPA) and docosahexaenoic acid (DHA) have been found to produce both cardioprotective and responses by modulating membrane phospholipids, thereby improving cardiac mitochondrial functions and energy production. Dietary supplementation of n-3 PUFAs has been found to reduce the endothelial cell apoptosis and mitochondrial dysfunction associated with oxidative stress. Additionally, it has the capacity to restore myocardial performance and vascular reactivity by counteracting the release of pro-inflammatory cytokines in vascular tissues and in the myocardium. In their review, Francesca Oppedisano et al. [13] have summarized the molecular mechanisms underlying the antioxidant and anti-inflammatory effects of n-3 PUFAs on vascular and cardiac tissues and their implication in the prevention and treatment of cardiovascular diseases.

Due to medical advances and lifestyle changes, the life expectancy of the population has increased. For this reason, it is important to achieve healthy aging by reducing the risk factors that cause age-related damage and pathologies. Through nutrition, one of the pillars of health, we are able to modify these factors by modulating the intestinal microbiota. In their bibliographic review, Elisa Sanchez-Morate et al. [14] show that diets such as the Mediterranean and Oriental diets exert healthy effects, mainly due to the high consumption of polyphenols and fibers, which interact with the intestinal bacteria, thereby generating beneficial effects on the body. Additionally, the low consumption of fats in these diets favors the state of the microbiota, thereby further contributing to the maintenance of good health [14].

In conclusion, this Special Issue addresses the roles that oxidative stress and inflammation play in different pathologies, such as ophthalmological, respiratory, and cardiovascular diseases as well as in obesity, cancer, and diabetes. In addition, without forgetting that pharmacological treatments are essential for their treatment, it has been revealed how natural products, diets, or certain foods could positively influence action against these diseases.

Author Contributions: Conceptualization, J.G.; software, K.S.; validation, J.G. and K.S.; resources, J.G. and K.S.; writing—original draft preparation, J.G.; writing—review and editing, K.S.; visualization, J.G. and K.S.; supervision, J.G. All authors have read and agreed to the published version of the manuscript.

Conflicts of Interest: The authors declare no conflict of interest.

References

1. Al Housseiny, H.; Singh, M.; Emile, S.; Nicoleau, M.; Wal, R.L.V.; Silveyra, P. Identification of Toxicity Parameters Associated with Combustion Produced Soot Surface Chemistry and Particle Structure by In Vitro Assays. *Biomedicines* **2020**, *8*, 345. [CrossRef] [PubMed]
2. Chen, C.-M.; Lu, H.-C.; Tung, Y.-T.; Chen, W. Antiplatelet Therapy for Acute Respiratory Distress Syndrome. *Biomedicines* **2020**, *8*, 230. [CrossRef] [PubMed]
3. Chistyakov, D.V.; Gancharova, O.S.; Baksheeva, V.E.; Tiulina, V.V.; Goriainov, S.V.; Azbukina, N.V.; Tsarkova, M.S.; Zamyatnin, J.A.A.; Philippov, P.P.; Sergeeva, M.G.; et al. Inflammation in Dry Eye Syndrome: Identification and Targeting of Oxylipin-Mediated Mechanisms. *Biomedicines* **2020**, *8*, 344. [CrossRef] [PubMed]
4. Bordoni, L.; Fedeli, D.; Piangerelli, M.; Pelikant-Malecka, I.; Radulska, A.; Samulak, J.J.; Sawicka, A.K.; Lewicki, L.; Kalinowski, L.; Olek, R.A.; et al. Gender-Related Differences in Trimethylamine and Oxidative Blood Biomarkers in Cardiovascular Disease Patients. *Biomedicines* **2020**, *8*, 238. [CrossRef] [PubMed]
5. Brown, T.; Sykes, D.; Allen, A.R. Implications of Breast Cancer Chemotherapy-Induced Inflammation on the Gut, Liver, and Central Nervous System. *Biomedicines* **2021**, *9*, 189. [CrossRef] [PubMed]
6. Matoba, K.; Takeda, Y.; Nagai, Y.; Yokota, T.; Utsunomiya, K.; Nishimura, R. Targeting Redox Imbalance as an Approach for Diabetic Kidney Disease? *Biomedicines* **2020**, *8*, 40. [CrossRef] [PubMed]
7. Methenitis, S.; Stergiou, I.; Antonopoulou, S.; Nomikos, T. Can Exercise-Induced Muscle Damage Be a Good Model for the Investigation of the Anti-Inflammatory Properties of Diet in Humans? *Biomedicines* **2021**, *9*, 36. [CrossRef] [PubMed]
8. Guinobert, I.; Blondeau, C.; Colicchio, B.; Oudrhiri, N.; Dieterlen, A.; Jeandidier, E.; Deschenes, G.; Bardot, V.; Cotte, C.; Ripoche, I.; et al. The Use of Natural Agents to Counteract Telomere Shortening: Effects of a Multi-Component Extract of *Astragalus mongholicus* Bunge and Danazol. *Biomedicines* **2020**, *8*, 31. [CrossRef] [PubMed]
9. Shahidullah, A.; Lee, J.-Y.; Kim, Y.-J.; Halimi, S.M.A.; Rauf, A.; Kim, H.-J.; Kim, B.-Y.; Park, W. Anti-Inflammatory Effects of Diospyrin on Lipopolysaccharide-Induced Inflammation Using RAW 264.7 Mouse Macrophages. *Biomedicines* **2020**, *8*, 11. [CrossRef] [PubMed]

10. Ma, S.; Tominaga, T.; Kanda, K.; Sugama, K.; Omae, C.; Hashimoto, S.; Aoyama, K.; Yoshikai, Y.; Suzuki, K. Effects of an 8-Week Protein Supplementation Regimen with Hyperimmunized Cow Milk on Exercise-Induced Organ Damage and Inflammation in Male Runners: A Randomized, Placebo Controlled, Cross-Over Study. *Biomedicines* **2020**, *8*, 51. [CrossRef]
11. la Russa, D.; Marrone, A.; Mandalà, M.; Macirella, R.; Pellegrino, D. Antioxidant/Anti-Inflammatory Effects of Caloric Restriction in an Aged and Obese Rat Model: The Role of Adiponectin. *Biomedicines* **2020**, *8*, 532. [CrossRef]
12. Tsukahara, T.; Haniu, H.; Uemura, T.; Matsuda, Y. Therapeutic Potential of Porcine Liver Decomposition Product: New Insights and Perspectives for Microglia-Mediated Neuroinflammation in Neurodegenerative Diseases. *Biomedicines* **2020**, *8*, 446. [CrossRef] [PubMed]
13. Oppedisano, F.; Macrì, R.; Gliozzi, M.; Musolino, V.; Carresi, C.; Maiuolo, J.; Bosco, F.; Nucera, S.; Zito, M.C.; Guarnieri, L.; et al. The Anti-Inflammatory and Antioxidant Properties of n-3 PUFAs: Their Role in Cardiovascular Protection. *Biomedicines* **2020**, *8*, 306. [CrossRef] [PubMed]
14. Sanchez-Morate, E.; Gimeno-Mallench, L.; Stromsnes, K.; Sanz-Ros, J.; Román-Domínguez, A.; Parejo-Pedrajas, S.; Inglés, M.; Olaso, G.; Gambini, J.; Mas-Bargues, C. Relationship between Diet, Microbiota, and Healthy Aging. *Biomedicines* **2020**, *8*, 287. [CrossRef] [PubMed]

biomedicines

MDPI

Article

Antioxidant/Anti-Inflammatory Effects of Caloric Restriction in an Aged and Obese Rat Model: The Role of Adiponectin

Daniele La Russa [1,2,*], Alessandro Marrone [2,3], Maurizio Mandalà [3], Rachele Macirella [3] and Daniela Pellegrino [2,3,*]

1 Department of Pharmacy, Health and Nutritional Sciences, University of Calabria, 87036 Rende, Italy
2 LARSO (Analysis and Research on Oxidative Stress Laboratory), University of Calabria, 87036 Rende, Italy; alessandro.marrone@unical.it
3 Department of Biology, Ecology and Earth Sciences, University of Calabria, 87036 Rende, Italy; m.mandala@unical.it (M.M.); rachele.macirella@unical.it (R.M.)
* Correspondence: daniele.larussa@unical.it (D.L.R.); danielapellegrino@unical.it (D.P.)

Received: 31 October 2020; Accepted: 23 November 2020; Published: 25 November 2020

Abstract: Caloric restriction (CR) represents a powerful intervention for extending healthspan and lifespan in several animal models, from yeast to primates. Additionally, in humans, CR has been found to induce cardiometabolic adaptations associated with improved health. In this study, we evaluated in an aged and obese rat model the effect of long-term (6 months) caloric restriction (−40%) on the oxidative/inflammatory balance in order to investigate the underlining mechanisms. In plasma, we analyzed the oxidative balance by photometric tests and the adiponectin/tumor necrosis factor-α-induced gene/protein 6 (TSG-6) levels by Western blot analysis. In the white adipose tissue, we examined the protein levels of AdipoR1, pAMPK, NFκB, NRF-2, and glutathione S-tranferase P1 by Western blot analysis. Our results clearly showed that caloric restriction significantly improves the plasmatic oxidative/inflammatory balance in parallel with a major increase in circulating adiponectin levels. Additionally, at the level of adipose tissue, we found a positive modulation of both anti-inflammatory and antioxidant pathways. These adaptations, induced by caloric restriction, with the achievement of normal weight, suggest that inflammatory and redox imbalance in obese aged rats appear to be more linked to obesity than to aging.

Keywords: caloric restriction; inflammation; oxidative balance; adiponectin; plasma; white adipose tissue

1. Introduction

Obesity prevalence is constantly growing worldwide in all age groups and represents a serious publichealth problem, given its close correlation with several chronic diseases [1,2]. Obesity is not always the result of an excessive intake of food and/or lack of physical activity, but it is also favored by other factors (stress, drugs, or hormonal metabolic alterations) that alter the physiological mechanisms capable of regulating the supply of energy in relation to consumption, as happens, for example, with advancing age. In particular, the age-related changes in body fat distribution (increase in abdominal obesity) and metabolism (insulin resistance and metabolic syndrome) represent key factors in a vicious cycle that can accelerate the aging process itself and the progression of age-related diseases [3,4]. Lines of evidence from several studies have shown that obesity adversely affects health status and life span through cellular processes in a manner similar to aging [3,4].

Aging is a complex, multifactorial process driven by both intrinsic (genetic) and extrinsic (environmental) factors. The aging process is linked to homeostasis deterioration characterized by an alteration of both oxidative and inflammatory states. The free radical theory of aging has been proposed since 1956 and highlights how the accumulation of oxidized biomolecules during chronic oxidative stress is the basis of the age-related structural and functional alterations of all types of cells [5,6]. Over the past decades, the close link between free radicals and aging has found corroboration in several studies [7–9], although some published papers appear to contradict this theory [10,11]. The aging process is also characterized by a chronic low-grade of inflammation, defined as inflamm-aging [12], with an upregulation of proinflammatory cytokines and inflammatory compounds, all of which have been shown to be involved in the pathogenesis of age-related diseases [13]. The theory of oxidation and inflammation of aging, termed oxi-inflamm-aging, was proposed to better define what occurs during the aging process [14,15].

Additionally, obesity is characterized by a redox/inflammatory imbalance that is probably due to the endocrine activity of adipose tissue via the production of several adipokines involved in the development of inflammation, oxidative stress, abnormal lipid metabolism, increased production of insulin, and insulin resistance [16–21]. In particular, visceral obesity is associated with the development of chronic metabolic diseases through a convergence of a chronic inflammatory state and enhanced production of reactive oxygen species [21]. Lines of evidence from several studies have shown that obesity adversely affects health status and life span through cellular processes in a manner similar to aging, and the link between these processes appears to be adiponectin [3,4]. This adipokine, mainly secreted from adipocytes, modulates a number of metabolic processes and represents a key molecule in maintaining the functionality of many organs [22]; it is also involved in the development and progression of several obesity-related malignancies such as breast cancer [23,24]. As adiponectin physiologically decreases with age [25] and obesity negatively affects the decline in adiponectin levels [26], it can be assumed that obesity alters the aging process through the regulation of adiponectin.

Caloric restriction (CR) is a dietary intervention with a chronic reduction of total calorie intake without incurring malnutrition. CR activates a complex series of events and represents a powerful intervention for extending healthspan and lifespan in several animal models, from yeast to primates [27]. Although the detailed mechanisms remain to be established, several sets of experimental data have confirmed that CR induces metabolic remodeling in several organs and tissues, including white adipose tissue (WAT). In particular, CR modulates the adipokine expression profile in rodent WAT [28,29]. WAT plays a central role in the regulation of both energy storage and expenditure and is also directly involved in the regulation of lifespan. The current knowledge on the molecular and cellular events associated with CR underline how the beneficial effects of this dietary intervention can be due to an improvement in the plasma and tissue redox inflammatory profile [30–32].

Given the close relationship between obesity and aging/age-related diseases, the present studyundertakes to determine the similarities in underlying mechanisms related to both obesity and aging, focusing our attention on the key role played by adiponectin. Since the use of old animals is very important to phenocopy the systemic aging context, we used an elderly and obese rat model, a useful model that mimics the weight gain due to aging that occurs in humans.

2. Materials and Methods

2.1. Animals

Experiments were performed on young (13–15 weeks old, $n = 6$) and aged (72 weeks old, $n = 12$) male Sprague–Dawley rats. Animals were housed in the animal care facility of the University of Calabria (Italy) in a 12:12 h light–dark cycle and temperature-controlled rooms (22 °C) and had free access to food and water. The old animals were then divided into two subgroups: (1) Control rats were continued on an ad libitum diet of a standard laboratory chow (ssniff diet V1535, German; metabolizable energy 3.057 Kcal/Kg), while (2) food-restriction rats were fed a diet of the same chow, restricted to 60% of the intake measured by weight in pairedcontrol chow-fed rats. The food restriction diet was carried on for a total period of 6 months, and thenthe aged animals (control and treated) were sacrificed at 24 months old. Water and food intakes were recorded every other day, while body mass was recorded monthly. Animals were euthanized with isoflurane (4%) followed by cervical transection and several tissueswere immediately removed: abdominal fat, kidney, blood, and skeletal muscle. All experiments were carried out in accordance with the European Guidelines for the care and use of laboratory animals (Directive 26/2014/EU) and were approved by the local ethical committee of the University of Calabria and by the Italian Ministry of Health (license n.295/2016-PR).

2.2. Measurement of Plasma Oxidative Status

Plasma oxidative status was evaluated through photometric measurement kits combined with a free radical analyzer system and a spectrophotometric device reader (FREE Carpe Diem, Diacron International, Grosseto, Italy), which are routinely used in our laboratory in both human and rat models [33–38]. The diacron-reactive oxygen metabolite (dROM) test was employed for analyzing the total amount of hydroperoxides in plasma samples. The normal range of the test results was 250–300 U.CARR (Carratelli Units), where 1 U.CARR corresponds to 0.8 mg/L of hydrogen peroxide. Total plasma antioxidant capacity was measured using a biological antioxidant capacity (BAP) test. Results are expressed in μmol/L of the reduced ferric ions.

2.3. Western Blot and Densitometric Analysis

White adipose tissue samples were lysed in ice-cold RIPA buffer containing a protease inhibitor cocktail (Sigma-Aldrich, Milan, Italy) and centrifuged for 20 min at 20,817× *g* at 4 °C. After removing the layer of lipids, supernatants were collected and the protein concentration was quantified using the Bradford method (Sigma, St Louis, MO, USA). For blood samples, after centrifuging for 15 min at 1500× *g* at 4 °C, plasma was collected and diluted (1:10 *v/v*) in ice-cold RIPA buffer containing a protease inhibitor cocktail (Sigma-Aldrich, Milan, Italy). The same amounts of total protein lysate were heated for 5 min in Laemmli buffer (SigmaAldrich, Milan, Italy), separated by sodium dodecyl sulfate polyacrylamide gel electrophoresis (SDSPAGE) in a Bio-Rad Mini Protean III machine and then electroblotted onto a nitrocellulose membrane (NitroBind, Maine Manufacturing, Maine, USA) using a mini transblot (BioRad Laboratories, Hercules, CA, USA). The gels for immunoblot analyses were transferred to a nitrocellulose membrane and incubated overnight at 4 °C, with primary antibodies diluted in TBS-T directed against AdipoR1, pAMPK, NFκB, NRF-2, GSTP1, TSG6, and adiponectin, followed by species-specific peroxidase-linked secondary antibodies (1:2000; Santa Cruz Biotechnology Inc., Dallas, TX, USA) for 1 h at room temperature. Immunodetection of protein bands was performed with an enhanced chemiluminescence kit (Western Blotting Luminol Reagent, Santa Cruz Biotechnology Inc.), and the membranes were exposed to X-ray films (Ultracruz Autoradiography Film, Santa Cruz Biotechnology Inc.). The films were then scanned, and densitometric analysis of the bands was performed using ImageJ software (1.52a version, National Institutes of Health, Bethesda, MD, USA). Beta actin and serum albumin were used as loading controls, respectively, for tissue and blood protein normalization.

2.4. Statistical Analysis

Data were analysed by one-way analysis of variance (ANOVA), followed by the Bonferroni multiple comparisons test using GraphPad/Prism version 5.01 statistical software (SAS Institute, Abacus Concept Inc., Berkeley, CA, USA. All the results are expressed as the mean ± SE.

3. Result

3.1. Effects of CR on Obesity and Plasmatic Oxidative Balance

In laboratory rodents, obesity is defined as the achievement of a 20% increase in body mass index [39]. In our obesity model, the aged rats (2 years old) showed a significant increase in body weight, greater than 45%, compared to young rats (13–15 weeks old). Furthermore, these aged specimens had a significant plasma oxidative imbalance, with a considerable increase in oxidative stress and a parallel and severe decrease in the antioxidant barrier. In our model, the calorie restriction (−40%) for 6 months determined a significant decrease in body weight (−34%) vs. control and, at the same time, significantly improved the oxidative balance with a remarkable decrease in oxidative stress, independent of changes in the plasmatic antioxidant barrier. The body weight data and the trend of both oxidative stress (d-ROMs) and antioxidant capacity efficiency (BAP) in plasma of young rats (Y), obese aged (OA), and aged undergoing calorie restriction (CRA) rats are reported in Figure 1.

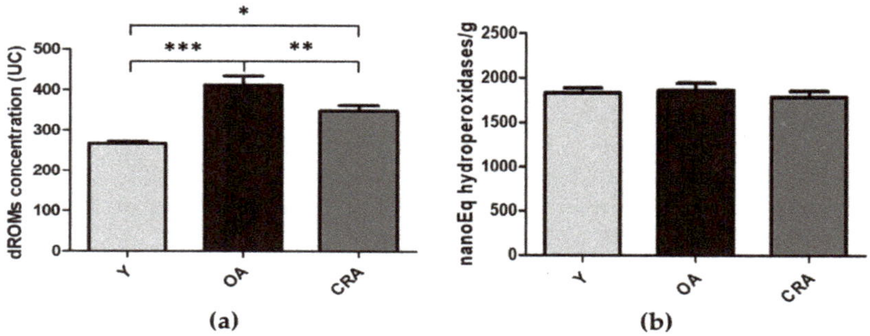

Figure 1. Plasmatic values of oxidative stress (d-ROMs) (**a**) and antioxidant capacity efficiency (BAP) (**b**) tests in young rats (Y), obese aged (OA), and aged undergoing calorie restriction (CRA)rats. Data are means ± SE of five determinations for each animal ($n = 6$). Statistical differences were evaluated by one-way ANOVA, followed by Bonferroni's multiple comparison test (* $p < 0.05$; ** $p < 0.001$; *** $p < 0.0001$).

3.2. *Effects of CR on Plasmatic Adiponectin Levels and Inflammation Markers*

To assess the possible role played by adiponectin in the antioxidant effect of CR, we evaluated its plasmatic protein levels through Western blotting analysis. In parallel, we also evaluated the plasmatic protein levels of TSG-6, a multifunctional protein associated with inflammation. Our results clearly indicate that the obesity condition associated with aging does change the circulating adiponectin levels and also induces a significant increase in TSG-6 levels, confirming the low-grade proinflammatory state found in both obesity and aging (Figure 2a). The caloric restriction determines an increase in the adiponectin plasma levels (doubled compared to both young and aged rats) and a significant reduction of the TSG-6 proinflammatory marker, which reverts to the values of the young rats (Figure 2b).

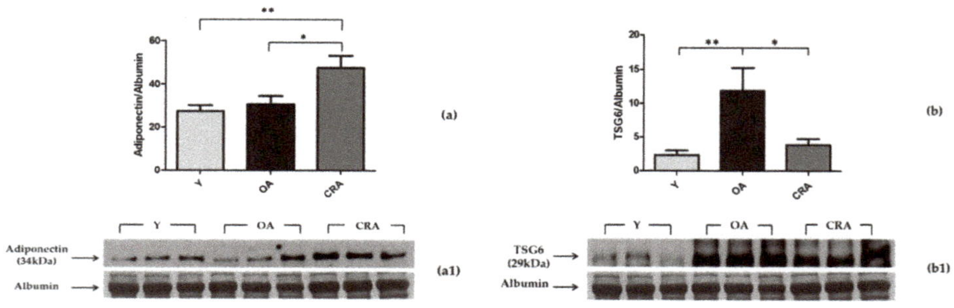

Figure 2. Western blotting of adiponectin (**a**) and TSG6 (**b**) in plasma samples of Y, OA, and CRA rats; (**a1**,**b1**) show the densitometric quantification of the blots. Protein loading was verified by plasmatic albumin level. Data are means ± SE of five determinations for each animal ($n = 6$). Statistical differences were evaluated by one-way ANOVA, followed by Bonferroni's multiple comparison test (* $p < 0.05$; ** $p < 0.001$).

3.3. *Effects of CR on AdipoR1–pAMPK–NFκB Pathway in Adipose Tissue*

Since adipose tissue represents a crucial junction in inflammatory processes and it is also a reserve of adipokines, we analyzed the AdipoR1–pAMPK–NFκB pathway at the level of adipose tissue. Through its receptor, adiponectin mediates AMPK activation (pAMPK), which is involved in the inhibition of NFκB activation and the suppression of inflammation. In our model, the obesity condition associated with aging determines an upregulation of AdipoR1, with a consequent increase of the AMPK active form in adipose tissue (Figure 3a,b). Despite the activation of this anti-inflammatory pathway, NFκB levels found in obese and aged subjects (control) were high compared to the young rats. CR, with the achievement of normal weight and the rise of both AdipoR1 and pAMPK, significantly inhibited NFκB expression (Figure 4) and consequently suppressed the proinflammatory state, which appears to be more linked to obesity than aging (Figure 2b).

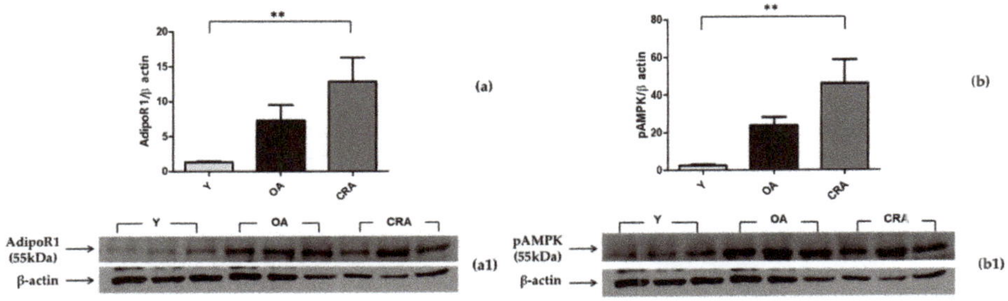

Figure 3. Western blotting of AdipoR1 (**a**) and AMPK activation (pAMPK) (**b**) in adipose tissue samples of Y, OA, and CRA rats; (**a1**,**b1**) show the densitometric quantification of the blots. Protein loading was verified by using the anti-β-actin antibody. Data are means ± SE of five determinations for each animal (n = 6). Statistical differences were evaluated by one-way ANOVA, followed by Bonferroni's multiple comparison test (** $p < 0.001$).

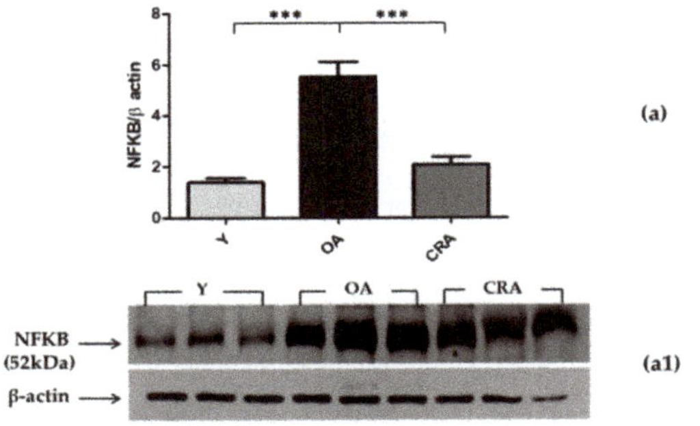

Figure 4. Western blotting of NFκB (**a**) in adipose tissue samples of Y, OA, and CRA rats; (**a1**) shows the densitometric quantification of the blots. Protein loading was verified by using the anti-β-actin antibody. Data are means ± SE of five determinations for each animal (n = 6). Statistical differences were evaluated by one-way ANOVA, followed by Bonferroni's multiple comparison test (*** $p < 0.0001$).

3.4. *Effects of CR on Antioxidant Enzymes in Adipose Tissue*

To analyze the oxidative imbalance linked to obesity detected at the plasma level, we evaluated two important cytoplasmatic antioxidant enzymes, SOD1 and GSTP1, in adipose tissue. SOD1, the most important preventive antioxidant, showed no significant changes in the three groups of rats (data not shown). Regarding the GSTP1 monomer (23 kDa), the form with antioxidant and proliferative activity, our results showed a significant increase in obese rats while it is reduced in CRArats (Figure 5a).

We also evaluated NRF2, a transcription factor physiologically present in the cytosol that migrates to the nucleus only under stress conditions, where it stimulates the expression of antioxidant genes. Our results clearly showed that in obese aged rats, the cytoplasmic fraction of NRF2 is significantly increased, while in CRA rats, it is significantly decreased (Figure 5b).

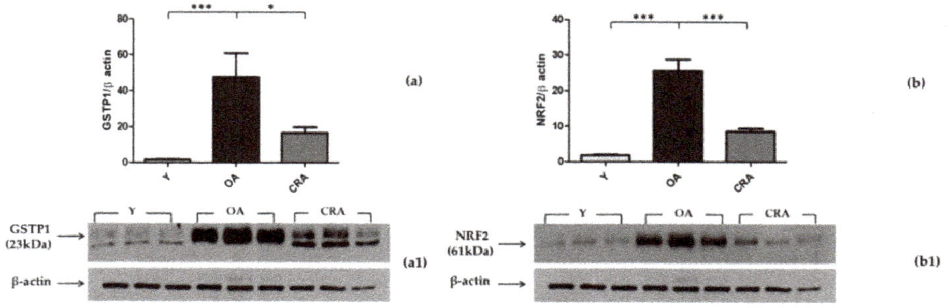

Figure 5. Western blotting of GSTP1(**a**) and NRF2(**b**) in adipose tissue samples of Y, OA, and CRA rats; (**a1**,**b1**) show the densitometric quantification of the blots. Protein loading was verified by using the anti-β-actin antibody. Data are means ± SE of five determinations for each animal (n = 6). Statistical differences were evaluated by one-way ANOVA, followed by Bonferroni's multiple comparison test (* $p < 0.05$; *** $p < 0.0001$).

4. Discussion

This study was designed to evaluate the effect of long-term (6 months) caloric restriction (−40%) on the oxidative/inflammatory balance in an aged and obese rat model and the putative role of adiponectin. Our results showed notable alterations in redox/inflammatory status in our aging obesity model compared to young rats and revealed that CR treatment improves the plasmatic and cellular capacity to neutralize oxidative insults and induces a significant reduction of proinflammatory markers. This improvement of the redox/inflammatory status during CR is connected with an important increase in adiponectin plasma levels, thus suggesting an important role of this adipokine in the antioxidant/anti-inflammatory properties of the organism. Additionally, at the level of adipose tissue, we found a positive modulation of both anti-inflammatory and antioxidant pathways.

During the aging process, there is often a gradual increase in body weight and, typically, the fat is redistributed from the subcutaneous to the abdominal deposits and the liver, and this phenotypic change can affect energy metabolism and systemic insulin resistance [40]. Aged rodents develop increased fat mass, with close similarities to aged humans [41], making these animals excellent experimental models for analyzing both obesity and aging. In our experimental model, age-related physiological weight gain leads to two-year-old rats with 45% increased body weight compared to the young animals and, therefore, with overt obesity [39]. These aged and obese specimens, according to the oxidation–inflammation theory of aging [14,15], showed a considerable increase in oxidative stress, a parallel and severe decrease in the antioxidant barrier, and a significant upregulation of TSG-6, a multifunctional protein associated with inflammation [42]. Our results clearly indicate that the obesity condition associated with aging induces oxidative/inflammatory stress situations, confirming the oxidative imbalance and low-grade proinflammatory state found in both obesity and aging [4]. In our aged and obese rat model, we did not detect changes in plasma adiponectin levels with respect to the young animals. Several factors may influence adiponectin levels and activity. In obesity, as the metabolic role of adipocytes changes, the secretion of adiponectin decreases in both humans and rodents, and this is associated with chronic inflammation [4,26,43]. Data on adiponectin levels and aging have revealed conflicting results; some authors have indicated that plasmatic adiponectin levels increase with advancing age [44], while others have reported no age-related changes in its levels [4,25].

Interestingly, in our model, the long-term caloric restriction reversed obesity, determining a significant decrease in body weight (−34%) and, in parallel, increasing the adiponectin plasma levels, which were doubled compared to both young and obese aged control rats. The increased adiponectin plasma levels led to the improvement of the proinflammatory state, with a severe reduction of the TSG-6 proinflammatory marker, which reverted to the values of the young rats. The protein TSG6, a critical anti-inflammatory cytokine detected in the context of many inflammatory diseases, is produced in response to inflammatory mediators, mostly after TNF-α stimulation [42]. The anti-inflammatory and cytoprotective effects of adiponectin have long been known [45–47], and caloric restriction is also considered a possible strategy to better body metabolic and inflammatory profiles [48,49]. The role played by adiponectin and caloric restriction in maintaining/restoring the oxidative balance is less clear. A wide number of studies have reported a negative correlation of adiponectin levels with markers of oxidative stress [50] and a cause–effect relationship between the metabolic syndrome and a deteriorated oxidative status related to the altered secretion of adipokines [51]. In addition, it has been suggested that oxidative stress can inhibit adiponectin expression in obesity, but the mechanism underlying this regulation is unclear [19]. Our results show a clear improvement in the plasma redox status with a remarkable decrease in oxidative stress, independent of changes in the plasmatic antioxidant barrier.

To investigate the mechanisms triggered by caloric restriction in the improvement of oxidative/inflammatory status in our model, we analyzed anti-inflammatory and antioxidant pathways at the level of adipose tissue, focusing on the key role played by adiponectin. Adipose tissue represents a crucial junction in inflammatory/oxidant processes, and it is also a reserve of adipokines. The biological activities of adiponectin are closely related to the activation of AMP-activated protein kinase (AMPK), a key enzyme in the regulation of cellular energy homeostasis and fatty acid metabolism [52,53]. Several authors have reported that AMPK plays an important role in the modulation of inflammation, and AMPK activators exert a protective effect in animal models of inflammatory diseases [45]. In addition, AMPK can inhibit ROS generation [53,54]. Recently, it has been suggested that adiponectin may control inflammation by upregulating AMPK phosphorylation and then reducing the ROS-initiated inflammatory response [54]. Moreover, in cellular models, adiponectin treatment linearly decreased the production of ROS [54]. Through its receptor, adiponectin exerts an anti-inflammatory response by AMPK activation (pAMPK), which is involved in the inhibition of NFκB activation and consequent TNF-α and IL-1β downregulation [45].

In our model, the obesity condition associated with aging determines an upregulation of AdipoR1, with a consequent increase of the AMPK active form in adipose tissue. Despite the activation of this anti-inflammatory pathway, the NFκB levels found were high compared to young rats. CR, with the achievement of normal weight, enhances the stimulation of both AdipoR1 and pAMPK, with significant inhibition of NFκB expression and, consequently, suppression of the proinflammatory state.

To better understand the tissue redox balance, we also focused on the expression of two important cytoplasmatic antioxidant enzymes, SOD1 and GSTP1, in adipose tissue. CR has been shown to positively affect tissue redox homeostasis by the enhancement of endogenous antioxidant systems [55]. In our model, the expression of SOD1, the most important preventive antioxidant, showed no significant changes in all groups of rats used, while the GSTP1 monomer, the form with antioxidant and proliferative activity, showed a negative modulation by CR treatment. We also evaluated the expression of NRF2, a transcription factor that is physiologically present in the cytosol that migrates to the nucleus only under stress conditions, where it stimulates the expression of antioxidant genes. Our results clearly show that in obese aged rats, the cytoplasmic fraction of NRF2 is significantly increased and that CR induces a substantial decrease, probably due to a translocation effect in the nucleus to modulate the expression of antioxidant genes.

Overall, our results highlight that the long-term caloric restriction leads to the achievement of normal weight and induces a number of adaptations that improve the redox/inflammatory status at both plasma and tissue levels, suggesting that inflammatory and redox imbalances in obese aged rats appear to be more linked to obesity than to aging.

Author Contributions: Conceptualization, D.P. and D.L.R.; methodology, D.P., D.L.R., and A.M.; software, D.P., D.L.R., and A.M.; validation, D.P. and D.L.R.; formal analysis, D.P., D.L.R., A.M., R.M., and M.M.; investigation, D.P., D.L.R., and A.M.; resources, D.P., D.L.R., and M.M.; data curation, D.P., D.L.R., and A.M.; writing—original draft preparation, D.P. and D.L.R.; writing—review and editing, D.P., D.L.R., and A.M.; visualization, D.P., D.L.R., A.M., R.M., and M.M.; supervision, D.P. and D.L.R.; project administration, D.P. and D.L.R.; funding acquisition, D.P. and M.M. All authors have read and agreed to the published version of the manuscript.

Funding: This research received no external funding.

Conflicts of Interest: The authors declare no conflict of interest.

References

1. Jones, A.R.; Tovee, M.J.; Cutler, L.R.; Parkinson, K.N.; Ells, L.J.; Araujo-Soares, V.; Pearce, M.S.; Mann, K.D.; Scott, D.; Harris, J.M.; et al. Health Effects of Overweight and Obesity in 195 Countries over 25 Years. *Yearb. Paediatr. Endocrinol.* **2018**. [CrossRef]
2. Cattaneo, A.; Monasta, L.; Stamatakis, E.; Lioret, S.; Castetbon, K.; Frenken, F.; Manios, Y.; Moschonis, G.; Savva, S.; Zaborskis, A.; et al. Overweight and obesity in infants and pre-school children in the European Union: A review of existing data. *Obes. Rev.* **2010**, *11*, 389–398. [CrossRef] [PubMed]
3. Salvestrini, V.; Sell, C.; Lorenzini, A. Obesity may accelerate the aging process. *Front. Endocrinol. (Lausanne)* **2019**, *10*. [CrossRef] [PubMed]
4. Jura, M.; Kozak, L.P. Obesity and related consequences to ageing. *Age (Omaha)* **2016**, *38*. [CrossRef]
5. Harman, D. Aging: A theory based on free radical and radiation chemistry. *J. Gerontol.* **1956**, *11*, 298–300. [CrossRef]
6. Remigante, A.; Morabito, R.; Marino, A. Natural antioxidants beneficial effects on anion exchange through band 3 protein in human erythrocytes. *Antioxidants* **2020**, *9*, 25. [CrossRef]
7. Barja, G. Free radicals and aging. *Trends Neurosci.* **2004**, *27*, 595–600. [CrossRef]
8. Gutteridge, J.M. Free radicals and aging. *Rev. Clin. Gerontol.* **1994**, *4*, 279–288. [CrossRef]
9. Liguori, I.; Russo, G.; Curcio, F.; Bulli, G.; Aran, L.; Della-Morte, D.; Gargiulo, G.; Testa, G.; Cacciatore, F.; Bonaduce, D.; et al. Oxidative stress, aging, and diseases. *Clin. Interv. Aging* **2018**, *13*, 757–772. [CrossRef]
10. Pérez, V.I.; Van Remmen, H.; Bokov, A.; Epstein, C.J.; Vijg, J.; Richardson, A. The overexpression of major antioxidant enzymes does not extend the lifespan of mice. *Aging Cell* **2009**, *8*, 73–75. [CrossRef]
11. Mele, J.; Van Remmen, H.; Vijg, J.; Richardson, A. Characterization of transgenic mice that overexpress both copper zinc superoxide dismutase and catalase. *Antioxidants Redox Signal.* **2006**, *8*, 628–638. [CrossRef] [PubMed]
12. Franceschi, C.; Ottaviani, E.; Olivieri, F.; De Benedictis, G.; Bonafè, M.; De Luca, M.; Valensin, S. Inflamm-aging. An evolutionary perspective on immunosenescence. *Ann. N. Y. Acad. Sci.* **2000**, *908*, 244–254. [CrossRef] [PubMed]
13. Vasto, S.; Candore, G.; Balistreri, C.R.; Caruso, M.; Colonna-Romano, G.; Grimaldi, M.P.; Listi, F.; Nuzzo, D.; Lio, D.; Caruso, C. Inflammatory networks in ageing, age-related diseases and longevity. *Mech. Ageing Dev.* **2007**, *128*, 83–91. [CrossRef]
14. Fuente, M.; Miquel, J. An Update of the Oxidation-Inflammation Theory of Aging: The Involvement of the Immune System in Oxi-Inflamm-Aging. *Curr. Pharm. Des.* **2009**, *15*, 3003–3026. [CrossRef] [PubMed]
15. De la Fuente, M. Editorial crosstalk between the nervous and the immune systems in health and sickness. *Curr. Pharm. Des.* **2014**, *20*, 4605–4607. [CrossRef]
16. Matsuda, M.; Shimomura, I. Increased oxidative stress in obesity: Implications for metabolic syndrome, diabetes, hypertension, dyslipidemia, atherosclerosis, and cancer. *Obes. Res. Clin. Pract.* **2013**, *7*. [CrossRef]
17. Manna, P.; Jain, S.K. Obesity, Oxidative Stress, Adipose Tissue Dysfunction, and the Associated Health Risks: Causes and Therapeutic Strategies. *Metab. Syndr. Relat. Disord.* **2015**, *13*, 423–444. [CrossRef]
18. Marseglia, L.; Manti, S.; D'Angelo, G.; Nicotera, A.; Parisi, E.; Di Rosa, G.; Gitto, E.; Arrigo, T. Oxidative stress in obesity: A critical component in human diseases. *Int. J. Mol. Sci.* **2015**, *16*, 378–400. [CrossRef]
19. Furukawa, S.; Matsuda, M.; Shimomura, I.; Fujita, T.; Shimabukuro, M.; Iwaki, M.; Yamada, Y.; Nakajima, Y.; Nakayama, O.; Makishima, M. Increased oxidative stress in obesity and its impact on metabolic syndrome. *J. Clin. Investig.* **2017**, *114*, 1752–1761. [CrossRef]
20. Włodarczyk, M.; Nowicka, G. Obesity, DNA damage, and development of obesity-related diseases. *Int. J. Mol. Sci.* **2019**, *20*, 1146. [CrossRef]

21. Dludla, P.V.; Nkambule, B.B.; Jack, B.; Mkandla, Z.; Mutize, T.; Silvestri, S.; Orlando, P.; Tiano, L.; Louw, J.; Mazibuko-Mbeje, S.E. Inflammation and oxidative stress in an obese state and the protective effects of gallic acid. *Nutrients* **2019**, *11*, 23. [CrossRef] [PubMed]
22. Fang, H.; Judd, R.L. Adiponectin regulation and function. *Compr. Physiol.* **2018**, *8*, 1031–1063. [CrossRef] [PubMed]
23. Naimo, G.D.; Gelsomino, L.; Catalano, S.; Mauro, L.; Andò, S. Interfering Role of ERα on Adiponectin Action in Breast Cancer. *Front. Endocrinol. (Lausanne)* **2020**, *11*, 66. [CrossRef] [PubMed]
24. Andò, S.; Naimo, G.D.; Gelsomino, L.; Catalano, S.; Mauro, L. Novel insights into adiponectin action in breast cancer: Evidence of its mechanistic effects mediated by ERα expression. *Obes. Rev.* **2020**, *21*. [CrossRef]
25. Li, J.-B.; Nishida, M.; Kaimoto, K.; Asakawa, A.; Chaolu, H.; Cheng, K.-C.; Li, Y.-X.; Terashi, M.; Koyama, K.I.; Amitani, H.; et al. Effects of aging on the plasma levels of nesfatin-1 and adiponectin. *Biomed. Rep.* **2014**, *2*, 152–156. [CrossRef]
26. Ukkola, O.; Santaniemi, M. Adiponectin: A link between excess adiposity and associated comorbidities? *J. Mol. Med.* **2002**, *80*, 696–702. [CrossRef]
27. Chung, K.W.; Kim, D.H.; Park, M.H.; Choi, Y.J.; Kim, N.D.; Lee, J.; Yu, B.P.; Chung, H.Y. Recent advances in calorie restriction research on aging. *Exp. Gerontol.* **2013**, *48*, 1049–1053. [CrossRef]
28. Chujo, Y.; Fujii, N.; Okita, N.; Konishi, T.; Narita, T.; Yamada, A.; Haruyama, Y.; Tashiro, K.; Chiba, T.; Shimokawa, I.; et al. Caloric restriction-Associated remodeling of rat white adipose tissue: Effects on the growth hormone/insulin-like growth factor-1 axis, sterol regulatory element binding protein-1, and macrophage infiltration. *Age (Omaha)* **2013**, *35*, 1143–1156. [CrossRef]
29. Fujii, N.; Narita, T.; Okita, N.; Kobayashi, M.; Furuta, Y.; Chujo, Y.; Sakai, M.; Yamada, A.; Takeda, K.; Konishi, T.; et al. Sterol regulatory element-binding protein-1c orchestrates metabolic remodeling of white adipose tissue by caloric restriction. *Aging Cell* **2017**, *16*, 508–517. [CrossRef]
30. Redman, L.M.; Smith, S.R.; Burton, J.H.; Martin, C.K.; Il'yasova, D.; Ravussin, E. Metabolic Slowing and Reduced Oxidative Damage with Sustained Caloric Restriction Support the Rate of Living and Oxidative Damage Theories of Aging. *Cell Metab.* **2018**, *27*, 805–815.e4. [CrossRef]
31. Calment, J.L. Aging, Adiposity, and Calorie Restriction. *JAMA* **2015**, *297*, 986–994.
32. Savas, H.B. Positive effects of meal frequency and calorie restriction on antioxidant systems in rats. *Nothern Clin. Istanbul* **2017**. [CrossRef] [PubMed]
33. Brunelli, E.; Domanico, F.; La Russa, D.; Pellegrino, D. Sex differences in oxidative stress biomarkers. *Curr. Drug Targets* **2014**, *15*. [CrossRef] [PubMed]
34. La Russa, D.; Brunelli, E.; Pellegrino, D. Oxidative imbalance and kidney damage in spontaneously hypertensive rats: Activation of extrinsic apoptotic pathways. *Clin. Sci.* **2017**, *131*, 1419–1428. [CrossRef] [PubMed]
35. Brunelli, E.; La Russa, D.; Pellegrino, D. Impaired oxidative status is strongly associated with cardiovascular risk factors. *Oxid. Med. Cell. Longev.* **2017**, *2017*. [CrossRef]
36. La Russa, D.; Giordano, F.; Marrone, A.; Parafati, M.; Janda, E.; Pellegrino, D. Oxidative Imbalance and Kidney Damage in Cafeteria Diet-Induced Rat Model of Metabolic Syndrome: Effect of Bergamot Polyphenolic Fraction. *Antioxidants* **2019**, *8*, 66. [CrossRef]
37. Russa, D.L.; Pellegrino, D.; Montesanto, A.; Gigliotti, P.; Perri, A.; Russa, A.L.; Bonofiglio, R. Oxidative Balance and Inflammation in Hemodialysis Patients: Biomarkers of Cardiovascular Risk? *Oxid. Med. Cell. Longev.* **2019**, *2019*, 1–7. [CrossRef]
38. Pellegrino, D.; La Russa, D.; Marrone, A. Oxidative imbalance and kidney damage: New study perspectives from animal models to hospitalized patients. *Antioxidants* **2019**, *8*, 594. [CrossRef]
39. Novelli, E.L.B.; Diniz, Y.S.; Galhardi, C.M.; Ebaid, G.M.X.; Rodrigues, H.G.; Mani, F.; Fernandes, A.A.H.; Cicogna, A.C.; Novelli Filho, J.L.V.B. Anthropometrical parameters and markers of obesity in rats. *Lab. Anim.* **2007**, *41*, 111–119. [CrossRef]
40. Kuk, J.L.; Saunders, T.J.; Davidson, L.E.; Ross, R. Age-related changes in total and regional fat distribution. *Ageing Res. Rev.* **2009**, *8*, 339–348. [CrossRef]
41. Huffman, D.M.; Barzilai, N. Role of visceral adipose tissue in aging. *Biochim. Biophys. Acta Gen. Subj.* **2009**, *1790*, 1117–1123. [CrossRef] [PubMed]
42. Milner, C.M.; Day, A.J. TSG-6: A multifunctional protein associated with inflammation. *J. Cell Sci.* **2003**, *116*, 1863–1873. [CrossRef] [PubMed]

43. Engin, A. Adiponectin-resistance in obesity. *Adv. Exp. Med. Biol.* **2017**, *960*, 415–441. [CrossRef] [PubMed]
44. Koh, S.J.; Hyun, Y.J.; Choi, S.Y.; Chae, J.S.; Kim, J.Y.; Park, S.; Ahn, C.M.; Jang, Y.; Lee, J.H. Influence of age and visceral fat area on plasma adiponectin concentrations in women with normal glucose tolerance. *Clin. Chim. Acta* **2008**, *389*, 45–50. [CrossRef]
45. Tilg, H.; Moschen, A.R. Adipocytokines: Mediators linking adipose tissue, inflammation and immunity. *Nat. Rev. Immunol.* **2006**, *6*, 772–783. [CrossRef]
46. Ouchi, N.; Walsh, K. Adiponectin as an anti-inflammatory factor. *Clin. Chim. Acta* **2007**, *380*, 24–30. [CrossRef]
47. Piao, C.; Park, J.H.; Lee, M. Anti-Inflammatory Therapeutic Effect of Adiponectin Gene Delivery Using a Polymeric Carrier in an Acute Lung Injury Model. *Pharm. Res.* **2017**, *34*, 1517–1526. [CrossRef]
48. Lettieri-Barbato, D.; Giovannetti, E.; Aquilano, K. Effects of dietary restriction on adipose mass and biomarkers of healthy aging in human. *Aging (Albany N.Y.)* **2016**, *8*, 3341–3355. [CrossRef]
49. Most, J.; Tosti, V.; Redman, L.M.; Fontana, L. Calorie restriction in humans: An update. *Ageing Res. Rev.* **2017**, *39*, 36–45. [CrossRef]
50. Frühbeck, G.; Catalán, V.; Rodríguez, A.; Ramírez, B.; Becerril, S.; Salvador, J.; Portincasa, P.; Colina, I.; Gómez-Ambrosi, J. Involvement of the leptin-adiponectin axis in inflammation and oxidative stress in the metabolic syndrome. *Sci. Rep.* **2017**, *7*. [CrossRef]
51. Gómez-Ambrosi, J.; Catalán, V.; Rodríguez, A.; Andrada, P.; Ramírez, B.; Ibáñez, P.; Vila, N.; Romero, S.; Margall, M.A.; Gil, M.J.; et al. Increased cardiometabolic risk factors and inflammation in adipose tissue in obese subjects classified as metabolically healthy. *Diabetes Care* **2014**, *37*, 2813–2821. [CrossRef] [PubMed]
52. Chandrasekar, B.; Boylston, W.H.; Venkatachalam, K.; Webster, N.J.G.; Prabhu, S.D.; Valente, A.J. Adiponectin blocks interleukin-18-mediated endothelial cell death via APPL1-dependent AMP-activated protein kinase (AMPK) activation and IKK/NF-κB/PTEN suppression. *J. Biol. Chem.* **2008**, *283*, 24889–24898. [CrossRef]
53. Steinberg, G.R.; Kemp, B.E. AMPK in health and disease. *Physiol. Rev.* **2009**, *89*, 1025–1078. [CrossRef] [PubMed]
54. Wang, F.; Liu, Y.; Yang, W.; Yuan, J.; Mo, Z. Adiponectin inhibits NLRP3 inflammasome by modulating the AMPK-ROS pathway. *Int. J. Clin. Exp. Pathol.* **2018**, *11*, 3338–3347. [PubMed]
55. Yanar, K.; Simsek, B.; Çaylı, N.; Övül Bozkır, H.; Mengi, M.; Belce, A.; Aydin, S.; Çakatay, U. Caloric restriction and redox homeostasis in various regions of aging male rat brain: Is caloric restriction still worth trying even after early-adulthood?: Redox homeostasis and caloric restriction in brain. *J. Food Biochem.* **2019**, *43*. [CrossRef]

biomedicines

MDPI

Article

Identification of Toxicity Parameters Associated with Combustion Produced Soot Surface Chemistry and Particle Structure by In Vitro Assays

Heba Al Housseiny [1], Madhu Singh [2], Shaneeka Emile [3], Marvin Nicoleau [4], Randy L. Vander Wal [2,5] and Patricia Silveyra [1,3,*]

1 Biobehavioral Laboratory, School of Nursing, The University of North Carolina at Chapel Hill, Chapel Hill, NC 27599, USA; hebaal@email.unc.edu

2 John and Willie Leone Family Department of Energy and Mineral Engineering, The Pennsylvania State University, University Park, PA 16801, USA; madhusingh@alumni.psu.edu (M.S.); ruv12@psu.edu (R.L.V.W.)

3 The Pennsylvania State University College of Medicine, Hershey, PA 17033, USA; snemile77@gmail.com

4 School of Medicine, Case Western Reserve University, Cleveland, OH 44106, USA; mnicoelea@fandm.edu

5 EMS Energy Institute, The Pennsylvania State University, University Park, PA 16801, USA

* Correspondence: patry@email.unc.edu

Received: 3 August 2020; Accepted: 8 September 2020; Published: 11 September 2020

Abstract: Air pollution has become the world's single biggest environmental health risk of the past decade, causing millions of yearly deaths worldwide. One of the dominant air pollutants is fine particulate matter ($PM_{2.5}$), which is a product of combustion. Exposure to $PM_{2.5}$ has been associated with decreased lung function, impaired immunity, and exacerbations of lung disease. Accumulating evidence suggests that many of the adverse health effects of $PM_{2.5}$ exposure are associated with lung inflammation and oxidative stress. While the physical structure and surface chemistry of $PM_{2.5}$ are surrogate measures of particle oxidative potential, little is known about their contributions to negative health effects. In this study, we used functionalized carbon black particles as surrogates for atmospherically aged combustion-formed soot to assess the effects of $PM_{2.5}$ surface chemistry in lung cells. We exposed the BEAS-2B lung epithelial cell line to different soot at a range of concentrations and assessed cell viability, inflammation, and oxidative stress. Our results indicate that exposure to soot with varying particle surface composition results in differential cell viability rates, the expression of pro-inflammatory and oxidative stress genes, and protein carbonylation. We conclude that particle surface chemistry, specifically oxygen content, in soot modulates lung cell inflammatory and oxidative stress responses.

Keywords: air pollution; soot; particulate matter; lung inflammation; functional groups

1. Introduction

Air pollution has become one of the greatest environmental health hazards to millions around the world and is primarily caused by years of industrialization and population growth, particularly in developing countries [1,2]. In the past decade, air pollution alone has been linked to 7 million annual deaths worldwide. The Global Burden of Disease Study identified air pollution as a risk factor for cardiovascular disease and respiratory infections, and it is estimated to have contributed to nearly 5 million premature deaths worldwide in 2017 alone [3,4].

Air pollutants are separated into two categories depending on the source of production. Primary pollutants such as heavy petroleum products (soot) and oxides of nitrogen (NOx) and sulfur (SOx) are emitted into the air by the combustion of fossil fuels, vehicle exhaust, natural fires, industrial practices, and natural dust [5]. Secondary pollutants are formed when primary pollutants react with other molecules in the atmosphere, altering their toxin absorption ability. Secondary pollutants include ozone, acid rain, and particulate air pollution [5].

Particulate matter (PM) is a complex mixture of volatile organic and inorganic compounds, including solid particles and liquid droplets, with different physicochemical properties and toxicity [6,7]. Carbon black, produced by an incomplete combustion of soot, comprises a significant portion of PM. The toxicity of PM is characterized by its size, surface chemistry, solubility, and ability to form reactive oxygen species. Fine PM size ranges from 2.5 μm to 10 μm in aerodynamic diameter ($PM_{2.5}$ to PM_{10}). Notably, $PM_{2.5}$ is known to exacerbate many pre-existing heart and respiratory diseases that increase the risk of death [8]. The finest particles, $PM_{2.5}$, have been reported to induce inflammation and oxidative stress in the respiratory tract, and they exacerbate respiratory and cardiovascular diseases including long-term chronic diseases such as cancer and asthma. Yet, the mechanisms underlying $PM_{2.5}$-induced inflammation are still unknown [8–12]. The mortality rate due to $PM_{2.5}$ is more prominent in the elderly, pregnant women, infants, and low-income populations [13,14]. Exposure to fine particles affects lower-income populations in which a significant proportion have an income below the poverty threshold, leading to environmental inequality and propagating economic burden [15,16].

Exposure of the nasal and lung epithelia to $PM_{2.5}$ triggers an inflammatory response within the respiratory system that, if not resolved, can contribute to chronic inflammation. This inflammatory response is characterized by the production of extracellular signaling proteins, including cytokines and chemokines secreted by epithelial and immune cells, and it plays a critical role in the lung's defense mechanism against oxidative stress [17]. Previous studies have described an increase in the expression of cellular pro-inflammatory cytokines such as interleukin 6 (IL-6) and interleukin 1 beta (IL-1β) following exposure to $PM_{2.5}$ [18–20]. Protein carbonylation has also been reported as a biomarker of oxidative stress-induced protein damage and has been associated with the development of cardiovascular and respiratory diseases [21,22]. A few studies have shown that protein carbonylation is increased in $PM_{2.5}$-treated human keratinocytes and rat epithelial lung cells [23]. Thus, while cytokine expression and protein carbonylation may serve as important biomarkers for numerous lung diseases, their role in $PM_{2.5}$-induced lung inflammation has not been extensively investigated in human cells.

Many of the adverse health effects of $PM_{2.5}$ exposure are hypothesized to be derived from oxidative stress, which is initiated by the formation of reactive oxygen species (ROS) within cells [24]. Although several studies have demonstrated the ROS potential and inflammatory action of diesel particulates from diesel engine combustion, the causative factors are less clear. Most studies use organics diluted and extracted from real exhaust particulates, and results reported may be skewed relative to cell exposure to the "complete" soot, i.e., $PM_{2.5}$ along with its heteroatoms and condensed fractions. It is increasingly being recognized that extracts of diesel soot are a poor representation of the full range of toxicity and mutagenic effects [25]. Rather, the particles, and specifically their surface chemistry, are thought to have considerable direct health impacts. Yet, no studies have assessed and quantified the effect of parameters such as particle size, morphology, and surface chemistry in the cellular response to combustion-formed $PM_{2.5}$ exposure. Therefore, we investigated these effects in human lung epithelial cells by using modified functionalized carbon blacks (soot) as surrogates for combustion-formed particulates. Our goal in using this approach was to understand the hierarchy of detrimental effects of soot from a combustion engine, subject to atmospheric aging, including the health effects of the primary particle itself, as compared to those of the functional groups on the carbonaceous backbone.

This work focuses on the identification of oxidative and pro-inflammatory factors induced as a response to exposure of human lung epithelial cells to synthetic soot in various surface chemistry forms. By exposing a male lung epithelial cell line (BEAS-2B) to lab-generated R-250 carbon black (nascent, nitric acid-treated, and ozone-treated carbon black), we tested the hypothesis that exposure to soot with different surface composition results in differential toxicity, inflammatory, and oxidative stress responses in human lung epithelial cells. We assessed the cell viability and expression of genes related to the inflammatory response and oxidative stress, including IL-1β, IL-6, superoxide dismutase

2 (SOD2), nuclear factor erythroid 2-related factor 2 (NFE2L2), and protein carbonylation levels at different time points and concentrations of soot. Our data indicate that the surface chemistry and concentration of soot, specifically higher oxygen content and concentration, play a critical role in the inflammatory and immune response initiated in the lung epithelium, and they are associated with a decrease in cell viability and an increase in protein carbonylation levels and expression of inflammatory cytokine genes.

2. Experimental Section

2.1. Synthesis and Characterization of Soot

Commercially produced carbon black (Regal 250, Cabot Corporation, Apharetta, GA, USA) was used as the model carbon black for its chemical purity and absence of organic content [25]. Synthetic soot was produced by functionalizing R250 carbon black via controlled oxidation by the methods described below. Four soot preparations were used for experiments:

(1) Nascent soot (S1): Unmodified, non-oxidized, R250. This commercially produced carbon black was used as the model nascent soot form given its chemical purity and absence of organic content;
(2) Nitric acid-treated soot (S2): Wet chemical treatment of R250 was conducted by treating 1 g of carbon black with 100 ml of laboratory-grade concentrated nitric acid (HNO_3, >90%) at 80 °C under reflux for 24 h, just below the acid's boiling point of 83 °C. The carbon–acid mixture was continuously stirred for uniform oxidation and functionalization. The mixture was maintained at a consistent simmer, and thereafter, it was washed with distilled water, filtered, and dried to obtain functionalized carbon black as synthetic soot;
(3) Ozone-treated soot (S3): Dry gaseous treatment of carbon black was performed via exposure to ozone (O_3) generated by subjecting oxygen (O_2) to ultraviolet (UV) light. Ozone, a reactive gas, interacts with the carbon at room temperature and mildly oxidizes it, thereby functionalizing the carbon in the process. This method is a comparatively mild oxidative treatment than the wet acid reflux;
(4) Nitric acid and heat-treated soot (S4): The powdered form of HNO_3-treated carbon black was subjected to isothermal heat treatment at 300 °C in a hot-wall furnace for 1 h under an inert (Ar) environment.

All synthetic soot preparations were further characterized for their atomic oxygen content and functional groups introduced onto the carbon black surface. Characterization was performed by X-ray photoelectron spectroscopy (XPS) and thermogravimetric analysis (TGA), as indicated below.

2.2. X-Ray Photoelectron Spectroscopy (XPS)

X-ray photoelectron spectroscopy was used to identify and quantify possible different functional groups on the carbon surface and their contribution to the total surface atomic oxygen. XPS is a surface analysis technique based on the photoelectric effect where incoming X-rays of a known wavelength (λ) are used to eject surface electrons. With the known total energy of a photon, the kinetic energy (KE) of the ejected electron is measured, and the binding energy (BE) is calculated. The BE of a core–shell electron is characteristic of the element from which it is ejected and is used to identify the elements present. XPS experiments were performed using a Physical Electronics VersaProbe II instrument equipped with a monochromatic Al kα x-ray source ($h\nu$ = 1486.7 eV) and a concentric hemispherical analyzer. Charge neutralization was performed using both low-energy electrons (<5 eV) and argon ions. The binding energy axis was calibrated using sputter-cleaned Cu foil (Cu $2p_{3/2}$ = 932.7 eV, Cu $2p_{3/2}$ = 75.1 eV). Peaks were charge referenced to the C-C band in the carbon 1s spectra at 284.5 eV. Quantification of the elements was done by curve-fitting of the high-resolution scan using the CasaXPS software.

2.3. *Thermogravimetric Analysis (TGA)*

A TA instruments Thermogravimetric Analyzer TA 5500 coupled with a Discovery Mass Spectrometer (MS) was used to analyze mass loss and the composition of the evolved gases. The temperature was ramped up at 5 °C/min in an inert atmosphere. Thermal analysis of the material gives a qualitative assessment of the volumetric uniformity of functionalization of the carbon; therefore, TGA is used as a bulk material characterization tool to complement the results observed by XPS. When subject to a steady temperature ramp, functional groups on the carbon oxidize (leave) at different temperatures. The subsequent mass loss curve can be used to qualitatively identify the oxygen functional groups present on the carbon blacks.

2.4. *Cell Culture and Soot Exposure*

Cells from the male bronchial epithelial cell line BEAS-2B (ATCC® CRL-9609™) were thawed and cultured in RPMI-1640 medium (Gibco), supplemented with 2 mM glutamine (Gibco), 10% (*v*/*v*) heat-inactivated fetal bovine serum (VWR), and 10,000 units of Penicillin–Streptomycin (Gibco). Cells were grown in a 75 cm^2 (T75) cell culture Flask (Corning) and incubated at 37 °C in a humidified chamber with 5% CO_2.

2.4.1. Cell and Soot Exposure for Cell Viability Assessment

For cell viability studies, BEAS-2B cells were plated in 24-well plates (Corning) at a density of 50,000 cells per well overnight prior to treatment with the soot preparations. The powder soot preparations were dissolved in a small amount of DMSO and then diluted in PBS. The final concentration of DMSO in the cell exposure medium was <1%. Moreover, the volume of soot solution added did not exceed 10% of the total media volume in the well. Cells were incubated with the soot preparations described above for either 6 h or 24 h at concentrations ranging from 1.56 μg/mL to 100 μg/mL at 37 °C in a humidified chamber with 5% CO_2.

2.4.2. Cell Culture and Soot Exposures for Gene Expression Assessment

To quantify the expression of inflammatory and oxidative stress genes, BEAS-2B cells were plated in 24-well plates (Corning) at a density of 50,000 cells per well overnight prior to treatment with the soot preparations. The powder soot preparations were dissolved in methanol (MeOH, negative control) and then diluted in PBS. The final concentration of MeOH in the cell exposure media was <0.5%. Moreover, the volume of soot solution added did not exceed 10% of the total media volume in the well. Cells were incubated for 6 h at 37 °C in a humidified chamber with 5% CO_2 with all soot preparations, at concentrations of 1.56 to 12.5 μg/mL for inflammatory genes expression and of 3.125 μg/mL for oxidative stress genes expression.

2.4.3. Cell Culture and Soot Exposures for Protein Carbonylation Assessment

For protein carbonylation studies, BEAS-2B cells were grown in a 75 cm^2 (T75) cell culture Flask (Corning) and incubated at 37 °C in a humidified chamber with 5% CO_2. To quantify protein carbonylation, cells were plated in 12-well plates (Corning) at a density of 100,000 cells per well overnight prior to treatment with the soot preparations. The powder soot preparations were dissolved in methanol (MeOH, negative control) and then diluted in PBS. The final concentration of MeOH in the cell exposure media was <1%. Moreover, the volume of soot solution added did not exceed 10% of the total media volume in the well. Cells were incubated for 24 h at 37 °C in a humidified chamber with 5% CO_2 with all the soot preparations at concentrations of 25 μg/mL.

2.5. *Cell Viability Assay*

Cell viability was assessed using the MultiTox-Fluor Multiplex Cytotoxicity Assay Kit (Promega, Madison WI, USA), according to the manufacturer's instructions at 6 h and 24 h post-exposure with the different soot preparations. The assay was tested for cell viability and cytotoxicity using specific positive controls: digitonin (toxicity) and ionomycin (necrosis).

2.6. RNA Purification and cDNA synthesis

After exposure to soot preparations, cells were harvested in TRizol (Life Technologies, Austin, TX, USA) and RNA was extracted using the Direct-zol kit (Zymo Research, Irvine, CA, USA) in the presence of DNAse. Total RNA was quantified by nanodrop measurement and stored at −80 °C until further analysis. For cDNA synthesis, 500 ng of RNA were retrotranscribed using the High Capacity cDNA kit (Life Technologies), following the manufacturer's protocol. The cDNA reactions were stored at −20 °C until further use.

2.7. Real-Time PCR

The expression of inflammatory and oxidative stress-related genes was measured in 40 ng of cDNA by Real-Time PCR with TaqMan™ assays (Life Technologies). The following probes were used: IL1B (assay Hs01555410), IL6 (assay Hs00174131), NFE2L2 (assay Hs00232352), and SOD2 (assay Hs00167309). A housekeeping gene 18S (assay Hs03003631, Life Technologies) was used as a normalization control from 2 ng of cDNA. The reactions were conducted in triplicate using the TaqMan™ Fast Advanced Master Mix in 10 μL of final volume, following the manufacturer's protocol. Expression results (Ct values) were monitored and extracted using the QuantStudio 12K Flex Software, and data were analyzed using the relative quantification method [26].

2.8. Total Protein Determination

After exposure to soot, cells were harvested in 150 μL of 20 mM Tris-HCl lysis buffer at pH 7.5. The total protein concentration in lysates was determined by the Bicinchoninic Acid (BCA) protein assay (Pierce), following the manufacturer's protocol, using bovine serum albumin as a standard.

2.9. Protein Carbonylation Assay

The high sensitivity Protein Carbonyl ELISA Kit (Enzo Life Sciences, Farmingdale, NY, USA; cat #ALX-850-312-KI01) was used to determine the concentration of protein carbonylation starting from a sample volume containing 200 μg of protein and following the manufacturer's protocol.

2.10. Statistical Analysis

Cell proliferation, gene expression, and protein carbonylation data are presented as means ± SE. Data were plotted, and statistical analyses were performed using the GraphPad Prism software (v.8.4.3). Interactions of treatment and concentration were determined by two-way ANOVA followed by Dunnett's post hoc test, and differences among treatment groups were analyzed by one-way ANOVA followed by Tukey's post hoc analysis with the GraphPad Prism software (v.8.4.3). Values of $p < 0.05$ were considered statistically significant.

3. Results

3.1. Characterization of Soot

An illustrative transmission electron micrograph (TEM) of a carbon black aggregate and primary particle is shown in Figure 1. After wet and dry chemical treatment, and prior to conducting cell exposures, the different soot preparations were characterized to determine their atomic oxygen content and functional groups introduced onto the carbon surface by XPS and TGA, as indicated below.

XPS was performed using survey and high-resolution scans, to identify the elements present on the surface of treated soot, specifically oxygen groups. As a baseline, nascent (untreated) carbon black (S1) was also subject to the same analytical procedure. Elements in each soot preparation were quantified via curve-fitting of the high-resolution scans using the commercial software CasaXPS. Table 1 shows the measured atomic percentages of the elements present in the analyzed soot. Table 2 gives the relative percentages of oxygen functional groups present in the soot samples. As expected, the oxygen content is higher in the acid-treated soot (S2) than the ozone-treated soot (S3) and acid + heat-treated soot (S4). Wet acid reflux treatment of carbon black resulted in ≈32 atomic % oxygen compared to a ≈10 atomic % from dry gaseous treatment, the latter being a relatively mild oxidant with oxidation performed at room temperature, explaining this difference in the type and degree of functionalization. Moreover, being the most reactive group, the -COOH functional group is selectively removed with heat treatment from the carbon black, significantly reducing the oxygen content to ≈12 at (%) overall as measured by XPS. TGA-MS revealed a negligible mass loss for the ozone-treated sample (S3) between 300 and 500 °C despite the curve fit value of ≈2 at (%) carboxylic assignment. Various factors account for this observation. First, lactone (i.e., ester) and carboxylic anhydride groups can also register as "carboxylic" groups by the XPS curve fit, given similar C1s binding energy. (Notably, these groups do not possess the labile hydrogen nor form an anionic state.) Possessing greater thermal stability, these groups do not decompose at 300 °C. Moreover, the 2 at (%) carboxylic content as extracted by deconvolution is near the minimal level detectable by this fitting procedure, which is estimated as ≈1 at (%). Correspondingly, ozone treatment is known to introduce minimal carboxylic (-COOH) functionality in carbons as well.

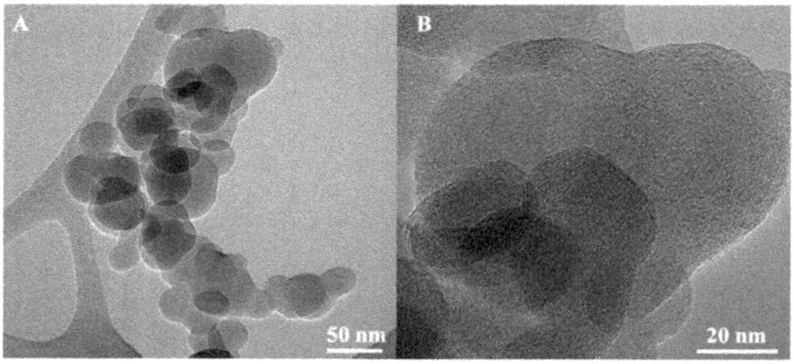

Figure 1. TEM image of a carbon black (**A**) aggregate and (**B**) primary particle.

Table 1. Elemental content measured as atomic percent for samples S1–S4. S1: nascent soot, S2: nitric acid-treated soot, S3: ozone-treated soot, S4: nitric acid and heat-treated soot.

Soot	Treatment	Measured Atomic [1] %			
		C	O	N	S
S1	None	97.2	1.3	–	0.9
S2	HNO_3	67.8	31.5	1.3	–
S3	Ozone	90	9.4	–	0.6
S4	HNO_3 + 300 °C	86.5	13.2	–	0.2

[1] C: carbon, O: oxygen, N: nitrogen, S: sulfur.

Table 2. Oxygen group percentages for samples S1–S4.

Soot	Treatment	Oxygen Groups %			
		C-O	C=O	O-C=O	Total O
S1	None	–	–	–	1.3
S2	HNO_3	10.2	4.9	9.4	34.0
S3	Ozone	2.2	1.4	2.4	8.3
S4	HNO_3 + 300 °C	7.3	3.8	0.5	12.1

3.2. Cell Viability and Cytotoxicity in BEAS-2B Cells Exposed to Synthetic Soot

BEAS-2B cell viability was measured at 6 and 24 h after exposure to soot preparations (Figures 2 and 3). A significant interaction of concentration and particle effect was found at both time points ($p < 0.0001$, two-way ANOVA). Treatment with ionomycin (positive control) resulted in a 95% reduction in cell viability after 6 h. When assessing independent effects, we found that after 6 h of treatment with S1 and S4 (soot with the lowest -COOH functional group content) (Table 2), there were no significant differences in cell viability at all the concentrations tested (Figure 2). Furthermore, the treatment of cells with soot containing the highest -COOH content (S2, S3) resulted in a reduction of viable cells in a dose-dependent manner. Treatment with S2 (9.4% -COOH content) resulted in a significant loss of cell viability at concentrations of 12.5 μg/mL and above. For S3 (2.4-COOH content), this effect was observed at a higher concentration (at least 50 μg/mL) (Figure 2).

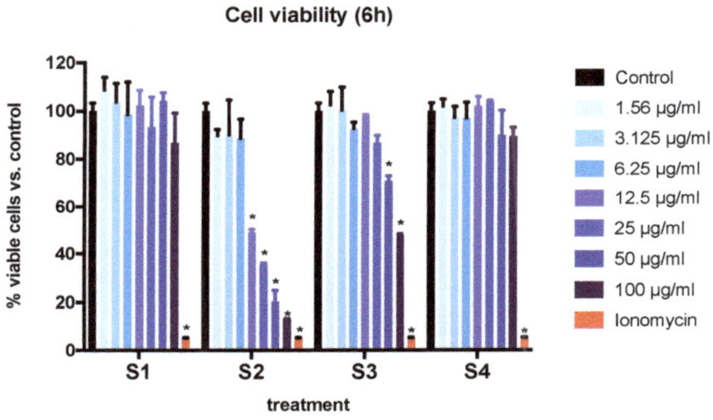

Figure 2. BEAS-2B cell viability expressed as percentage of viable cells at 6 h after exposure to four different soot preparations (S1–S4). The bars summarize data from three independent experiments ($n = 3$ replicates per experiment) with results normalized to control (cells exposed to DMSO). Data are expressed as mean ± SEM. * $p < 0.001$ (Dunnett's post hoc multiple comparisons test). Two-way ANOVA interaction: $p < 0.0001$, $F(21, 40) = 7.640$; concentration effect: $p < 0.0001$, $F(7, 40) = 25.67$); soot-type effect ($p < 0.0001$, $F(3, 40) = 69.91$. For a description of S1–S4, see Section 2.

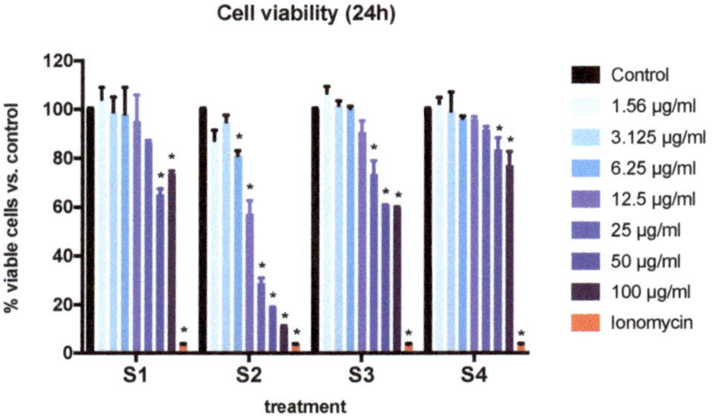

Figure 3. BEAS-2B cell viability expressed as percentage of viable cells after exposure to four different soot preparations for 24 h. The graph summarizes data from three independent experiments ($n = 3$ replicates per experiment), with results normalized to control cells (exposed to DMSO). Data are expressed as mean ± SEM. * $p < 0.001$ (Dunnett's post hoc multiple comparisons test). Two-way ANOVA interaction: $p < 0.0001$, $F(21, 36) = 11.59$; concentration effect: $p < 0.0001$, $F(7, 36) = 100.4$; soot type effect ($p < 0.0001$, $F(3, 36) = 127.6$). For a description of S1–S4, see Section 2.

At the 24-h time point, the exposure of cells to S1 and S4 at a concentration of 50 μg/mL or above induced a significant reduction in cell viability ($p < 0.001$) (Figure 3). The effect was observed at a much lower concentration (6.25 μg/mL and above) for S2, the soot with the highest -COOH content. Finally, the effect was observed at a concentration of 25 μg/mL or higher for S3 (Figure 3).

3.3. *Expression of Pro-Inflammatory Genes in Cells Exposed to Synthetic Soot*

To assess the ability of the different soot to induce an inflammatory response in BEAS-2B cells, we conducted real-time PCR experiments on extracts from cells exposed to S1–S4. To avoid significant cell death, we selected concentrations below 12.5 μg/mL and the 6-h time point based on the results obtained in Figure 2. We measured the expression of two pro-inflammatory cytokines (IL-1β and IL-6) that have been previously reported to increase in response to particulate matter exposure in human bronchial epithelial cells [20,27]. We limited our focus to IL-6 and IL-1β to compare the inflammatory effects of all soot preparations on IL-6 and IL-1β expression to these previously established outcomes. A significant interaction of concentration and particle effects was observed after 6 h of exposure to S1–S4 for both genes (IL-1β, $p = 0.022$; IL6, $p < 0.0001$, two-way ANOVA) (Figures 4 and 5).

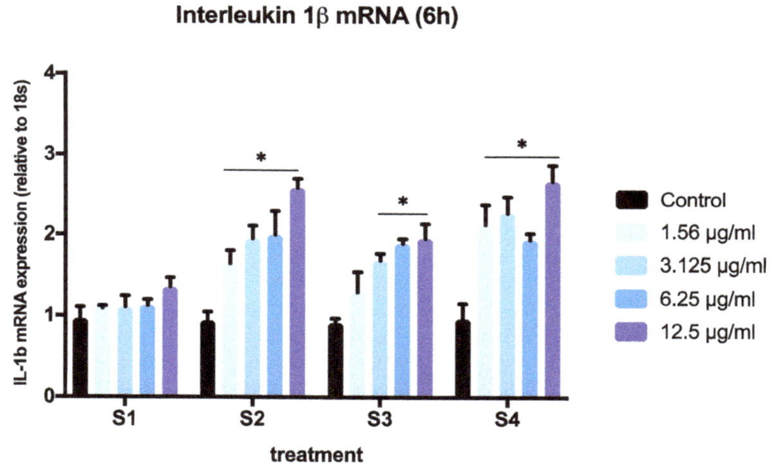

Figure 4. Expression of human interleukin-1 mRNA (IL1B) (relative to 18S expression) in BEAS-2B cell after exposure to soot preparations for 6 h. The graph summarizes data from three independent experiments ($n = 3$ replicates per experiment), with results normalized to controls (exposed to methanol) and expressed as mean ± SEM. Two-way ANOVA interaction: $p = 0.0109$, $F (12, 71) = 2.415$; concentration effect: $p < 0.0001$, $F (4, 71) = 30.51$; soot type effect ($p < 0.0001$, $F (3, 71) = 15.48$). * $p < 0.05$, different from control (Dunnett's multiple comparison's test). For a description of S1–S4, see Section 2.

The expression of IL-1β was significantly increased in a dose-dependent manner, when cells where exposed to S2, S3, or S4 at concentrations above 3.125 μg/mL (Figure 4). At the lowest concentration tested (1.56 μg/mL), only soot with a higher total oxygen content and C=O groups (S2 and S4) induced significant changes in IL-1β expression (Figure 4). A comparison of IL-1β expression in cells exposed to all soot at the highest concentration (12.5 μg/mL) revealed a significant effect of functionalized particles (S2, S3, S4) vs. nascent particles ($p < 0.05$, one-way ANOVA) (Figure 6A). This effect was also observed at concentrations as low as 3.125 μg/mL (Figure 6B).

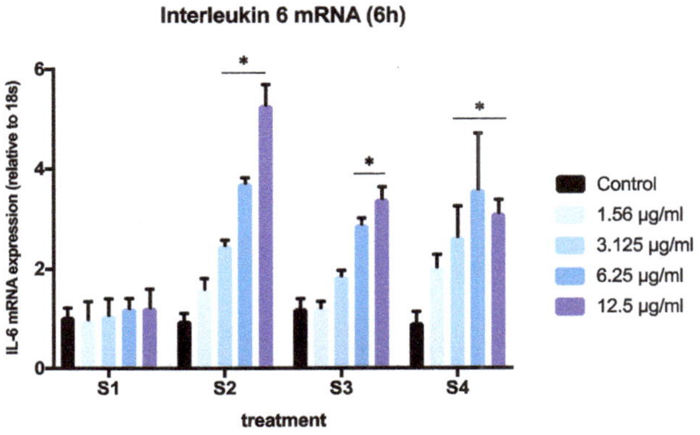

Figure 5. Expression of human interleukin-6 mRNA (IL6) (relative to 18S expression) in BEAS-2B cell after exposure to soot preparations for 6 h. The graph summarizes data from three independent experiments ($n = 3$ replicates per experiment), with results normalized to controls (exposed to methanol) and expressed as mean ± SEM. Two-way ANOVA interaction: $p < 0.0001$, F (12, 61) = 5.563 concentration effect: $p < 0.0001$, F (4, 61) = 36.99; soot type effect ($p < 0.0001$, F (3, 61) = 22.84). * $p < 0.05$, different from control (Dunnett's multiple comparison's test). For a description of S1–S4, see Section 2.

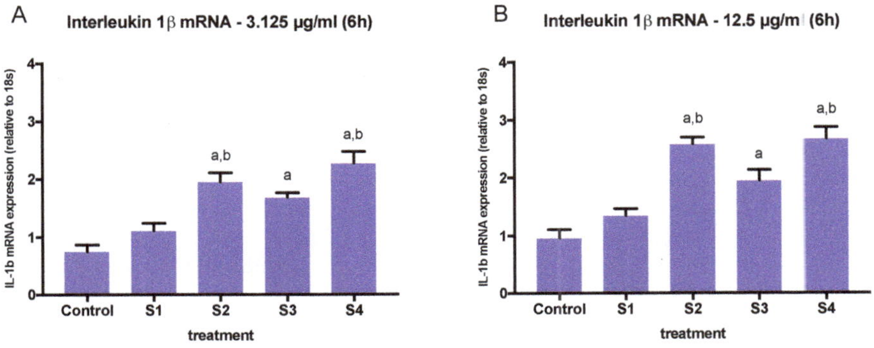

Figure 6. Human IL-1β mRNA (IL1B) expression (relative to 18S expression) in BEAS-2B cells treated with S1–S4 soot at 3.125 µg/mL (**A**) or 12.5 µg/mL (**B**) for 6 h. The graphs summarize data from three independent experiments ($n = 3$ replicates per experiment), with results normalized to controls (exposed to methanol) and expressed as mean ± SEM. a: different from control, b: different from S1 ($p < 0.05$). One-way ANOVA ($p < 0.001$, F (4, 20) = 20.47).

Similarly, the expression of IL-6 was significantly higher in cells exposed to functionalized soot (S2, S3, S4) at 6.25 µg/mL and 12.5 µg/mL, and it was significantly higher at 3.125 µg/mL only in cells exposed to S2 (Figure 5). When comparing the effects of different soot exposure at the highest concentration (12.5 µg/mL), we found significant differences among particles, with S2 inducing a significantly higher IL-6 mRNA expression than S3 and S4 (Figure 7A), and all three functionalized soot stimulating higher expression than the nascent (S1) particle ($p < 0.05$). In contrast, when comparing the effects of different soot at 3.125 µg/mL, the IL-6 response mimicked that of IL-1β (Figure 7B).

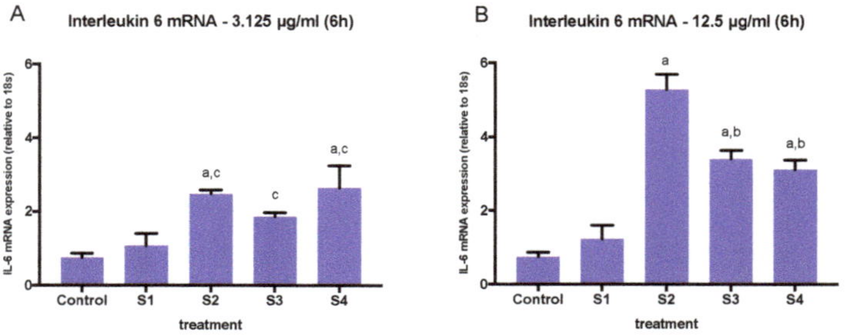

Figure 7. Human IL-6 mRNA (IL6) expression (relative to 18s) in BEAS-2B cells treated with S1–S4 soot at 3.125 μg/mL (**A**) or 12.5 μg/mL (**B**) for 6 h. The graphs summarize data from three independent experiments ($n = 3$ replicates per experiment), with results normalized to controls (exposed to methanol) and expressed as mean ± SEM. a: different from control and S1 ($p < 0.001$), b: different from S2 ($p < 0.05$), c: different from control. One-way ANOVA ($p < 0.001$, $F(3, 8) = 25.7$).

3.4. Expression of Oxidative Stress-Related Genes in Cells Exposed to Synthetic Soot

To assess the ability of the different soot preparations to induce the expression of oxidative stress-related genes in BEAS-2B cells, we conducted real-time PCR experiments on extracts from cells exposed to S1, S2, S3, and S4. We selected a concentration of 3.125 μg/mL at a 6-h time point considering that all soot preparations elicited changes in IL-6 and IL-1β gene expression at this concentration (Figure 4), while minimizing cell death (Figure 2). We measured the expression of two genes related to oxidative stress (SOD2 and NFE2L2), as previous studies have observed that $PM_{2.5}$-induced oxidation alters the expression of these genes in respiratory tract cells [28]. Both NFE2L2 and SOD2 are critical molecules in the lung's defense mechanism against oxidative stress, and their disruption enhances susceptibility to airway inflammation [29,30].

A significant interaction of particle effects on SOD2 and NFE2L2 expression (SOD2, $p = <0.0001$; NFE2L2, $p = 0.0001$, one-way ANOVA) was observed after 6 h of exposure to all soot particles at 3.125 μg/mL. SOD2 expression was significantly downregulated in cells exposed to S2, S3, and S4, but not S1 (Figure 8A). Cell exposure to S2 and S3 resulted in the most significant downregulation in SOD2 expression, both being the highest in O-C=O content compared to S1 and S4 (Table 2). Similarly, the expression of NFE2L2 was downregulated by cell exposure to all soot preparations, including S1, with the greatest effect observed in S2 and S3 exposure (Figure 8B). Comparison of SOD2 and NFE2L2 expression in cells exposed to all soot preparations at 3.125 μg/mL revealed a significant effect of functionalized particles (S1, S2, S3, S4) vs. control particles.

3.5. Protein Carbonylation in Cells Exposed to Synthetic Soot

To assess the ability of the soot preparations to alter protein carbonylation, we measured carbonylation levels in protein extracts from BEAS-2B cells exposed to S1, S2, S3, and S4 at a concentration of 25 μg/mL at a 24-h time point. We chose this concentration because it is the minimum concentration that results in a reduction in cell viability at this time point. The exposure of cells to S2 and S4, i.e., the soot with the highest oxygen, C-O, and C=O content, resulted in the greatest increase in total of protein carbonylation compared to S1 and S3 (Figure 9). Interestingly, the increase of protein carbonylation triggered by S2 and S4 mimics the effects observed on IL-1β expression at 12.5 μg/mL at 6 h of exposure.

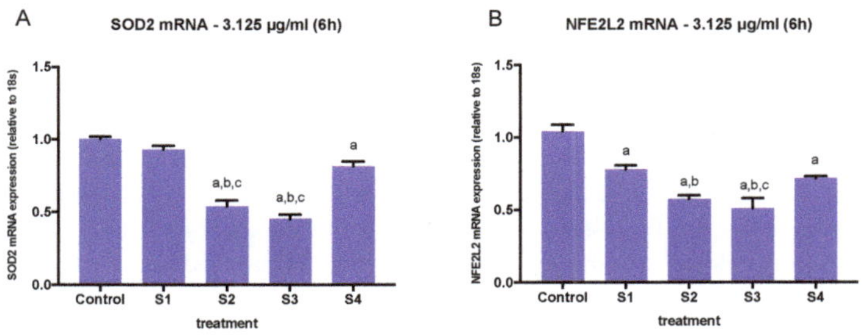

Figure 8. Expression of oxidative stress genes (relative to 18S expression) in BEAS-2B cells treated with S1–S4 soot at 3.125 ug/mL for 6 h. (**A**) Superoxide dismutase 2 (SOD2) mRNA. (**B**) Nuclear factor erythroid 2-related factor 2 (NFE2L2) mRNA. The graphs summarize data from three independent replicates, with gene expression results normalized to controls (exposed to DMSO) and expressed as mean ± SEM. a: different from control, b: different from S1, c: different from S4. One-way ANOVA ($p < 0.05$).

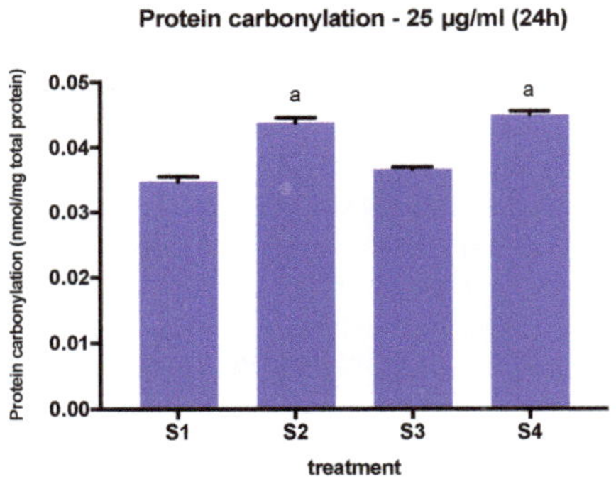

Figure 9. Protein carbonylation levels in BEAS-2B cells treated with S1–S4 soot at 25 ug/mL for 24 h. Results are expressed as nmol/mg of total protein. a: different from S1 and S3. One-way ANOVA ($p < 0.001$, $F(3, 12) = 63.07$).

4. Discussion

Air pollution is a significant health hazard that is associated with the worsening of cardiopulmonary disease and reduction of life expectancy. It is estimated that over 90% of the world population is exposed to higher than recommended levels of ambient air pollution, including outdoor particle pollution such as $PM_{2.5}$ [31]. Decades of epidemiological and toxicological research have demonstrated that exposure to $PM_{2.5}$ is detrimental to lung health and contributes significantly to the development and exacerbation of a multitude of lung diseases [32]. Nonetheless, the cellular and molecular mechanisms driving these outcomes remain poorly understood, and the influence of physicochemical characteristics of soot particles in these mechanisms has not been yet explored. Accumulating evidence from in vivo and in vitro studies using environmental samples or purified $PM_{2.5}$ mixtures have indicated that the lung epithelium responds to particle exposures in a dose- and time-dependent manner, by activating redox responses, initiating and/or exacerbating inflammation, and causing DNA damage and epigenetic alterations [14]. In this study, rather than evaluating the effects of purified particles from environmental samples, we investigated the effects of exposing lung epithelial cells to synthetic soot. We assessed the effects of particles directly on oxidative stress and inflammatory responses to understand the contributions of their surface chemistry vs. the carbonaceous soot backbone itself. Our data revealed that surface chemistry, and specifically oxygen and carboxylic acid content, contributes to cell death, the expression of inflammatory and oxidative stress genes, and protein oxidative damage (carbonylation) in human lung epithelial cells in a concentration and time-dependent way.

Many of the adverse health effects of $PM_{2.5}$ exposure are hypothesized to be derived from oxidative stress and inflammation, which is initiated by the formation of reactive oxygen species (ROS) and expression of pro-inflammatory genes within cells [33]. Although several studies have demonstrated the ROS potential and inflammatory action of diesel particulates from diesel engines [34], the causative factors are less clear. Most studies assessing these effects have used organics diluted and extracted from real exhaust particulates, and the results reported may be skewed relative to cell exposure to the "complete" soot, i.e., particulate matter along with its heteroatoms and condensed fractions. It is increasingly being recognized that extracts of diesel soot are a poor representation of the full range of toxicity [35]. Rather, the particles and, in particular, their surface chemistry have considerable direct impacts. To understand and potentially quantify the effect of parameters such as particle size, morphology, and chemistry, this study used surface-modified carbon black being a close substitute in its make and morphology. Functionalized carbon black is a surrogate for soot to understand the hierarchy of detrimental effects of soot from a combustion engine, i.e., the health effects of the primary particle itself as compared to those of the functional groups on the carbonaceous backbone. We chose carbon black to be able to control the extent of functionalization introduced and study the cell response by selectively modifying the material to exclude acidic functional groups. Exposure of a human lung epithelial cell line to model soot that closely resembles real combustion-generated soot in structure, particle size, and chemistry allowed us to identify and associate specific outcomes with particle physicochemical characteristics.

To our knowledge, this is the first study to examine the effects of surface particle chemistry and nanostructure on human lung epithelial responses. Prior studies using purified environmental samples have reported limited and often contradictory outcomes. Moreover, the majority of in vitro studies testing for toxicity use washing soot extracts that convolve condensed organics on the particles with extracted organics from the particle, ignoring the fixed particle surface chemistry. This has complicated the toxicity assessment of engine exhaust products, which is mainly due to our limited understanding of the specific contributions of different soot components. Our study provides new information on the contributions of surface chemistry to the particle's cytotoxicity. Our data indicate that both oxygen content and functional groups enhance the particle's ability to induce cell death. We demonstrate here that particles with the highest surface oxygen percentage and carboxylic acid content impair cell viability at lower concentrations than those with lower oxygen and carboxylic acid content. In addition, we show that this effect is also concentration- and time-dependent. Higher exposure times (24 h vs. 6 h) resulted in a significantly lower number of viable cells for a given concentration in particles with lower carboxylic acid content (S1, S4), but not in those with higher content (S2, S3).

It has been recently shown that exposure to $PM_{2.5}$ below the current U.S. Environmental Protection Agency standards is associated with increased mortality [36]. This suggests that the inhalation of soot at very low concentrations may induce cellular damage that accumulates over time. While it is not possible to determine how closely the concentrations tested in this study reflect those of actual in vivo exposures in the human lung epithelium, we aimed to use concentrations that do not cause significant cytotoxicity when determining the contributions of particle chemistry on inflammation and oxidative stress effects. Thus, we examined the expression of two pro-inflammatory markers known to be expressed by lung epithelial cells (IL-1β and IL-6) [37] in BEAS-2B cells exposed for 6 h to soot at concentrations that were not toxic and did not have major effects on cell viability (12.5 μg/mL or lower). Our results demonstrate that the presence of functional groups in the particle's surface was sufficient to induce an inflammatory response, as indicated by the stimulation of IL-1β and IL-6 gene expression by S2, S3, and S4, but not S1. Moreover, this effect was dose-dependent, indicating a potential mechanism involving the activation of pattern recognition receptors [38]. These receptors are known for recognizing specific ligands such as pathogen- and damage-associated molecular patterns, which are endogenous ligands derived from stressed cells [39]. The activation of pattern recognition receptors such as Toll-like-receptors in response to PM exposure results in the release of cytokines and chemokines to attract immune cells to the site of injury [40,41]. At the highest concentration tested (12.5 μg/mL), we did not observe a differential effect on IL-1β expression among different soot preparations. However, the expression of IL-6 mRNA was significantly higher in cells exposed to S2. This soot not only presents the higher oxygen atomic content, but also the higher percentage of -COOH, C=O, and C-O groups. In a previous study, 100 μg/mL ultrafine carbon black was observed to increase mRNA and protein expressions of IL-1β and IL-6 in primary rat epithelial lung cells, but IL-6 protein expression was delayed compared to IL-6 mRNA expression, and IL-1β mRNA and protein expression were not correlated [42]. Other studies have shown that IL-1β mRNA levels do not necessarily reflect IL-1β protein secretion [43]. Furthermore, it has been observed that endotoxin contamination, a component of some environmental PM preparations, may cause an intracellular accumulation of cytokines, including IL-1β [44], although previous findings indicate that endotoxin is usually found on coarse PM [45]. To further investigate the inflammatory effects of the synthetic soot, future studies should also examine the expression of IL-8 and TNF-α, as these genes have been implicated in numerous human lung diseases [46,47] and found to be upregulated in human bronchial epithelial cells exposed to PM [48,49].

In addition to studying the inflammatory response triggered by soot exposure, we examined the expression of SOD2 and NFE2L2, which play a critical role in antioxidant defense mechanisms against ROS. We used a concentration that did not significantly reduce cell viability (3.125 μg/mL) but was enough to elicit an inflammatory response by altering IL-6 and IL-1β gene expression. We found that the presence of functional groups in the particles' surface was sufficient to alter the expression of both SOD2 and NFE2L2, as indicated by the gene expression changes in cells exposed to S1, S2, S3, and S4. Interestingly, SOD2 mRNA expression was significantly lower in cells exposed to all soot variants, including S1, but NFE2L2 gene expression was not significantly affected in cells treated with S1. The expression of SOD2 and NFE2L2 was the lowest in cells exposed to S2 and S3, the highest total oxygen carboxylic acid-containing soot, indicating a potential role of these groups in the inhibition of these gene's expression.

Combined, these findings suggest that $PM_{2.5}$ toxicity induces a decrease in the expression of antioxidant response genes SOD2 and NFE2L2. Under physiologic conditions, ROS generation is minimized by antioxidant proteins, but an overproduction of ROS disturbs the antioxidant defense system, leading to oxidative stress [30]. ROS are produced by the reduction of molecular oxygen and the formation of superoxide anions. Superoxides are precursors to most ROS but are metabolized by SOD2 to hydrogen peroxide (H_2O_2). Catalase (CAT) serves as a protective enzyme that breaks down H_2O_2 and eliminates ROS formation. Some studies have shown that exposure to $PM_{2.5}$ induces a loss of SOD2 and CAT activity, leading to an accumulation of ROS [24]. $PM_{2.5}$ has also been observed to downregulate protein kinase B (Akt) signaling, which is a known modulator of SOD2 and NFE2L2, decreasing the expression of SOD2 and NFE2L2 [49,50]. Another study observed that NFE2L2 expression in human BEAS-2B bronchial epithelial cells is downregulated when cells are subjected to high concentrations of $PM_{2.5}$ or repeated exposure protocols [51].

An impairment in the antioxidant defense mechanism by the downregulation of SOD2 and NFE2L2 increases the expression of IL-1β and IL-6, inducing an inflammatory response, as observed in our findings [52]. Based on our data, a decrease in SOD2 and NFE2L2 gene expression is associated with a significant increase in IL-1β and IL-6, particularly in cells treated with S2 and S4, potentiating an inflammatory response as expected. The high oxygen content of S2 and S4 makes them potential good oxidants that can cause changes in oxygen saturation and can react with molecular oxygen to form H_2O_2 and the most potent form of ROS, hydroxyl radicals. Exposure to $PM_{2.5}$ can downregulate CAT activity, causing an overaccumulation of these ROS, resulting in production and oxidative stress, increasing the inflammatory response [53]. While S3 (O_3 treated $PM_{2.5}$) did not cause the most significant increase in IL-1 β and IL-6 gene expression, S3 along with S2 did cause the most significant decrease in SOD2 and NFE2L2 gene expression. O_3 generates ROS, including H_2O_2, thus exerting similar effects to soot with higher oxygen content [54]. Overall, more research is needed to elucidate the mechanisms by which the expression of antioxidant enzymes and transcription factors relates to oxidative stress responses induced by soot with varying surface chemistry.

Carbonylation is an irreversible protein modification induced by oxidative stress and is associated with chronic inflammation. Thus, we examined protein carbonylation as a potential biomarker of oxidative stress induced by exposure to $PM_{2.5}$ in our studies. Protein carbonylation is a well-used biomarker for studying numerous human diseases, including Alzheimer's disease, diabetes, and chronic lung disease. Despite this, very little is known about $PM_{2.5}$-induced protein carbonylation and its role in oxidative stress. We exposed BEAS-2B cells for 24 h to soot preparations at a concentration that elicited changes in cell viability at 24 h (25 μg/mL) but no cell death. Protein carbonylation has been previously observed to increase in human keratinocytes exposed to $PM_{2.5}$ at 50 μg/mL at a 24-h time point [23], indicating that changes in protein carbonylation require higher concentrations of PM than those required to elicit changes in gene expression. We found that that protein carbonylation was significantly higher in cells exposed to S2 and S4 compared to cells exposed to S1 and S3, thus following a similar trend observed in IL-1β and IL-6 gene expression. Targets of carbonylation are dependent on the oxidative environment of the cell and abundance of ROS. In the NFE2L2/Kelch-like ECH-associated protein 1 (KEAP1) mechanism, cytoplasmic KEAP1 binds NFE2L2, targeting it for proteasomal degradation. When carbonylated, KEAP1 releases NFE2L2, which translocates to the nucleus and, along with other transcription factors, binds to antioxidant response elements to produce cytoprotective proteins [22].

Our study has several limitations. First, while our characterization of lung epithelial cellular responses to synthetically modified soot revealed important contributions of surface chemistry, we used a submerged monolayer culture model wherein cells have been removed from their physiological conditions, including interactions with neighboring cells in the airway epithelium. Therefore, our studies will need to be replicated and investigated by alternative methods such as exposures in air–liquid interface cell cultures, using cell lines and primary cells of the lung and nasal epithelia, and using in vivo exposure models. Second, the BEAS-2B cell line is derived from an adult male individual; therefore, our results do not reflect the potential effects of sex/gender and/or age in the observed responses. Considering the known differential effects of air pollution exposure in men and women [55], and in individuals of different age groups and disease status [56], it will be important to expand these investigations to models that are representative of such populations. Third, while according to the literature, a particle concentration of 100 μg/mL corresponds to approximately 16μg/cm^2 if all the suspended particles are deposited on the cells on the surface of the plates [57], we have not directly measured the proportion of particles that were in contact with cultured cells in our experiments. Finally, we have reported a differential reduction on the percent of viable cells as well as changes in mRNA expression of selected inflammatory and oxidative stress-related genes upon exposures, although in the current study, we have not evaluated changes in cytokine protein expression, the activity of oxidative stress enzymes, nor mechanisms previously associated with $PM_{2.5}$ responses, including mitochondrial damage, apoptosis, autophagy, DNA damage, and epigenetic changes [52,58–60].

Our study has potential implications for environmental health. Vehicular traffic and consequent engine exhaust and industrial emissions are among the top contributors to outdoor pollution that results in millions of annual causalities worldwide. In light of the recent COVID-19 outbreak, one pilot (unpublished) study highlighted that an increase of only 1 μg/m^3 in $PM_{2.5}$ is associated with an 8% increase in the COVID-19 death rate [61]. While particle air pollution regulations are currently based on mass, the discussion is ongoing as to whether to include particle number concentration as a pseudo-surrogate for particle surface area. The results from our study reflect the impact of particle surface chemistry and physical structure as direct operative factors in health impacts, suggesting that such factors should be considered when developing environmental policies. These physicochemical properties are relatable to combustion conditions and fuel, indicating that precautions for exposure to small particles from various sources may be improved, and corresponding improvements in mitigation strategies may be more rapidly engineered.

In summary, we report that particle surface chemistry contributes to the cellular and molecular responses exerted in lung epithelial cells. We show that higher oxygen content and carboxylic acid functional groups in soot result in greater cell damage and death and cause the cells to react by activating inflammatory responses. These effects are exacerbated by soot concentration and exposure time. Together, our results demonstrate the role of particle surface chemistry as a direct operative factor impacting health. This physicochemical property is relatable to combustion conditions and fuel type. Thus, precautions for exposure to other soot types with similar surface (oxygen) chemistry may be improved, enabling better assessment from other anthropogenic sources and thereby formulating effective mitigation strategies to tackle this problem worldwide.

5. Conclusions

We conclude that particle surface chemistry, and specifically oxygen content and the presence of carboxylic acid groups in soot, differentially affect inflammatory and oxidative stress responses in human lung epithelial cells.

Author Contributions: Conceptualization, R.L.V.W., P.S.; methodology, H.A.H., S.E., M.S., M.N., R.L.V.W., P.S.; formal analysis, H.A.H., S.E., M.S., M.N., R.L.V.W., P.S.; investigation, H.A.H., S.E., M.S., M.N., R.L.V.W., P.S.; writing—original draft preparation, H.A.H., M.S., R.L.V.W., P.S.; writing—review and editing, H.A.H., S.E., M.S., R.L.V.W., P.S.; supervision, R.L.V.W., P.S.; validation, H.A.H., R.L.V.W., P.S.; visualization, H.A.H., R.L.V.W., P.S.; project administration, R.L.V.W., P.S.; funding acquisition, R.L.V.W., P.S. All authors have read and agreed to the published version of the manuscript.

Funding: This research was funded by the Pennsylvania State University Human Health & the Environment Seed Grant (R.L.V., P.S.), and the National Heart Lung and Blood Institute of the National Institutes of Health under award number HL133520 (PS).

Conflicts of Interest: The authors declare no conflict of interest. The funders had no role in the design of the study; in the collection, analyses, or interpretation of data; in the writing of the manuscript, or in the decision to publish the results.

References

1. Zhang, R.; Wang, G.; Guo, S.; Zamora, M.; Ying, Q.; Lin, Y.; Wang, W.; Hu, M.; Wang, Y. Formation of Urban Fine Particulate Matter. *Chem. Rev.* **2015**, *115*, 3803–3855. [CrossRef] [PubMed]
2. Dai, L.; Zanobetti, A.; Koutrakis, P.; Schwartz, J.D. Associations of fine particulate matter species with mortality in the united states: A multicity time-series analysis. *Environ. Health Perspect.* **2014**, *122*, 837–842. [CrossRef] [PubMed]
3. Lelieveld, J.; Pozzer, A.; Pöschl, U.; Fnais, M.; Haines, A.; Münzel, T. Loss of life expectancy from air pollution compared to other risk factors: A worldwide perspective. *Cardiovas. Res.* **2020**. [CrossRef]
4. Babatola, S.S. Global burden of diseases attributable to air pollution. *J. Public Health Afr.* **2018**, *9*, 813. [CrossRef]
5. Schwarze, P.E.; Ovrevik, J.; Låg, M.; Refsnes, M.; Nafstad, P.; Hetland, R.B.; Dybing, E. Particulate matter properties and health effects: Consistency of epidemiological and toxicological studies. *Hum. Exp. Toxicol.* **2006**, *25*, 559–579. [CrossRef] [PubMed]
6. Bell, M.L.; Dominici, F.; Ebisu, K.; Zeger, S.L.; Samet, J.M. Spatial and temporal variation in PM2.5 chemical composition in the United States for health effects studies. *Environ. Health Perspect.* **2007**, *115*, 989–995. [CrossRef]
7. Cassee, F.R.; Héroux, M.E.; Gerlofs-Nijland, M.E.; Kelly, F.J. Particulate matter beyond mass: Recent health evidence on the role of fractions, chemical constituents and sources of emission. *Inhal. Toxicol.* **2013**, *25*, 802–812. [CrossRef]
8. Xing, Y.F.; Xu, Y.H.; Shi, M.H.; Lian, Y.X. The impact of PM2.5 on the human respiratory system. *J. Thorac. Dis.* **2016**, *8*, E69–E74. [CrossRef]

9. Liu, Q.; Xu, C.; Ji, G.; Shao, W.; Zhang, C.; Gu, A.; Zhao, P. Effect of exposure to ambient PM2.5 pollution on the risk of respiratory tract diseases: A meta-analysis of cohort studies. *J. Biomed. Res.* **2017**, *31*, 130–142. [CrossRef]
10. Du, Y.; Xu, X.; Chu, M.; Guo, Y.; Wang, J. Air particulate matter and cardiovascular disease: The epidemiological, biomedical and clinical evidence. *J. Thorac. Dis.* **2016**, *8*, E8–E19. [CrossRef]
11. Li, D.; Li, Y.; Li, G.; Zhang, Y.; Li, J.; Chen, H. Fluorescent reconstitution on deposition of PM 2.5 in lung and extrapulmonary organs. *Proc. Natl. Acad. Sci. USA* **2019**, *116*, 2488–2493. [CrossRef] [PubMed]
12. Bourdrel, T.; Bind, M.A.; Béjot, Y.; Morel, O.; Argacha, J.F. Cardiovascular effects of air pollution. *Arch. Cardiovasc. Dis.* **2017**, *110*, 634–642. [CrossRef] [PubMed]
13. Huynh, M.; Woodruff, T.J.; Parker, J.D.; Schoendorf, K.C. Relationships between air pollution and preterm birth in California. *Paediatr. Perinat. Epidemiol.* **2006**, *20*, 454–461. [CrossRef] [PubMed]
14. Salvi, S.; Holgate, S.T. Mechanisms of particulate matter toxicity. *Clin. Exp. Allergy* **1999**, *29*, 1187–1194. [CrossRef]
15. Martinelli, N.; Girelli, D.; Cigolini, D.; Sandri, M.; Ricci, G.; Rocca, G.; Olivieri, O. Access rate to the emergency department for venous thromboembolism in relationship with coarse and fine particulate matter air pollution. *PLoS ONE* **2012**, *7*. [CrossRef] [PubMed]
16. De Oliveira, B.F.A.; Ignotti, E.; Artaxo, P.; Do Nascimento Saldiva, P.H.; Junger, W.L.; Hacon, S. Risk assessment of PM2.5 to child residents in Brazilian Amazon region with biofuel production. *Environ. Health A Glob. Access Sci. Source* **2012**, *11*, 1–11. [CrossRef]
17. Chung, K.F. Cytokines in chronic obstructive pulmonary disease. *Eur. Respir. J.* **2001**, *18*, 50–59. [CrossRef]
18. Delfino, R.J.; Staimer, N.; Tjoa, T.; Arhami, M.; Polidori, A.; Gillen, D.L.; George, S.C.; Shafer, M.M.; Schauer, J.J.; Sioutas, C. Associations of primary and secondary organic aerosols with airway and systemic inflammation in an elderly panel cohort. *Epidemiology* **2010**, *21*, 892–902. [CrossRef]
19. Xu, F.; Qiu, X.; Hu, X.; Shang, Y.; Pardo, M.; Fang, Y.; Wang, J.; Rudich, Y.; Zhu, T. Effects on IL-1B signaling activation induced by water and organic extracts of fine particulate matter (PM2.5) *in vitro*. *Environ. Pollut.* **2018**, *237*, 592–600. [CrossRef]
20. Fujii, T.; Hayashi, S.; Hogg, J.C.; Vincent, R.; Van Eeden, S.F. Particulate matter induces cytokine expression in human bronchial epithelial cells. *Am. J. Respir. Cell Mol. Biol.* **2001**, *25*, 265–271. [CrossRef]
21. Dalle-Donne, I.; Giustarini, D.; Colombo, R.; Rossi, R.; Milzani, A. Protein carbonylation in human diseases. *Trends Mol. Med.* **2003**, *9*, 169–176. [CrossRef]
22. Dalle-Donne, I.; Aldini, G.; Carini, M.; Colombo, R.; Rossi, R.; Milzani, A. Protein carbonylation.; cellular dysfunction.; and disease progression. *J. Cell Mol. Med.* **2006**, *10*, 389–406. [CrossRef] [PubMed]
23. Piao, M.J.; Ahn, M.J.; Kang, K.A.; Ryu, Y.S.; Hyun, Y.J.; Shilnikova, K.; Zhen, A.X.; Jeong, J.W.; Choi, Y.H.; Kang, H.K.; et al. Particulate matter 2.5 damages skin cells by inducing oxidative stress, subcellular organelle dysfunction, and apoptosis. *Arch. Toxicol.* **2018**, *92*, 2077–2091. [CrossRef] [PubMed]
24. Aztatzi-Aguilar, O.; Valdés-Arzate, A.; Debray-García, Y.; Calderón-Aranda, E.; Uribe-Ramirez, M.; Acosta-Saavedra, L.; Gonsebatt, M.E.; Maciel-Ruiz, J.A.; Petrosyan, P.; Mugica-Alvarez, V.; et al. Exposure to ambient particulate matter induces oxidative stress in lung and aorta in a size- and time-dependent manner in rats. *Toxicol. Res. Appl.* **2018**, *2*. [CrossRef]
25. Figueiredo, J.L.; Pereira, M.F. The role of surface chemistry in catalysis with carbons. *Catal. Today* **2010**, *150*, 2–7. [CrossRef]
26. Livak, K.J.; Schmittgen, T.D. Analysis of relative gene expression data using real-time quantitative PCR and the 2(-Delta Delta C(T)) Method. *Methods* **2001**, *25*, 402–408. [CrossRef]
27. Longhin, E.; Holme, J.A.; Gualtieri, M.; Camatini, M.; Øvrevik, J. Milan winter fine particulate matter (wPM2.5) induces IL-6 and IL-8 synthesis in human bronchial BEAS-2B cells, but specifically impairs IL-8 release. *Toxicol. Vitr.* **2018**, *52*, 365–373. [CrossRef]
28. Hong, Z.; Guo, Z.; Zhang, R.; Xu, J.; Dong, W.; Zhuang, G.; Deng, C. Airborne Fine Particulate Matter Induces Oxidative Stress and Inflammation in Human Nasal Epithelial Cells. *Tohoku J. Exp. Med.* **2016**, *239*, 117–125. [CrossRef]
29. Rangasamy, T.; Guo, J.; Mitzner, W.A.; Roman, J.; Singh, A.; Fryer, A.D.; Yamamoto, M.; Kensler, T.W.; Tuder, R.M.; Georas, S.N.; et al. Disruption of Nrf2 enhances susceptibility to severe airway inflammation and asthma in mice. *J. Exp. Med.* **2005**, *202*, 47–59. [CrossRef]

30. Cui, Y.; Chen, G.; Yang, Z. Mitochondrial superoxide mediates PM2.5-induced cytotoxicity in human pulmonary lymphatic endothelial cells. *Environ. Pollut.* **2020**, *263*. [CrossRef]
31. World Health Organization. Ambient Air Pollution: A Global Assessment of Exposure and Burden of Disease. World Health Organization. 2016. Available online: http://apps.who.int/iris/bitstream/10665/250141/1/9789241511353-eng.pdf (accessed on 6 August 2020).
32. Cohen, A.J.; Brauer, M.; Burnett, R.; Anderson, H.R.; Frostad, J.; Estep, K.; Balakrishnan, K.; Brunekreef, B.; Dandona, L.; Dandona, R.; et al. Estimates and 25-year trends of the global burden of disease attributable to ambient air pollution: An analysis of data from the Global Burden of Diseases Study 2015. *Lancet* **2017**, *389*, 1907–1918. [CrossRef]
33. Pope, C.A.; Bhatnagar, A.; McCracken, J.P.; Abplanalp, W.; Conklin, D.J.; O'Toole, T. Exposure to Fine Particulate Air Pollution Is Associated With Endothelial Injury and Systemic Inflammation. *Circ. Res.* **2016**, *119*, 1204–1214. [CrossRef] [PubMed]
34. Steiner, S.; Bisig, C.; Petri-Fink, A.; Rothen-Rutishauser, B. Diesel exhaust: Current knowledge of adverse effects and underlying cellular mechanisms. *Arch. Toxicol.* **2016**, *90*, 1541–1553. [CrossRef] [PubMed]
35. Steiner, S.; Heeb, N.V.; Czerwinski, J.; Comte, P.; Mayer, A.; Petri-Fink, A.; Rothen-Rutishauser, B. Test-methods on the test-bench: A comparison of complete exhaust and exhaust particle extracts for genotoxicity/mutagenicity assessment. *Environ. Sci. Technol.* **2014**, *48*, 5237–5244. [CrossRef] [PubMed]
36. Shi, L.; Zanobetti, A.; Kloog, I.; Coull, B.A.; Koutrakis, P.; Melly, S.J.; Schwartz, J.D. Low-Concentration PM2.5 and Mortality: Estimating Acute and Chronic Effects in a Population-Based Study. *Environ. Health Perspect.* **2016**, *124*, 46–52. [CrossRef]
37. Gioda, A.; Fuentes-Mattei, E.; Jimenez-Velez, B. Evaluation of cytokine expression in BEAS cells exposed to fine particulate matter (PM2.5) from specialized indoor environments. *Int. J. Environ. Health Res.* **2011**, *21*, 106–119. [CrossRef]
38. Bauer, R.N.; Diaz-Sanchez, D.; Jaspers, I. Effects of air pollutants on innate immunity: The role of Toll-like receptors and nucleotide-binding oligomerization domain-like receptors. *J. Allergy Clin. Immunol.* **2012**, *129*, 14–26. [CrossRef]
39. Bianchi, M.E. DAMPs, PAMPs and alarmins: All we need to know about danger. *J. Leukoc. Biol.* **2007**, *81*, 1–5. [CrossRef]
40. Lafferty, E.I.; Qureshi, S.T.; Schnare, M. The role of toll-like receptors in acute and chronic lung inflammation. *J. Inflamm.* **2010**, *7*, 57. [CrossRef]
41. Bach, N.S.; Låg, M.; Øvrevik, J. Toll like receptor-3 priming alters diesel exhaust particle-induced cytokine responses in human bronchial epithelial cells. *Toxicol. Lett.* **2014**, *228*, 42–47. [CrossRef]
42. Totlandsdal, A.I.; Refsnes, M.; Låg, M. Mechanisms involved in ultrafine carbon black-induced release of IL-6 from primary rat epithelial lung cells. *Toxicol. Vitr.* **2010**, *24*, 10–20. [CrossRef] [PubMed]
43. Watkins, L.R.; Hansen, M.K.; Nguyen, K.T.; Lee, J.E.; Maier, S.F. Dynamic regulation of the proinflammatory cytokine, interleukin-1beta: Molecular biology for non-molecular biologists. *Life Sci.* **1999**, *65*, 449–481. [CrossRef]
44. Monn, C.; Becker, S. Cytotoxicity and induction of proinflammatory cytokines from human monocytes exposed to fine (PM2.5) and coarse particles (PM10-2.5) in outdoor and indoor air. *Toxicol. Appl. Pharmacol.* **1999**, *155*, 245–252. [CrossRef] [PubMed]
45. Pavilonis, B.T.; Anthony, T.R.; O'Shaughnessy, P.T.; Humann, M.J.; Merchant, J.A.; Moore, G.; Thorne, P.S.; Weisel, C.P.; Sanderson, W.T. Indoor and outdoor particulate matter and endotoxin concentrations in an intensely agricultural county. *J. Expo. Sci. Environ. Epidemiol.* **2013**, *23*, 299–305. [CrossRef] [PubMed]
46. McNamara, M.; Thornburg, J.; Semmens, E.; Ward, T.; Noonan, C. Coarse particulate matter and airborne endotoxin within wood stove homes. *Indoor Air* **2013**, *23*, 498–505. [CrossRef] [PubMed]
47. Lundblad, L.K.; Thompson-Figueroa, J.; Leclair, T.; Sullivan, M.J.; Poynter, M.E.; Irvin, C.G.; Bates, J.H. Tumor necrosis factor-alpha overexpression in lung disease: A single cause behind a complex phenotype. *Am. J. Respir. Crit. Care Med.* **2005**, *171*, 1363–1370. [CrossRef]
48. Pease, J.E.; Sabroe, I. The role of interleukin-8 and its receptors in inflammatory lung disease: Implications for therapy. *Am. J. Respir. Med.* **2002**, *1*, 19–25. [CrossRef]
49. Cooper, D.M.; Loxham, M. Particulate matter and the airway epithelium: The special case of the underground? *Eur. Respir. Rev.* **2019**, *28*, 190066. [CrossRef]

50. Deng, X.; Rui, W.; Zhang, F.; Ding, W. PM2.5 induces Nrf2-mediated defense mechanisms against oxidative stress by activating PIK3/AKT signaling pathway in human lung alveolar epithelial A549 cells. *Cell Biol. Toxicol.* **2013**, *29*, 143–157. [CrossRef]
51. Leclercq, B.; Kluza, J.; Antherieu, S.; Sotty, J.; Alleman, L.Y.; Perdrix, E.; Loyens, A.; Coddeville, P.; Guidice, J.-M.L.; Marchetti, P.; et al. Air pollution-derived PM2.5 impairs mitochondrial function in healthy and chronic obstructive pulmonary diseased human bronchial epithelial cells. *Environ. Pollut.* **2018**, *243*, 1434–1449. [CrossRef]
52. Cho, C.C.; Hsieh, W.Y.; Tsai, C.H.; Chen, C.Y.; Chang, H.F.; Lin, C.S. In Vitro and In Vivo Experimental Studies of $PM_{2.5}$ on Disease Progression. *Int. J. Environ. Res. Public Health* **2018**, *15*, 1380. [CrossRef] [PubMed]
53. Park, H.S.; Kim, S.R.; Lee, Y.C. Impact of oxidative stress on lung diseases. *Respirology* **2009**, *14*, 27–38. [CrossRef]
54. Bocci, V.; Valacchi, G.; Corradeschi, F.; Aldinucci, C.; Silvestri, S.; Paccagnini, E.; Gerli, R. Studies on the biological effects of ozone: 7. Generation of reactive oxygen species (ROS) after exposure of human blood to ozone. *J. Biol. Regul. Homeost. Agents* **1998**, *12*, 67–75. [PubMed]
55. Bell, M.L.; Son, J.Y.; Peng, R.D.; Wang, Y.; Dominici, F. Ambient PM2.5 and Risk of Hospital Admissions: Do Risks Differ for Men and Women? *Epidemiology* **2015**, *26*, 575–579. [CrossRef] [PubMed]
56. Chen, R.; Yin, P.; Meng, X.; Liu, C.; Wang, L.; Xu, X.; Ross, J.A.; Tse, L.A.; Zhao, Z.; Kan, H.; et al. Fine Particulate Air Pollution and Daily Mortality. A Nationwide Analysis in 272 Chinese Cities. *Am. J. Respir. Crit. Care Med.* **2017**, *196*, 73–81. [CrossRef]
57. Gerlofs-Nijland, M.E.; Totlandsdal, A.I.; Tzamkiozis, T.; Leseman, D.L.; Samaras, Z.; Låg, M.; Schwarze, P.; Ntziachristos, L.; Cassee, F.R. Cell toxicity and oxidative potential of engine exhaust particles: Impact of using particulate filter or biodiesel fuel blend. *Environ. Sci. Technol.* **2013**, *47*, 5931–5938. [CrossRef] [PubMed]
58. Li, N.; Sioutas, C.; Cho, A.; Schmitz, D.; Misra, C.; Sempf, J.; Wang, M.; Oberley, T.; Froines, J.; Nel, A. Ultrafine particulate pollutants induce oxidative stress and mitochondrial damage. *Environ. Health Perspect.* **2003**, *111*, 455–460. [CrossRef]
59. Zhu, X.M.; Wang, Q.; Xing, W.W.; Long, M.H.; Fu, W.L.; Xia, W.R.; Jin, C.; Guo, N.; Xu, D.Q.; Xu, D.G. PM2.5 induces autophagy-mediated cell death via NOS2 signaling in human bronchial epithelium cells. *Int. J. Biol. Sci.* **2018**, *14*, 557–564. [CrossRef]
60. Longhin, E.; Holme, J.A.; Gutzkow, K.B.; Arlt, V.M.; Kucab, J.E.; Camatini, M.; Gualtieri, M. Cell cycle alterations induced by urban PM2.5 in bronchial epithelial cells: Characterization of the process and possible mechanisms involved. *Part. Fibre Toxicol.* **2013**, *10*, 63. [CrossRef]
61. Wu, X.; Nethery, R.C.; Sabath, B.M.; Braun, D.; Dominici, F. Exposure to air pollution and COVID-19 mortality in the United States: A nationwide cross-sectional study. Preprint. *medRxiv* **2020**. [CrossRef]

biomedicines

MDPI

Article

Inflammation in Dry Eye Syndrome: Identification and Targeting of Oxylipin-Mediated Mechanisms

Dmitry V. Chistyakov [1,*], Olga S. Gancharova [1], Viktoriia E. Baksheeva [1], Veronika V. Tiulina [1,2], Sergei V. Goriainov [3], Nadezhda V. Azbukina [4], Marina S. Tsarkova [2], Andrey A. Zamyatnin, Jr. [1,5], Pavel P. Philippov [1], Marina G. Sergeeva [1], Ivan I. Senin [1] and Evgeni Yu. Zernii [1,5,*]

1 Belozersky Institute of Physico-Chemical Biology, Lomonosov Moscow State University, 119992 Moscow, Russia; olgancharova@belozersky.msu.ru (O.S.G.); vbaksheeva@belozersky.msu.ru (V.E.B.); tyulina_nika@list.ru (V.V.T.); zamyat@belozersky.msu.ru (A.A.Z.J.); pf@belozersky.msu.ru (P.P.P.); mg.sergeeva@gmail.com (M.G.S.); senin@belozersky.msu.ru (I.I.S.)
2 Skryabin Moscow State Academy of Veterinary Medicine and Biotechnology, 109472 Moscow, Russia; marina.tsarkova@gmail.com
3 Shared Research and Education Center of the Peoples' Friendship University of Russia (RUDN University), 117198 Moscow, Russia; goryainovs@list.ru
4 Faculty of Bioengineering and Bioinformatics, Moscow Lomonosov State University, 119234 Moscow, Russia; ridernadya@gmail.com
5 Institute of Molecular Medicine, Sechenov First Moscow State Medical University, 119991 Moscow, Russia
* Correspondence: chistyakof@gmail.com (D.V.C.); zerni@belozersky.msu.ru (E.Y.Z.); Tel.: +7-495-939-4332 (D.V.C.); +7-495-939-2344 (E.Y.Z.)

Received: 21 July 2020; Accepted: 8 September 2020; Published: 11 September 2020

Abstract: Dry eye syndrome (DES) is characterized by decreased tear production and stability, leading to desiccating stress, inflammation and corneal damage. DES treatment may involve targeting the contributing inflammatory pathways mediated by polyunsaturated fatty acids and their derivatives, oxylipins. Here, using an animal model of general anesthesia-induced DES, we addressed these pathways by characterizing inflammatory changes in tear lipidome, in correlation with pathophysiological and biochemical signs of the disease. The decline in tear production was associated with the infiltration of inflammatory cells in the corneal stroma, which manifested one to three days after anesthesia, accompanied by changes in tear antioxidants and cytokines, resulting in persistent damage to the corneal epithelium. The inflammatory response manifested in the tear fluid as a short-term increase in linoleic and alpha-linolenic acid-derived oxylipins, followed by elevation in arachidonic acid and its derivatives, leukotriene B4 (5-lipoxigenase product), 12-hydroxyeicosatetraenoic acid (12-lipoxigeanse product) and prostaglandins, D2, E2 and F2α (cyclooxygenase products) that was observed for up to 7 days. Given these data, DES was treated by a novel ophthalmic formulation containing a dimethyl sulfoxide-based solution of zileuton, an inhibitor of 5-lipoxigenase and arachidonic acid release. The therapy markedly improved the corneal state in DES by attenuating cytokine- and oxylipin-mediated inflammatory responses, without affecting tear production rates. Interestingly, the high efficacy of the proposed therapy resulted from the synergetic action of its components, namely, the general healing activity of dimethyl sulfoxide, suppressing prostaglandins and the more specific effect of zileuton, downregulating leukotriene B4 (inhibition of T-cell recruitment), as well as upregulating docosahexaenoic acid (activation of resolution pathways).

Keywords: dry eye syndrome; inflammation; oxidative stress; corneal damage; tear lipidome; 5-lipoxigenase; leukotriene B4; prostaglandins; dimethyl sulfoxide; zileuton

---

1. Introduction

Dry eye syndrome (DES; also known as dry eye, dry eye disease, or keratoconjunctivitis sicca) is a common multifactorial ocular surface disease, characterized by decreased production/increased evaporation of the tear, resulting in its hyperosmolarity and instability of the tear film [1]. DES affects up to 40% of the adult population and manifests as eye irritation, hyperemia, glare, eye fatigue, and blurred vision [2,3]. Etiologically, alterations in tear homeostasis are associated with dysfunction of the lachrymal and/or Meibomian glands (such as in Sjögren syndrome and Meibomian Gland Dysfunction (MGD)) as well as a number of other factors, including contact lens wearing, adverse effects of various medications, complications of ocular surgery and general anesthesia [1,4–7].

In DES pathogenesis, the reduced tear production and/or alterations in the tear composition results in the loss of lubricating, nourishing and protective qualities of tears against the ocular surface tissues [8]. The most critical consequences of this desiccating stress are ocular surface inflammation and damage, which in severe cases can cause blindness, due to corneal scarring, opacification or ulceration [3]. Consistently, the generally accepted treatment of DES involves not only using lubricating eye drops and ointments, but also topical anti-inflammatory therapy [9,10]. Unfortunately, the administration of common ocular anti-inflammatory medications, such as corticosteroid eye drops or cyclosporine, is associated with a number of adverse effects in patients with dry eye, which generally limits their employment [11]. Thus, there is a great demand for a new safe and effective anti-inflammatory therapy for DES.

The solution to this problem requires an understanding of the mechanisms underlying inflammation in DES, which can be selectively targeted. Currently, it is recognized that an inflammatory reaction in DES is triggered by cytokines (such as interleukin (IL) 1 beta and tumor necrosis factor alpha (TNF-α)) secreted in tear fluid (TF) during the early stages of the disease. Indeed, hyperosmolarity of the tear film stimulates an inflammatory cascade, resulting in the release of these cytokines by limbal epithelial cells [12]. In addition, the desiccating stress leads to compensatory reflex stimulation of the lachrymal gland, which may activate a neurogenic inflammatory cytokine response [3,8]. These events induce maturation and an increase in the density of antigen-presenting dendritic cells in the cornea, subsequent activation of T-cells and their recruitment to the ocular surface (including conjunctiva and lacrimal glands) and release of additional effector cytokines in the TF, thereby causing further damage to the corneal epithelium [3,13]. These processes are accompanied by infiltration of the cornea by leucocytes and other immune cells [3,14]. Consistently, DES can be treated by using drugs blocking the activation of T cells (i.e., lifitegrast, LFA-1 antagonist) or inhibiting cytokine production by these cells (i.e., cyclosporine, suppressor of calcineurin regulated transcription of cytokine genes), as well as using cytokine receptor inhibitors [13,15,16]. Inflammatory changes in DES are also associated with oxidative stress of the ocular surface tissues, stemming from TF deficiency. Indeed, TF contains low molecular weight antioxidants (glutathione, ascorbic acid, and others) and reactive oxygen species (ROS) scavenging enzymes (glutathione reductase, glutathione peroxidase, superoxide dismutase, etc.) thereby providing local antioxidant defense [17,18]. Accordingly, the inflammatory component of DES can be attenuated by the topical administration of antioxidants [6,19].

The separate classes of molecules that contribute to inflammatory responses in DES and can be targeted in its prospective therapy are polyunsaturated fatty acids (PUFAs) and their derivative oxylipins, representing multipotent lipid mediators of inflammation. Oxylipins are biosynthesized from PUFAs via multiple oxidative reactions catalyzed by specific enzymes (cyclooxygenase (COX), lipoxygenase (LOX) or cytochrome P450 monooxygenase (CYP)) or proceeding in an enzyme-independent manner in the presence of ROS [20]. Previously, it was suggested that chronic inflammation in DES is associated with an imbalance between omega-3 (docosahexaenoic acid (DHA) and eicosapentaenoic acid (EPA)) and omega-6 (arachidonic acid (AA)) PUFAs, which lead to the hyperproduction of proinflammatory lipid mediators (omega-6 derivative oxylipins, such as prostaglandins) and underproduction of proresolving (omega-3 derivative oxylipis) molecules [21]. Consistently, DES patients were characterized by upregulation of prostaglandin (PG) E2 in TF, the levels of which correlated with their symptom grades [21–23]. Interestingly, selective inhibition of COX-2, responsible for PGE2 biosynthesis, reduced the levels of pro-inflammatory cytokines in DES apparently via the attenuating effect of PGE2 on antigen-presenting dendritic cells [24], indicating the existence of interrelation between inflammatory pathways in DES. Although COX suppression seems to be a promising route in DES therapy, the well-acknowledged inhibitors of cyclooxygenases, non-steroidal anti-inflammatory drugs (NSAIDs), are not recommended in patients with DES, due to a number of severe side effects [25,26]. Thus, it is important to develop an alternative approach to selective targeting of the oxylipin-dependent inflammatory pathways, based on an understanding of the dynamic changes of the full spectrum of these lipid mediators in DES.

Previously, we developed a rabbit model of DES, closely reproducing the pathogenesis of the human disease [27]. In this model, DES is induced by exposure of the animals to general anesthesia, which diminishes the production of basal and reflex tears and decreases the stability of the tear film thereby inducing common signs of the disease [4,28]. In a more recent study, we adopted a quantitative UPLC-MS/MS-based approach to identify and characterize baseline patterns of lipid mediators in the TF of healthy rabbits and demonstrated that they did not differ significantly from that of human TF [29]. Here, we employed these approaches to characterize TF lipidomic changes in DES, focusing on PUFAs, oxylipins and phospholipid derivatives contributing to the regulation of inflammation, and to find correlations between these changes and the pathophysiological and biochemical signs of the disease. Based on the data obtained, we proposed a novel complex anti-inflammatory therapy, targeting the specific oxylipin-mediated mechanisms revealed in DES. Using subsequent morphological, biochemical and lipidomic studies, this therapy was found to markedly improve the corneal state in DES by selective suppression of its inflammatory component, without affecting tear production rates.

2. Experimental Section

2.1. Materials

Anesthetic preparation containing 50 mg/mL tiletamine and 50 mg/mL zolazepam was from Virbac (Carros, France). Xylazine hydrochloride was from Nita-Farm (Saratov region, Russia). Ultragrade Tris was from Amresco (Solon, OH, USA). Phosphate-buffered saline (PBS) was from Thermo Fisher Scientific (Waltham, MA, USA). Zileuton, DMSO, hemoglobin, luminol, hydrogen peroxide solution, and Trolox (6-hydroxy-2,5,7,8-tetramethylchroman-2-carboxylic acid) were from Sigma-Aldrich (St. Louis, MO, USA). Reagents for histological examination were from Biovitrum (Moscow, Russia). Bicinchoninic acid (BCA) assay kit was from Sigma-Aldrich. Glutathione peroxidase and superoxide dismutase assay kits were from Randox (Crumlin, UK). Tumor necrosis factor alpha (TNF-α) and interleukin 10 (IL-10) assay kits were from Immunotex (Stavropol, Russia). The Schirmer's test tear strips were from Contacare Ophthalmics and Diagnostics (Vadodara, Gujarat, India.). The deuterated oxylipins standards 6-keto PGF1α-d4, TXB2-d4, PGF2α-d4, PGE2-d4, PGD2-d4, LTC4-d5, LTB4-d4, 5(S)-HETE-d8, 12(S)-HETE-d8, 15(S)-HETE-d8, Oleoyl Ethanolamide-d4, EPA-d5, DHA-d5, and AA-d8 were from Cayman Chemical (Ann Arbor, MI, USA). Solid-phase lipid extraction cartridge Oasis® PRIME HLB was obtained from Waters, Eschborn, Germany. Other reagents and suppliers used in this study were from Sigma-Aldrich, Amresco, or Serva (Heidelberg, Germany) and were at least of reagent grade. All buffers and other solutions were prepared using ultrapure water.

2.2. Experimental Animals and Ethics Statement

The study involved a total of 102 healthy New Zealand white rabbits (6 months old, weight of 2.3 to 3 kg) purchased from a certified farm (Krolinfo, Moscow region, Russia). The rabbits were housed in individual cages (795 × 745 × 1776 mm^3) under normal conditions (12 h light/12 h dark, 22–25 °C, 55–60% humidity) with free access to food and water. The daily monitoring of health status of all animals involved ophthalmological exam, inspection of habitus, derma and mucous membranes as well as monitoring of heart/respiratory rates and body temperature. No adverse events were observed during the course of the study. The humane euthanasia of the animals intended for histological analysis of the anterior segment of the eye was performed by an overdose of the anesthetic (for general anesthesia conditions, see next section). The eyeballs of the animals were enucleated postmortem. Otherwise, the animals were rehabilitated for three days and returned to the farm. The animals were treated according to the 8th edition "Guide for the Care and Use of Laboratory Animals" of the National Research Council and "Statement for the Use of Animals in Ophthalmic and Visual Research" of The Association for Research in Vision and Ophthalmology (ARVO). The study was approved by the Belozersky Institute of Physico-chemical Biology Animal Care and Use Committee (Protocol number 1/2016, 12 January 2016).

2.3. Experimental Model

The experiments were performed using a single-blind method. The rabbits were divided into 17 groups, 6 animals in each group (Table 1), and treated as described in Section 3. DES was induced by introducing rabbits into prolonged general anesthesia as described in previous studies [6,30]. Particularly, the animals were placed in prone position in a restraining device and subjected to repeating intramuscular injection of anesthetic preparation containing 1:2 mixture of 50 mg/mL tiletamine/zolazepam and 20 mg/mL xylazine hydrochloride to achieve continuous narcotic sleep for 6 h. For the anti-inflammation therapy, the animals received conjunctival instillations of the eye drops, consisting of either 50% dimethyl sulfoxide (DMSO) in normal saline (0.90% *w*/*v* of NaCl), or the same solution containing 0.5 mg/mL (0.05% (*w*/*v*)) zileuton. The eye drops were prepared under sterile conditions. Each of the formulations was administrated 1 drop 3 times daily in each eye for up to 7 days, starting from the day of DES induction.

Table 1. Parameters of the experimental groups.

Group	Treatment	Analysis	Time of Analysis
1	-	Histology	0 h (control)
2	-	Histology	6 h
3	-	Histology	1 d [1]
4	-	Histology	3 d
5	-	Histology	7 d
6	-	Schirmer's test	0 h, 6 h, 1 d, 3 d, 7 d
7	-	Biochemistry [1]	0 h, 6 h, 1 d, 3 d, 7 d
8	-	Lipidomics [2]	0 h, 6 h, 1 d, 3 d, 7 d
6	DMSO	Histology	1 d
7	DMSO	Histology	3 d
8	DMSO	Histology	7 d
9	DMSO/zileuton	Histology	1 d
10	DMSO/zileuton	Histology	3 d
11	DMSO/zileuton	Histology	7 d
12	DMSO	Schirmer's test	1 d, 3 d, 7 d
13	DMSO	Biochemistry [1]	1 d, 3 d, 7 d
14	DMSO	Lipidomics [2]	1 d, 3 d, 7 d
15	DMSO/zileuton	Schirmer's test	1 d, 3 d, 7 d
16	DMSO/zileuton	Biochemistry [1]	1 d, 3 d, 7 d
17	DMSO/zileuton	Lipidomics [2]	1 d, 3 d, 7 d

[1] Measurement of total protein concentration, total antioxidant activity, antioxidant enzyme activity, and cytokine concentration in TF; [2] UPLC-MS/MS of lipid mediators (PUFAs, oxylipins and phospholipid derivatives) in TF; d: day.

2.4. Histological Analysis

Histological analysis of the cornea was performed essentially as described earlier [6,31,32]. Briefly, the eyeball was enucleated immediately postmortem and fixed in 10% neutral buffered formalin in phosphate buffer (pH 7.4) for 24 h at room temperature. The cornea and iris were trimmed out, dehydrated (absolute isopropanol, 7 portions × 5 h) and embedded in Histomix paraffin medium. Eight 3-micron thick serial nasotemporal cross-sections of each cornea were obtained and mounted on glass slides. The sections were then deparaffinized (xylene, 5 min, two times), hydrated, and stained with Carazzi's hematoxylin and 0.5% eosin Y. Stained sections were dehydrated by 96% ethanol and xylene, cleared in BioClear tissue clearing agent, mounted into BioMount synthetic medium, and examined using Leica DM4000 microscope with Leica DFC Camera (Leica, Wetzlar, Germany) or Zeiss AxioVert.A1 microscope with Axiocam IC C5 camera (Carl Zeiss, Oberkochen, Germany). Processing of the microphotographs was performed using the AxioVision 8.0 and ZEN 2 lite ZEISS Microscope Software (Carl Zeiss, Oberkochen, Germany) and Adobe Photoshop CS6 Extended (Adobe Systems, San Jose, CA, USA) software.

2.5. Schirmer's Test

Tear secretion in animals was measured without topical or general anesthesia according to the following procedure [6,30]. Schirmer's test tear strips were placed under the lower eyelid the restrained animal for 5 min, and the length of the moistened paper (in mm) was recorded. The procedure was repeated at least three times, and the average values were calculated.

2.6. TF Collection

The collection of TF for analytical purposes was performed in separate groups of animals (Table 1). For biochemical analysis, TF was obtained according to the Schirmer's test procedure, except for the strip was allowed to get moistened for exactly 20 mm. Fifteen millimeters-long fragments of the strip were then cut off, extracted with 150 μL of PBS for 30 min and the resulting solution was collected and stored until the biochemical analysis (see Sections 2.7–2.9) at −80 °C [6]. To collect TF samples for lipidomic analysis [29] (see Sections 2.10 and 2.11), the strip was allowed to get moistened reaching exactly 15 mm, the procedure was repeated with 3 strips and 15 mm fragments of each strip were cut off, transferred to a plastic tube with 1 mL of anhydrous methanol containing 0.1% *v/v* BHT and stored at −80 °C.

2.7. Total Protein Concentration Measurement

The concentration of total protein in TF samples was measured using BCA assay. Colorimetric reaction was monitored with Synergy H4 Hybrid plate reader (Biotek, Winooski, VT, USA). The calibration curve was plotted using standard solutions of bovine serum albumin in PBS.

2.8. Total Antioxidant Activity Analysis

The total antioxidant activity in TF was analyzed using hemoglobin/H_2O_2/luminol system [6,33,34]. Briefly, the TF samples were diluted 1:4 by PBS and added to the reaction mixture, containing 0.01 mM luminol and 0.5 mM hemoglobin. The reaction was initiated in the presence of 6 μM H_2O_2 and chemiluminescence of the samples was monitored every one second for 10 min using Glomax-Multi Detection System luminometer (Promega, Madison, WI, USA). The results were calculated in the Trolox equivalent after measuring chemiluminescence of standard solutions, containing 1–8 μM Trolox in PBS.

2.9. Antioxidant Enzymes Activity and Cytokine Concentration Analysis

The activities of superoxide dismutase and glutathione peroxidase and the contents of TNF-α and IL-10 in TF samples were measured without their additional dilution using the respective commercially available kits. The colorimetric reactions were monitored using Synergy H4 Hybrid Reader (Biotek, Winooski, VT, USA).

2.10. Lipid Extraction

The extraction of lipids for UPLC-MS/MS analysis was performed exactly as described in our resent study [29]. Briefly, TF samples were mixed with 2 ng of deuterated internal standard solutions and centrifuged (12,000× *g*, 3 min). The supernatants were mixed with 0.1% acetic acid (6 mL) and loaded onto solid-phase lipid extraction cartridge, which was washed with 15% methanol, 0.1% formic acid (2 mL), and the lipids were eluted with 500 μL of anhydrous methanol and subsequently with 500 μL of acetonitrile. The obtained TF extracts were concentrated by evaporation, reconstituted in 50 μL of 90% methanol and stored at −80 °C.

2.11. UPLC-MS/MS Analysis

TF lipids were analyzed in the obtained extracts using 8040 series UPLC-MS/MS mass spectrometer (Shimadzu, Japan) in multiple-reaction monitoring mode at a unit mass resolution for both the precursor and product ions [29,35]. The lipids separation was performed by reverse-phase UPLC on Phenomenex C8 column (0.4 mL/min, sample temperature of 5 °C). The compounds were eluted with 10–95% acetonitrile gradient in 0.1% (*v*/*v*) formic acid and subjected to MS analysis using electrospray ionization (in both positive and negative ion modes). The molecular ions were fragmentized by collision-induced dissociation in the gas phase and analyzed by tandem (MS/MS) mass spectrometry. The selected lipids were identified and quantified by comparing their mass-spectrometric and chromatographic data with those obtained for the corresponding oxylipins standards (see Section 2.1.) using Lipid Mediator Version 2 software (Shimadzu, Japan).

2.12. Statistical Analysis

The line charts in the figures represent mean ± SEM. Statistical significance was assessed using the repeated measure ANOVA (for analysis within the groups) and one way ANOVA (for analysis between the groups) with post-hoc pairwise comparisons using Tukey's test. The probability of less than 0.05 was considered significant.

3. Results

3.1. Dynamics of Inflammation in DES: Tear Production and Morphological Changes in the Cornea

To characterize the inflammatory responses associated with DES, a control group and four experimental groups of animals were created (groups 1–5, Table 1). To induce DES, the animals within all the experimental groups were exposed to six hours of general anesthesia in accordance with the approach developed in our previous study [6]. Using this setup, we assessed the dynamics of the pathological process in DES, focusing on its inflammatory component. To this end, we performed a histopathological examination of corneas obtained from animals euthanized immediately after anesthesia (at the sixth hour), as well as on days one, three and seven. To complete DES characterization, the intensity of tear production was analyzed in a separate group of animals (group 6, Table 1) using a standardized Schirmer's test.

It was found that tear production decreased two-fold immediately after anesthesia and was completely restored only on day three (Figure 1a). These changes were associated with pronounced morphological changes in the cornea, involving denudation of the corneal stroma, which had already appeared during the period of narcotic sleep, as a result of a large number of deaths of the corneal epithelial cells (Figure 1b, C0). The denudation was preserved focally on day one (Figure 1b, C1). On the remainder of the surface, the epithelium was non-homogenous, consisting of different numbers of layers. Notably, at this stage, the epithelium was abundantly infiltrated by inflammatory cells, mainly granulocytes. Such infiltrates were even found in the areas, where its structure was not significantly altered. The corneal stroma also contains a granulocyte infiltrate. Moderate areas of denudation and multiple epithelial lesions, together with the signs of inflammatory infiltration in the stroma but without intraepithelial infiltration, remained on day three (Figure 1b, C3). In addition, at this time-point, the stroma contained activated keratocytes and exhibited remodeling processes. The signs of inflammation were not entirely resolved until the seventh day after DES induction (Figure 1b, C7). Meanwhile, sporadic areas of denudation remained until day seven, when they were surrounded by reepithelialization rolls along the edges, indicating a developed healing process.

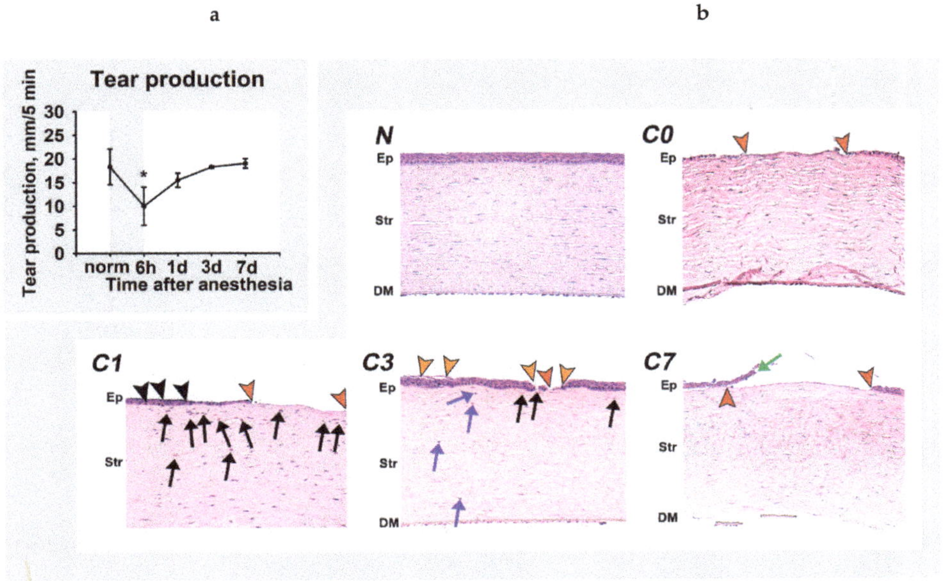

Figure 1. Dynamic changes in tear secretion and corneal morphology in general anesthesia-induced DES. (**a**) The results of standardized Schirmer's tests performed in animals at 6th hour, 1st day, 3rd day or 7th day after their exposure to 6-h general anesthesia. $* p < 0.05$ compared with the values measured in the control group. (**b**) Representative microscopic images of hematoxylin and eosin-stained cross-sections of the corneas obtained at 6th hour (C0), 1st day (C1), 3rd day (C3) and 7th day (C7) after exposure of the animals to general anesthesia. The image of the normal cornea is also presented (N). Stromal denudation (complete absence of the corneal epithelium) areas (red arrowheads), loci of desquamation/destruction of the epithelial layer (orange arrowheads), and sites of reepithelialization (green arrows; the detachment of the new epithelium from the stroma represents an artifact stemmed from histological processing) are indicated. The inflammatory changes include granulocytic infiltration of the corneal epithelium (intraepithelial granulocytes; black arrowheads) and stroma (black arrows), and postinflammatory signs of regeneration (activation of stromal keratocytes) at the ex-sites of the infiltration (blue arrows). Ep: epithelium; Str: stroma; DM: Descemet's membrane and endothelium. Hematoxylin and eosin staining, magnification 200×. The central areas of the cornea are presented. Gaps, cracks and folds of preparations are of an artificial origin.

We concluded that the pathological process in our DES model involved ocular surface inflammation, reaching a maximum on day one after anesthesia, which was accompanied by a decline in tear production and prolonged corneal damage.

3.2. *Dynamics of Inflammation in DES: Biochemistry and Lipidomics of the Tear Fluid*

To understand the mechanisms underlying the inflammatory reactions observed on the ocular surface, we next examined biochemical markers of the associated inflammatory pathways, focusing on lipid mediators (Figure 2). The analysis was performed on TF, which is known to be responsible for nourishing the cornea and maintaining the immune responses of the ocular surface [29]. TF was collected using Schirmer's strips in experimental group 8 (Table 1), following the aforementioned timeline and analyzed by a high-performance, quantitative mass-spectrometric approach, developed in our recent studies [29]. In parallel, TF samples (group 7, Table 1) were analyzed for total protein content, characteristic proinflammatory (TNF-α) and anti-inflammatory (IL-10) cytokines and antioxidant molecules (total antioxidant activity (low molecular weight antioxidants), superoxide dismutase and glutathione peroxidase), which were previously characterized as markers of anesthesia-induced DES [6].

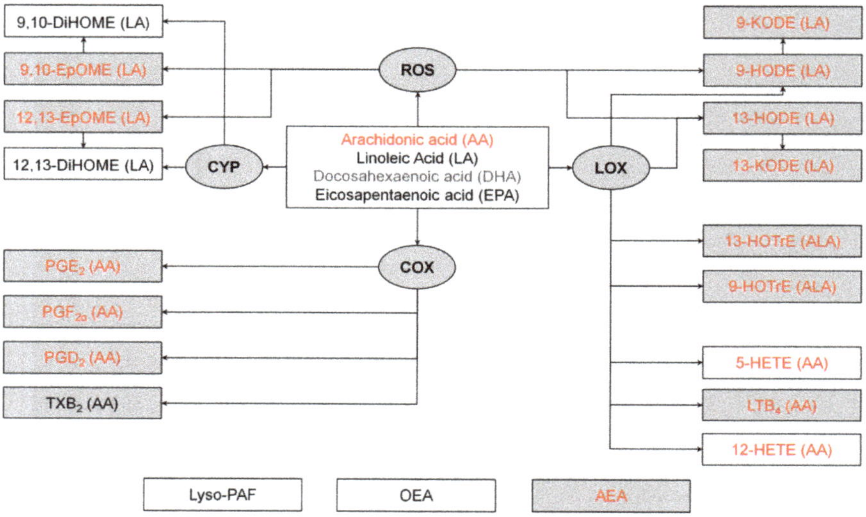

Figure 2. Mechanisms of biosynthesis of lipid mediators. Metabolites of arachidonic acid (AA), linoleic acid (LA) and alpha-linolenic acid (ALA) are divided into the groups synthesized via lipoxygenase (LOX), cyclooxygenas (COX), cytochrome P450 monooxygenase (CYP) or reactive oxygen species (ROS) dependent pathways. The other abbreviations are as follows: AEA, N-arachidonoylethanolamine; DHA, docosahexaenoic acids; 9,10-DiHOME, 9,10-dihydroxyoctadecamonoenoic acid; 12,13-DiHOME, 12,13-dihydroxyoctadecamonoenoic acid; EPA, eicosapentaenoic acid; 9,10-EpOME, 9,10-epoxyoctadecamonoenoic acid; 12,13-EpOME, 12,13-epoxyoctadecamonoenoic acid; 9-HODE, 9-hydroxyoctadecadienoic acid; 13-HODE, 13-hydroxyoctadecadienoic acid; 9-KODE, 9-oxo-octadecadienoic acid; 13-KODE, 13-oxo-octadecadienoic acid; LTB4, leukotriene B4; lyso-PAF, lyso-platelet-activating factor; OEA, oleoylethanolamine; PGD2, prostaglandin D2; PGE2, prostaglandin E2; PGF2α, prostaglandin F2α. The mediators altered in DES and affected by the proposed anti-inflammatory therapy (see below) are indicated in red and gray colors, respectively.

It was noted that the pathological process reflected in TF as a rapid decline of the total antioxidant activity and moderate upregulation of glutathione peroxidase (day one) as well as a more delayed suppression of superoxide dismutase, manifested on day three (Figure 3). The observed alterations were accompanied by inflammatory changes, such as an increase in total protein concentration and a decrease in IL-10 content, without having a significant effect on TNF-α. Importantly, these changes were most pronounced on day one, which concurred with histological findings (see Figure 1).

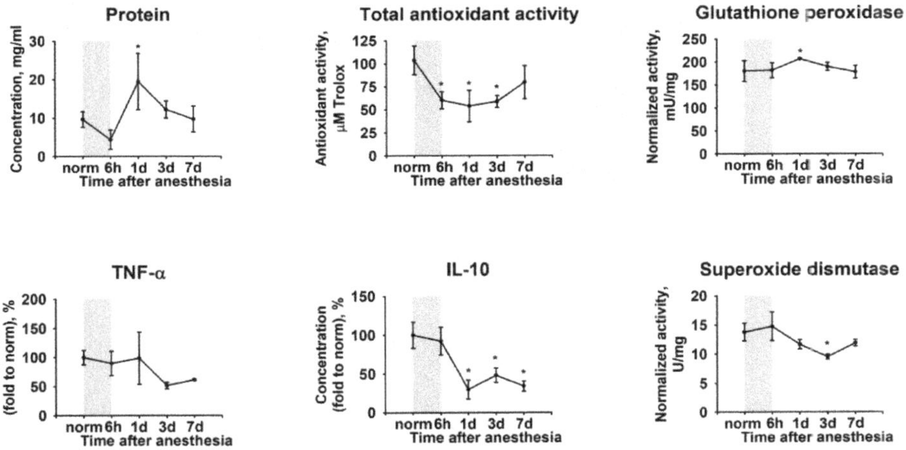

Figure 3. Dynamic changes in biochemical properties of TF in DES. The animals were exposed to general anesthesia for 6 h (shown as gray box). TF samples were collected before (norm) and immediately after (6 h) the general anesthesia as well as on 1, 3, and 7 day post-exposure. The samples were analyzed for total protein, TNF-α, IL-10, as well as total antioxidant activity (in Trolox equivalent) and activity of glutathione peroxidase and superoxide dismutase using the respective assays. * $p < 0.05$ as compared to parameters of TF of the intact (control) animals.

A UPLC-MS/MS analysis of TF samples revealed a total of 23 lipid mediators, including three PUFAs (AA, DHA and EPA), 18 oxylipins and three phospholipid derivatives (OEA, AEA, Lyso-PAF) (Figure 4; full names and biosynthesis pathways for all lipids detected in the study are presented in Figure 2). The identified oxylipins were assigned to five subgroups, namely cyclooxygenase (COX)-dependent derivatives of AA (PGD2, PGE2, PGF2α, TXB2), cytochrome p450 (CYP)-dependent derivatives of LA (9,10-DiHOME/9,10-EpOME and 12,13-DiHOME/12,13-EpOME), as well as lipoxygenase (LOX)-dependent derivatives of AA (5-HETE, 12-HETE, and LTB4), LA (9-HODE/9-KODE and 13-HODE/13-KODE) and ALA (9-HOTrE, 13-HOTrE). The detected lipid mediators exhibited different behavior in DES. Thus, the most prolonged change in TF content was observed for AA and its COX-dependent (PGD2, PGE2, PGF2α) and LOX-dependent (LTB4, 5-HETE, 12-HETE) products, most of which exhibited sustained growth until the seventh day after the anesthesia. The significant increase in LTB4 was accompanied by an increase and a subsequent decrease in the TF content of its precursor 5-HETE. In turn, the LOX/oxidative stress-dependent derivatives of LA (9-HODE/9-KODE and 13-HODE/13-KODE), LOX-dependent derivatives of ALA (9-HOTrE, 13-HOTrE), CYP derivatives of LA (9,10-EpOME and 12,13-EpOME) as well as the phospholipid derivative AEA demonstrated a short-term increase on day one indicating the critical significance of this time-point as the peak of the oxidative and inflammatory response. Finally, no significant DES-dependent changes were observed in the case of DHA and EPA, as well as OEA and Lyso-PAF.

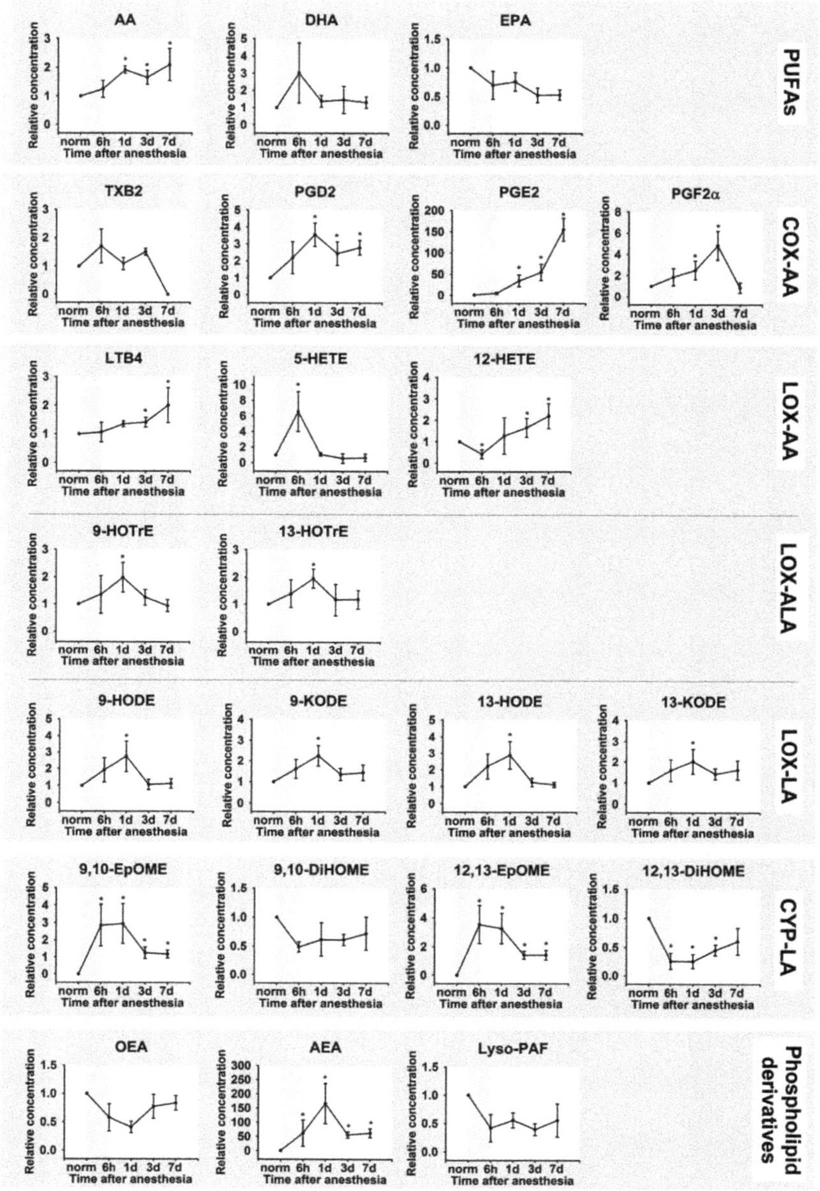

Figure 4. Dynamic changes in TF content of lipid mediators in DES. The animals were exposed to general anesthesia for 6 h (shown as gray box). TF samples were collected before (norm) and immediately after (6 h) the general anesthesia as well as on 1, 3, and 7 day post-exposure. The concentrations of the lipid mediators (phospholipid derivatives, PUFAs and oxylipins) in TF were measured using quantitative UPLC-MS/MS analysis. * $p < 0.05$ as compared to the parameters of TF of the intact (control) animals. The identified oxylipins are divided into subgroups according to their precursors (AA, ALA, LA, phospholipids) and major biosynthetic pathways, involving COX, LOX, or CYP.

Considered together, these data demonstrate that anesthesia-induced DES is associated with oxidative stress and inflammatory response, with the latter being governed mainly by AA and its derivative oxylipins, namely 5-HETE/LTB4 (5-LOX products) and 12-HETE (12-LOX product) as well as COX-dependent prostaglandins (PGD2, PGE2, PGF2α).

3.3. Selective Targeting of Inflammation in DES: Rationale for the Drug Formulation

The obtained lipidomic data indicated that ocular inflammation in DES was governed mainly by two pathways, which depend on AA release and involve its processing by 5/12-LOX and COX. Thus, its targeting may include compounds dampening these pathways. The common COX inhibitors, NSAIDs, are efficacious in relieving different forms of ocular inflammation, but they can exacerbate DES by causing severe side effects [25,26]. Therefore, we focused on alternative methods of treatment, such as targeting LOX-dependent pathways. For this purpose, we chose zileuton (N-(1-Benzo(b)thien-2-ylethyl)-N-hydroxyurea), an anti-asthmatic drug, selectively inhibiting 5-LOX and thereby suppressing the generation of leukotrienes, including LTB4 [36]. An important benefit of zileuton is that it also inhibits AA release and, consequently, downregulates prostaglandins [37].

Given that zileuton (a low water-soluble drug) had never been employed in ophthalmology, a new formulation was developed for its administration in the form of eye drops, containing dimethyl sulfoxide (DMSO). DMSO was selected as it is low toxic [38,39], high tissue permeable, and facilitates the penetration of other compounds through biological membranes [40,41]. The use of up to 50% DMSO was recognized as not causing any adverse reactions upon topical administration in the eye [38,42]. Since maximum solubility of zileuton in 50% solution of DMSO in PBS was reported to be 0.5 mg/mL [43], we settled on the formulation of complete eye drops, consisting of 0.5 mg/mL zileuton in normal saline, containing 50% DMSO. According to the results of clinical examinations performed by an experienced veterinarian (co-author of this study), this dosage was well tolerated by both healthy rabbits and the animals with DES. Thus, no signs of local (i.e., in the cornea, conjunctiva, iris or eyelids) or systemic reactions were registered. It should be emphasized that the formulation was not regarded as final, but it was approved for primary verification of the proposed anti-inflammatory approach.

3.4. Selective Targeting of Inflammation in DES: A Morphological Study

To trial the suggested anti-inflammatory therapy, DES was induced in six experimental groups of animals (groups 6–11, Table 1), which subsequently received instillations of the complete zileuton/DMSO eye drops (zileuton groups) or 50% DMSO in normal saline (DMSO groups). One drop of each of these forms was administrated three times daily in each eye for up to seven days and the animals were euthanized on days one, three and seven following the anesthesia for histological analysis.

Schirmer's tests performed on similar groups of animals receiving the same instillations of zileuton/DMSO or DMSO (groups 12 and 15, Table 1), revealed no effect of the therapy on tear production (Figure 5a). Yet, already on the first day after the anesthesia, the corneas of zileuton groups exhibited pronounced histological signs of epithelial recovery, such as reepithelization rolls (Figure 5b, Z1). The area of denudation was minimal, as single-layer epithelium covered a significant part of the surface, which was drastically in contrast to the untreated samples. Importantly, at this time-point, the cornea exhibited almost no inflammatory infiltrate both in epithelium and stroma. On day three, the epithelium was restored across most of the cornea: the stromal denudation areas were rare and their size did not exceed single cells (Figure 5b, Z3). The newly formed epithelium had a thickness of several layers, although it did not reach the full-size characteristic of normal tissue. These samples exhibited no edema and acute inflammation, but there were signs of the completed inflammatory process and subsequent regeneration, such as an increased number of activated keratocytes at the corresponding sites. Finally, on day seven, the cornea of the rabbits which received zileuton (Figure 5b, Z7) was indistinguishable from the tissue of the healthy animals (Figure 5b, N).

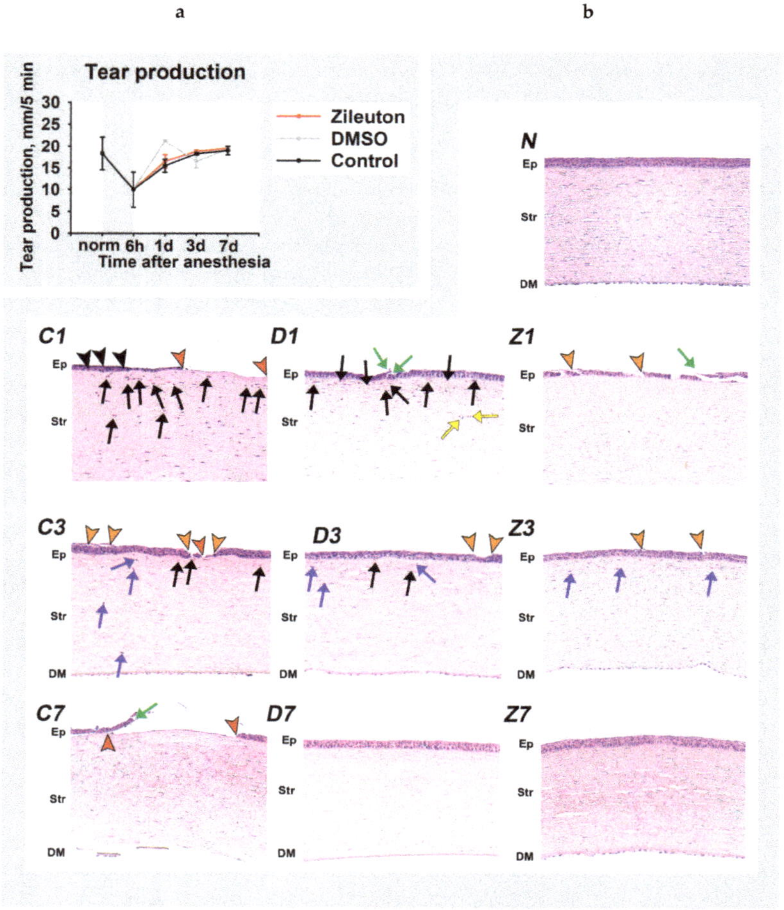

Figure 5. Dynamic changes in tear secretion and corneal morphology in DES in the course of anti-inflammatory therapy. The animals were exposed to general anesthesia for 6 h (shown as gray box) and subsequently received instillations of the eye drops containing 50% DMSO (D1, D3, D7) or 50% DMSO with 0.5% zileuton (Z1, Z3, Z7) for 7 days. (**a**) The results of standardized Schirmer's tests performed at 6th hour, 1st day, 3rd day or 7th day after the exposure. (**b**) Representative microscopic images of hematoxylin and eosin-stained cross-sections of the corneas at 1st (D1, Z1), 3rd (D3, Z3) and 7th (D7, Z7) day after exposure. The image of the normal cornea is also presented (N). Stromal denudation (complete absence of the corneal epithelium) areas (red arrowheads), loci of desquamation/destruction of the epithelial layer (orange arrowheads), and sites of reepithelialization (green arrows) are indicated. The inflammatory changes include granulocytic infiltration in the corneal epithelium (intraepithelial granulocytes; black arrowheads) and stroma (black arrows), neovascularization (yellow arrows), and postinflammatory signs of regeneration (activation of stromal keratocytes) at the ex-sites of the infiltration (blue arrows). Ep: epithelium; Str: stroma; DM: Descemet's membrane and endothelium. Hematoxylin and eosin staining, magnification 200×. The central areas of the cornea are presented. Gaps, cracks and folds of preparations are of an artificial origin.

Interestingly, some of these effects can be attributed to DMSO, as animals of the DMSO group also exhibited accelerated recovery from the anesthesia-induced lesions. Thus, on day one after anesthesia, their cornea contained far fewer denudation areas and signs of intraepithelial infiltration by granulocytes (Figure 5b, D1). However, on days one to three, its stroma was still infiltrated by granulocytes (Figure 5b, D1, D3), whereas in the zileuton group, these infiltrations were completely absent (Figure 5b, Z1, Z3). Furthermore, in the DMSO group, the stroma contained newly formed capillaries (signs of neovascularization), characteristic of keratitis (Figure 5b, D1). Although these animals exhibited early signs of regeneration, these were less prominent than in the zileuton group. Overall, DMSO enhanced corneal healing and produced a moderate anti-inflammatory effect, while zileuton effectively reduced stromal infiltration by granulocytes, neovascularization and other manifestations of acute inflammation.

Overall, we concluded that the treatment using zileuton/DMSO-containing eye drops can markedly improve the corneal state in DES, by selective suppression of its inflammatory component without affecting tear production rates.

3.5. Selective Targeting of Inflammation in DES: Biochemistry and Lipidomics of the Tear Fluid

To address the mechanisms underlying the observed therapeutic effects, we next analyzed alterations in biochemical properties and the lipid content of TF, associated with zileuton/DMSO treatment. To this end, TF was collected in animals from two DES groups (groups 13–14 and 16–17, Table 1) receiving either complete eye drops (zileuton groups) or DMSO alone (DMSO groups). The therapy using zileuton/DMSO had almost no impact on the antioxidant activity of the TF but prevented the increase in total protein concentration in the TF (Figure 6). These effects could be associated with DMSO activity, as a similar picture was observed in the DMSO group. Yet only the therapy with eye drops containing zileuton upregulated the anti-inflammatory cytokine IL-10 and attenuated the decline in activity of the superoxide dismutase.

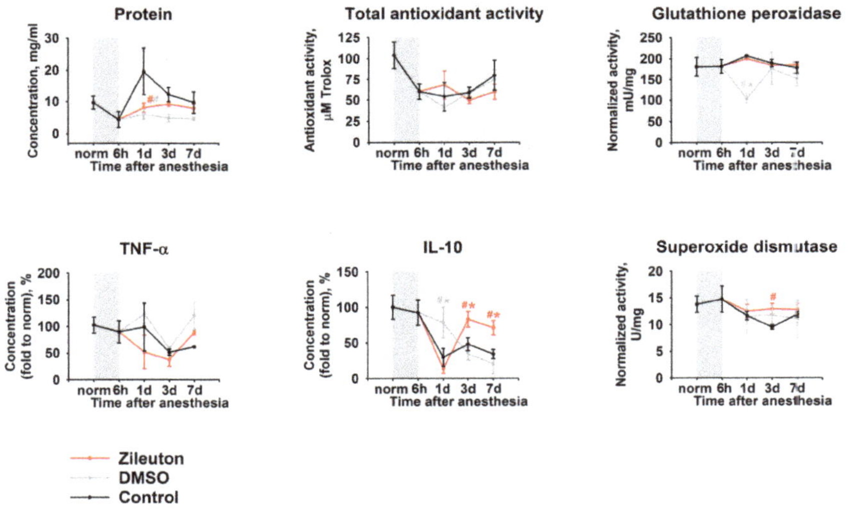

Figure 6. Dynamic changes in biochemical properties of TF in DES in the course of anti-inflammatory therapy. The animals were exposed to general anesthesia for 6 h (shown as gray box) and subsequently received instillations of the eye drops containing 50% DMSO (gray) or 50% DMSO with 0.5% zileuton (red), 1 drop 3 times daily in each eye for 7 days. TF samples were collected before (norm) and immediately after (6 h) general anesthesia as well as on 1, 3, and 7 day post-exposure. The samples were analyzed for total protein, TNF-α, IL-10, total antioxidant activity (in Trolox equivalent) and activity of glutathione peroxidase and superoxide dismutase using the respective assays. # $p < 0.05$ as compared to parameters of TF of the untreated animals with DES (black). * $p < 0.05$ as compared to parameters of TF of the animals from the DMSO or zileuton group.

These findings were consistent with the results of the UPLC-MS/MS analysis of lipid mediators of TF in animals of the same groups, confirming the antioxidant and pronounced anti-inflammatory activity of the proposed therapy (Figure 7). Thus, zileuton/DMSO treatment prevented an increase in AA and its derivatives, prostaglandins (PGD2, PGE2, PGF2α) and LTB4, whereas the contents of 5-HETE and 12-HETE were much less affected. In addition, the therapy suppressed short-term elevations in the content of LOX/oxidative stress-dependent derivatives of LA (9-HODE/9-KODE and 13-HODE/13-KODE), LOX-dependent derivatives of ALA (9-HOTrE, 13-HOTrE), CYP derivatives of LA (9,10-EpOME and 12,13-EpOME) and the phospholipid derivative AEA.

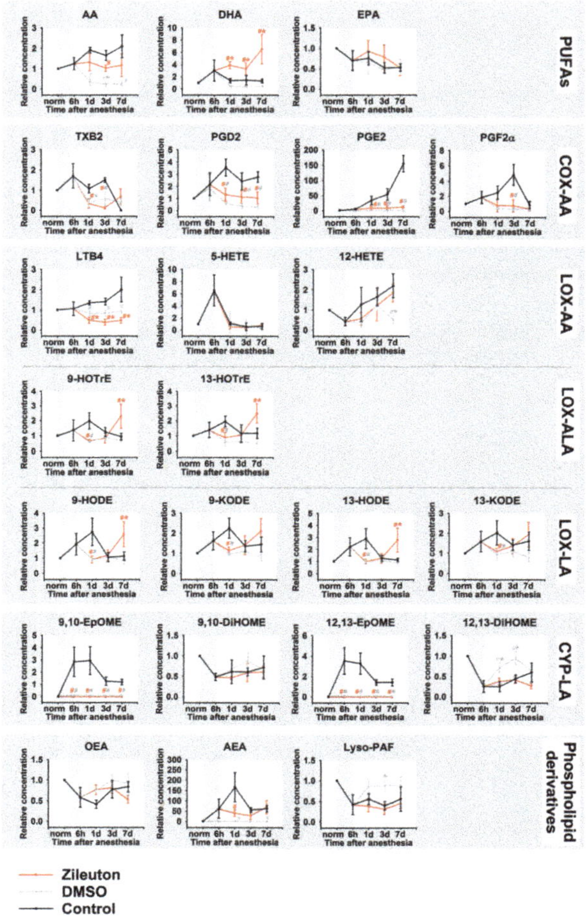

Figure 7. Dynamic changes in TF content of lipid mediators in DES in the course of anti-inflammatory therapy. The animals were exposed to general anesthesia for 6 h (shown as gray box) and subsequently received instillations of the eye drops containing 50% DMSO (gray) or 50% DMSO with 0.5% zileuton (red), one drop three times daily in each eye for 7 days. TF samples were collected before (norm) and immediately after (6 h) the general anesthesia as well as on 1, 3, and 7 day post-exposure. The concentrations of the lipid mediators (phospholipid derivatives, PUFAs and oxylipins) in TF were measured using quantitative UPLC-MS/MS analysis. # $p < 0.05$ as compared to parameters of TF of the untreated animals with DES (black). * $p < 0.05$ as compared to parameters of TF of the animals from the DMSO or zileuton group.

Interestingly, some of these effects were similar among the zileuton and DMSO groups, thereby demonstrating for the first time the broad anti-inflammatory activity of DMSO. However, LTB4, the main product of 5-LOX, was faster and more potently downregulated in the zileuton group and its level was even less than among healthy animals. Furthermore, zileuton treatment generally increased the TF content of anti-inflammatory mediator DHA, whereas DMSO had no effect in this regard. It should be added that the animals from the zileuton group also exhibited increased content of oxylipins 9-/13-HOTrE and 9-/13-HODE on the seventh day apparently representing delayed or compensatory response on the therapy.

Overall, based on the data obtained, we can conclude that the high efficacy of the proposed complex therapy is a result of the synergetic action of two components of the eye drops, namely the general healing property of DMSO and the more specific anti-inflammatory effects of zileuton.

4. Discussion

Our study represents the first comprehensive characterization of inflammatory mechanisms in DES mediating by PUFAs and their derivatives, oxylipins, which was performed in a time-dependent manner, considering the alterations in tear production rates, as well as the pathophysiological and biochemical (oxidative stress, cytokine response) signs of the disease. Importantly, it is these mechanisms that are most commonly impacted by the currently approved anti-inflammatory drugs (such as dexamethasone or NSAIDs) and represent the prospective targets for novel specific therapies. Generally, the nomenclature of inflammatory mediators in rabbit tears identified in this study (23 lipids), accords with our recent findings regarding human TF [29]. A number of attempts have been made to examine alterations in the TF content of PUFAs/oxylipins in DES, both in animal and human studies, but most of them have focused on single mediators, such as three PUFAs (AA, DHA and EPA) and two prostaglandins (PGE2 and PGD2). Thus, it was found that the ratio of ω-6 (AA) to ω-3 (DHA + EPA) fatty acids is increased in DES patients [21], which concurs with our observations (see Figure 3). Furthermore, a number of works reported DES-associated growth of the TF level of PGE2, which is recognized as a hallmark of the disease [21–23,44]. Consistently, in our experiments, PGE2 exhibited the most pronounced elevation among the identified mediators (see Figure 3). To date, the most detailed study of lipid mediators in DES has focused on eicosanoids, which were profiled in the TF of healthy individuals, in comparison with MGD patients, by means of an MS-based approach [45]. The reliable disease-associated increase was found in relation to six compounds, including 5-HETE and LTB4, which were similarly increased in our DES model. Furthermore, our results complement these data well, since we detected a significant increase in two more prostaglandins, PGD2 and PGF2α, as well as 12-HETE. Overall, taking into account our findings and the existing literature data, we can conclude that an inflammatory response in DES is governed mainly by AA and its derivative oxylipins 5-HETE and LTB4 (5-LOX products), 12-HETE (12-lipoxigeanse product) as well as PGD2, PGE2 and PGF2α (cyclooxygenase products). Notably, in our experiments, most of the aforementioned lipids demonstrated a prolonged increase not reaching their maximum even after seven days of observation, which correlates with their permanent elevations in human DES patients, exhibiting chronic inflammation.

It should be added that among the changes in AA derivatives, there was an increase in AEA (anandamide), a product of the non-oxidative metabolism of AA-containing phospholipid N-arachidonoyl phosphatidylethanolamine. AEA is an endocannabinoid, exhibiting proinflammatory activity as it was found to exacerbate endotoxin-induced uveitis, enhancing the clinical score of intraocular inflammation and increasing the amount of leukocyte and protein concentration in the aqueous humor [46]. Our results represent the first indication of the participation of AEA in the inflammatory response associated with DES, recognizing this compound as one of the promising targets for use in an anti-inflammatory therapy for the disease.

In contrast to AA and its products, six LA derivatives, namely 9-HODE/9-KODE, 13-HODE/13-KODE, and 9,10-EpOME/12,13-EpOME, exhibited a pronounced but short-term increase, manifested only on day one after general anesthesia. In fact, this time-point represents a critical period not only for the inflammatory reaction but also for oxidative responses in our DES model. Thus, on day one, the most pronounced granulocytic infiltration in the corneal stroma, maximal protein concentration in TF and the most prominent cytokine alterations were accompanied by minimal antioxidant activity in TF, indicating the development of oxidative stress. We suggest that increased levels of 9-HODE/9-KODE and 13-HODE/13-KODE may reflect non-enzymatic oxidation of LA by ROS. Indeed, these compounds are well-recognized markers of oxidative stress [47,48]. Similarly, biosynthetic pathways for 9,10-EpOME and 12,13-EpOME, which are produced by neutrophils and macrophages and mediate different inflammatory effects, may involve non-enzymatic oxidation [20,49,50]. It was suggested that inflammatory changes on the ocular surface in DES are related to chronic oxidative stress, accompanied by reduced local antioxidant activity [51,52]. For instance, superoxide dismutase downregulation was shown to be associated with inflammation in the lacrimal glands and decreased tear secretion [53], and we observed a decrease in superoxide dismutase activity in DES. Thus, the quenching of the oxidative stress by topical administration of antioxidants may represent a powerful strategy in the treatment of the disease (including its inflammatory component), which was confirmed in our recent study [6].

In addition to AA and LA derivatives, we detected two products of ALA, 9-HOTrE and 13-HOTrE, to be elevated in the acute phase of inflammation (day one). Notably, 9-HOTrE can be produced from ALA by 5-LOX and glutathione peroxidase [54]. Moreover, these enzymes can catalyze the production of AA into 9-HODE [54], another oxylipin increased in the acute phase. In our biochemical experiments, glutathione peroxidase was found to be moderately upregulated in day one, which supports the importance of the aforementioned cascades in DES. Thus, in summary, we detected four LOX-5-dependent oxylipins elevated in the early (9-HODE and 9-HOTrE) and late (5-HETE and LTB4) phases of anesthesia-induced DES. Based on these data, we proposed that the inflammatory response, associated with the disease, can be efficiently treated by the topical administration of zileuton, the only specific inhibitor of 5-LOX, approved by the US FDA [36,55]. The choice of zileuton was especially justified, as it was previously shown to inhibit the release of AA and, consequently, to downregulate prostaglandins [37], which, according to our data, contributed most to the development of prolonged inflammation in DES. Zileuton is a low water-soluble drug which has never been employed in ophthalmology, to the best of our knowledge. Yet, topical administration of zileuton (500 μg) dissolved in 100% DMSO was previously employed in animal studies for the treatment of ear edema [56]. In this study, we used eye drops containing 0.5 mg/mL solution of zileuton in 50% DMSO. Such concentration of DMSO was recognized as not causing any adverse reactions upon topical administration in the eye [38,42]. Indeed, according to our observations, the resulting eye drops were generally well tolerated by the animals. It should be noted that the described composition of the eye drop was approved only for primary verification of the proposed anti-inflammatory approach in this study. Further studies are required for careful optimization of the dosage of the proposed zileuton/DMSO-based prodrug.

The suggested treatment produced an unexpectedly prominent therapeutic benefit, preventing granulocytic infiltration and other signs of inflammation, and accelerating corneal healing by at least three days. The underlying mechanisms involved selective inhibition of inflammation without affecting the antioxidant activity and tear-producing rates. Interestingly, some of the observed benefits can be attributed to DMSO. Indeed, this compound was previously shown to exhibit its own therapeutic activity in the eye by facilitating corneal healing and exhibiting anti-inflammatory effects [57–60]. The mechanisms underlying these benefits may be related to the downregulation of PGE2 [61]. A similar effect of DMSO was observed in our model (see Figure 6). Yet, we have found that DMSO suppressed several other pathways indicating its broader biological action. For example, it significantly reduced the activity of glutathione peroxidase, which may partially underlie the suppression of 9-HODE and 9-HOTrE content in TF [54], seen in our experiments. Downregulation of 9-HODE and 13-HODE may inhibit monocyte activation, reduce pain syndrome and produce other therapeutic effects in DES [62,63].

Currently, the intravesical instillation of 50% aqueous solution DMSO (RIMSO-50®) is approved by the FDA for the treatment of interstitial cystitis. Furthermore, DMSO is used as a cosolvent in several other FDA-approved products, including Onyx® (injection into brain arteriovenous malformation), Viadur® (subcutaneous implantation) and Pennasid® (topical administration). Although in early studies the ocular effects of DMSO were considered contradictory and there was no systematic examination of DMSO-based formulations in ophthalmic clinical trials, today, growing evidence confirms the feasibility of this compound as a cosolvent in topical medication for the treatment of a wide range of ophthalmological conditions, including superficial keratitis, blepharoconjunctivitis, blepharitis and glaucoma [64–67]. Considered together, these data justify the future trialing safety and efficacy of a 50% DMSO-based solution of zileuton.

Despite the prominent healing activity of DMSO, the introduction of zileuton has led to a substantial improvement in the therapeutic benefit of the eye drops. Thus, according to our histological data, in the DMSO group, the signs of inflammation, such as infiltration by granulocytes and neovascularization, remained one to three days after general anesthesia, whereas in the zileuton group, these signs were absent (see Figure 5b). Indeed, zileuton produced additional, more specific anti-inflammatory effects. The first specific effect was the pronounced upregulation of IL-10, the anti-inflammatory cytokine previously found to be associated with DES [68]. Interestingly, a similar effect of zileuton against IL-10 was demonstrated in other inflammation-related disorders [69]. The second specific effect of zileuton was the downregulation of the proinflammatory mediator, LTB4. This oxylipin was shown to govern ocular inflammation, being secreted by the corneal, conjunctival and Meibomian gland epithelium in response to lipopolysaccharide action [70]. A specific increase in the TF concentration of LTB4 was also induced by contact lens wearing, a common ethological factor in DES [71]. Given that LTB4 was established as a key factor in recruiting effector T cells [72,73], its downregulation by zileuton might specifically suppress the T-cell response in DES (see Introduction section). The third specific effect of zileuton was the pronounced upregulation of the anti-inflammatory mediator, DHA. Previously, the deficiency of DHA and EPA was found to correlate with the clinical manifestations of DES [21]. Consistently, the daily supplementation of these ω-3 PUFAs was found to reduce or reverse the symptoms of DES in different species including humans [74–76]. DHA is a well-recognized precursor of proresolving lipid mediators, controlling epithelial wound healing, inflammatory cell migration and nerve regeneration [21]. Thus, the treatment with zileuton-containing eye drops might affect the resolution of the inflammatory response in DES by promoting the release of DHA and its derivative resolvins.

Overall, we can conclude that the high efficacy of the proposed complex therapy resulted from the synergetic action of its components, DMSO and zileuton. The general healing activity of DMSO includes the downregulation of prostaglandins. Meanwhile, zileuton suppresses cytokine-dependent inflammatory mechanisms, apparently restrains the T-cell response via selective inhibition of LTB4 and promotes resolution pathways by upregulating DHA. Thus, these compounds act synergistically, encompassing virtually all aspects of the mechanism underlying the inflammatory response in DES. Based on these data, we suggest that the proposed therapeutic approach can be considered in future as one of the promising methods of DES treatment.

Author Contributions: Conceptualization, D.V.C., P.P.P., M.G.S., I.I.S. and E.Y.Z.; methodology, D.V.C. and I.I.S.; software, N.V.A.; validation, M.S.T. and M.G.S.; formal analysis, D.V.C. and V.E.B.; investigation, D.V.C., V.V.T., O.S.G., V.E.B., S.V.G., N.V.A., and I.I.S.; resources, A.A.Z.J., and E.Y.Z.; data curation, M.S.T. and A.A.Z.J.; writing—original draft, E.Y.Z.; writing—review and editing, D.V.C., P.P.P. and E.Y.Z.; visualization, V.E.B., O.S.G., and D.V.C.; supervision, M.S.T., P.P.P., M.G.S. and E.Y.Z.; project administration, E.Y.Z.; funding acquisition, E.Y.Z. All authors have read and agreed to the published version of the manuscript.

Funding: This research was funded by the Russian Science Foundation, grant number 16-15-00255.

Acknowledgments: The authors acknowledge the Preclinical Clinical Study Centre, "RUDN University Program 5-100", for their service with UPLC-MS/MS analysis.

Conflicts of Interest: The authors declare no conflict of interest. The funders had no role in the design of the study; in the collection, analyses, or interpretation of data; in the writing of the manuscript, or in the decision to publish the results.

Abbreviations

AA	Arachidonic acid
AEA	N-arachidonoylethanolamine
ALA	Alpha-linolenic acid
BCA	Bicinchoninic acid
COX	Cyclooxygenases
CYP	Cytochrome P450 monooxygenases
DES	Dry eye syndrome
DHA	Docosahexaenoic acids
DMSO	Dimethyl sulfoxide
9,10-DiHOME	9,10-dihydroxyoctadecamonoenoic acid
12,13-DiHOME	12,13-dihydroxyoctadecamonoenoic acid
EPA	Eicosapentaenoic acid
9,10-EpOME	9,10-epoxyoctadecamonoenoic acid
12,13-EpOME	12,13-epoxyoctadecamonoenoic acid
9-HODE	9-hydroxyoctadecadienoic acid
13-HODE	13-hydroxyoctadecadienoic acid
IL-1	Interleukin-1
IL-10	Interleukin-10
IL-1β	Interleukin-1 beta
9-KODE	9-oxo-octadecadienoic acid
13-KODE	13-oxo-octadecadienoic acid
LTB4	Leukotriene B4
LA	Linoleic acid
LOX	Lipoxygenase
lyso-PAF	Lyso-Platelet-Activating Factor (1-O-hexadecyl-sn-glyceryl-3-phosphorylcholine)
MGD	Meibomian gland dysfunction
NSAID	Nonsteroidal anti-inflammatory drug
OEA	Oleoylethanolamine ((Z)-N-(2-Hydroxyethyl)octadec-9-enamide)
PBS	Phosphate-buffered saline
PUFA	Polyunsaturated fatty acid
PGD2	Prostaglandin D2
PGE2	Prostaglandin E2
PGF2α	Prostaglandin F2 alpha
ROS	Reactive oxygen species
TF	Tear fluid
TNF-α	Tumor necrosis factor alpha
UPLC-MS/MS	Ultra performance liquid chromatography-tandem mass spectrometry

References

1. Bron, A.J.; De Paiva, C.S.; Chauhan, S.K.; Bonini, S.; Gabison, E.E.; Jain, S.; Knop, E.; Markoulli, M.; Ogawa, Y.; Perez, V.; et al. TFOS DEWS II pathophysiology report. *Ocul. Surf.* **2017**, *15*, 438–510. [CrossRef] [PubMed]
2. Stapleton, F.; Alves, M.; Bunya, V.Y.; Jalbert, I.; Lekhanont, K.; Malet, F.; Na, K.-S.; Schaumberg, D.; Uchino, M.; Vehof, J.; et al. TFOS DEWS II Epidemiology Report. *Ocul. Surf.* **2017**, *15*, 334–365. [CrossRef] [PubMed]
3. Yamaguchi, T. Inflammatory Response in Dry Eye. *Investig. Opthalmol. Vis. Sci.* **2018**, *59*, DES192–DES199. [CrossRef] [PubMed]
4. Malafa, M.M.; Coleman, J.E.; Bowman, R.W.; Rohrich, R.J. Perioperative Corneal Abrasion: Updated Guidelines for Prevention and Management. *Plast. Reconstr. Surg.* **2016**, *137*, 790e–798e. [CrossRef] [PubMed]

5. Kara-Junior, N.; De Espíndola, R.F.; Filho, J.V.; Rosa, C.P.; Ottoboni, A.; Silva, E.D. Ocular risk management in patients undergoing general anesthesia: An analysis of 39,431 surgeries. *Clinics* **2015**, *70*, 541–543. [CrossRef]
6. Zernii, E.Y.; Gancharova, O.S.; Baksheeva, V.E.; Golovastova, M.O.; Kabanova, E.I.; Savchenko, M.S.; Tiulina, V.V.; Sotnikova, L.F.; Zamyatnin, J.A.A.; Philippov, P.P.; et al. Mitochondria-Targeted Antioxidant SkQ1 Prevents Anesthesia-Induced Dry Eye Syndrome. *Oxid. Med. Cell. Longev.* **2017**, *2017*, 9281519. [CrossRef]
7. Baksheeva, V.E.; Gancharova, O.S.; Tiulina, V.V.; Iomdina, E.N.; Zamyatnin, J.A.A.; Philippov, P.P.; Zernii, E.Y.; Senin, I.I. Iatrogenic Damage of Eye Tissues: Current Problems and Possible Solutions. *Biochemistry* **2018**, *83*, 1563–1574. [CrossRef]
8. The Definition and Classification of Dry Eye Disease: Report of the Definition and Classification Subcommittee of the International Dry Eye Workshop. *Ocul. Surf.* **2007**, *5*, 75–92. [CrossRef]
9. Skalicky, S.E.; Petsoglou, C.; Gurbaxani, A.; Fraser, C.L.; McCluskey, P. New Agents for Treating Dry Eye Syndrome. *Curr. Allergy Asthma Rep.* **2012**, *13*, 322–328. [CrossRef]
10. Zernii, E.Y.; Baksheeva, V.E.; Yani, E.V.; Philippov, P.P.; Senin, I.I. Therapeutic Proteins for Treatment of Corneal Epithelial Defects. *Curr. Med. Chem.* **2019**, *26*, 517–545. [CrossRef]
11. Messmer, E.M. The Pathophysiology, Diagnosis, and Treatment of Dry Eye Disease. *Dtsch. Aerzteblatt Online* **2015**, *112*, 71–82. [CrossRef] [PubMed]
12. Li, D.Q.; Luo, L.; Chen, Z.; Kim, H.S.; Song, X.J.; Pflugfelder, S.C. JNK and ERK MAP kinases mediate induction of IL-1beta, TNF-alpha and IL-8 following hyperosmolar stress in human limbal epithelial cells. *Exp. Eye Res.* **2006**, *82*, 588–596. [CrossRef] [PubMed]
13. Perez, V.L.; Pflugfelder, S.C.; Zhang, S.; Shojaei, A.; Haque, R. Lifitegrast, a Novel Integrin Antagonist for Treatment of Dry Eye Disease. *Ocul. Surf.* **2016**, *14*, 207–215. [CrossRef]
14. Lin, H.; Li, W.; Dong, N.; Chen, W.; Liu, J.; Chen, L.; Yuan, H.; Geng, Z.; Liu, Z. Changes in Corneal Epithelial Layer Inflammatory Cells in Aqueous Tear–Deficient Dry Eye. *Investig. Opthalmol. Vis. Sci.* **2010**, *51*, 122–128. [CrossRef]
15. Matsuda, S.; Koyasu, S. Mechanisms of action of cyclosporine. *Immunopharmacology* **2000**, *47*, 119–125. [CrossRef]
16. Colligris, B.; Alkozi, H.A.; Pintor, J. Recent developments on dry eye disease treatment compounds. *Saudi J. Ophthalmol.* **2013**, *28*, 19–30. [CrossRef]
17. Saijyothi, A.V.; Fowjana, J.; Madhumathi, S.; Rajeshwari, M.; Thennarasu, M.; Prema, P.; Angayarkanni, N. Tear fluid small molecular antioxidants profiling shows lowered glutathione in keratoconus. *Exp. Eye Res.* **2012**, *103*, 41–46. [CrossRef]
18. Crouch, R.K.; Goletz, P.; Snyder, A.; Coles, W.H. Antioxidant Enzymes in Human Tears. *J. Ocul. Pharmacol. Ther.* **1991**, *7*, 253–258. [CrossRef]
19. Dogru, M.; Kojima, T.; Simsek, C.; Tsubota, K. Potential Role of Oxidative Stress in Ocular Surface Inflammation and Dry Eye Disease. *Investig. Opthalmol. Vis. Sci.* **2018**, *59*, DES163–DES168. [CrossRef]
20. Gabbs, M.; Leng, S.; Devassy, J.G.; Monirujjaman, M.; Aukema, H.M. Advances in Our Understanding of Oxylipins Derived from Dietary PUFAs. *Adv. Nutr.* **2015**, *6*, 513–540. [CrossRef]
21. Walter, S.D.; Gronert, K.; McClellan, A.L.; Levitt, R.C.; Sarantopoulos, K.D.; Galor, A. omega-3 Tear Film Lipids Correlate with Clinical Measures of Dry Eye. *Investig. Ophtamol. Vis. Sci.* **2016**, *57*, 2472–2478. [CrossRef] [PubMed]
22. Shim, J.; Park, C.; Lee, H.S.; Park, M.S.; Lim, H.T.; Chauhan, S.; Dana, R.; Lee, H.; Lee, H.K. Change in Prostaglandin Expression Levels and Synthesizing Activities in Dry Eye Disease. *Ophthalmology* **2012**, *119*, 2211–2219. [CrossRef] [PubMed]
23. Lekhanont, K.; Sathianvichitr, K.; Pisitpayat, P.; Anothaisintawee, T.; Soontrapa, K.; Udomsubpayakul, U. Association between the levels of prostaglandin E2 in tears and severity of dry eye. *Int. J. Ophthalmol.* **2019**, *12*, 1127–1133. [CrossRef] [PubMed]
24. Ji, Y.W.; Seo, Y.; Choi, W.; Yeo, A.; Noh, H.; Kim, E.K.; Lee, H.K. Dry Eye-Induced CCR7+CD11b+ Cell Lymph Node Homing Is Induced by COX-2 Activities. *Investig. Opthalmol. Vis. Sci.* **2014**, *55*, 6829–6838. [CrossRef] [PubMed]
25. Rigas, B.; Huang, W.; Honkanen, R. NSAID-induced corneal melt: Clinical importance, pathogenesis, and risk mitigation. *Surv. Ophthalmol.* **2020**, *65*, 1–11. [CrossRef] [PubMed]

26. Guidera, A.C.; I Luchs, J.; Udell, I.J. Keratitis, ulceration, and perforation associated with topical nonsteroidal anti-inflammatory drugs. *Ophthalmology* **2001**, *108*, 936–944. [CrossRef]
27. Zernii, E.Y.; Golovastova, M.O.; Baksheeva, V.E.; Kabanova, E.; Ishutina, I.E.; Gancharova, O.S.; Gusev, A.E.; Savchenko, M.S.; Loboda, A.P.; Sotnikova, L.F.; et al. Alterations in tear biochemistry associated with postanesthetic chronic dry eye syndrome. *Biochemistry* **2016**, *81*, 1549–1557. [CrossRef]
28. White, E.; Crosse, M.M. The aetiology and prevention of peri-operative corneal abrasions. *Anaesthesia* **1998**, *53*, 157–161. [CrossRef]
29. Chistyakov, D.V.; Azbukina, N.V.; Astakhova, A.A.; Goriainov, S.V.; Chistyakov, V.V.; Tiulina, V.V.; Baksheeva, V.E.; Kotelin, V.I.; Fedoseeva, E.V.; Zamyatnin, A.A., Jr.; et al. Comparative lipidomic analysis of inflammatory mediators in the aqueous humor and tear fluid of humans and rabbits. *Metabolomics* **2020**, *16*, 27. [CrossRef]
30. Zernii, E.Y.; Baksheev, V.E.; Kabanova, E.I.; Tiulina, V.V.; Golovastova, M.O.; Gancharova, O.S.; Savchenko, M.S.; Sotikova, L.F.; Zamyatnin, J.A.A.; Filippov, P.P.; et al. Effect of General Anesthesia Duration on Recovery of Secretion and Biochemical Properties of Tear Fluid in the Post-Anesthetic Period. *Bull. Exp. Biol. Med.* **2018**, *165*, 269–271. [CrossRef]
31. Zernii, E.Y.; Gancharova, O.S.; Tiulina, V.V.; Zamyatnin, J.A.A.; Philippov, P.P.; Baksheeva, V.E.; Senin, I.I. Mitochondria-targeted antioxidant SKQ1 protects cornea from oxidative damage induced by ultraviolet irradiation and mechanical injury. *BMC Ophthalmol.* **2018**, *18*, 336. [CrossRef] [PubMed]
32. Chistyakov, D.; Azbukina, N.; Goriainov, S.; Gancharova, O.; Tiulina, V.; Baksheeva, V.; Iomdina, E.; Philippov, P.; Sergeeva, M.; Senin, I.; et al. Inflammatory metabolites of arahidonic acid in tear fluid in UV-induced corneal damage. *Biomed. Khidm.* **2019**, *65*, 33–40. [CrossRef] [PubMed]
33. Baksheeva, V.E.; Tiulina, V.V.; Tikhomirova, N.K.; Gancharova, O.S.; Komarov, S.V.; Philippov, P.P.; Zamyatnin, J.A.A.; Senin, I.I.; Zernii, E.Y. Suppression of Light-Induced Oxidative Stress in the Retina by Mitochondria-Targeted Antioxidant. *Antioxidants* **2018**, *8*, 3. [CrossRef]
34. Chistyakov, D.V.; Baksheeva, V.E.; Tiulina, V.V.; Goriainov, S.V.; Azbukina, N.V.; Gancharova, O.S.; Arifulin, E.A.; Komarov, S.V.; Chistyakov, V.V.; Tikhomirova, N.K.; et al. Mechanisms and Treatment of Light-Induced Retinal Degeneration-Associated Inflammation: Insights from Biochemical Profiling of the Aqueous Humor. *Int. J. Mol. Sci.* **2020**, *21*, 704. [CrossRef] [PubMed]
35. Chistyakov, D.V.; Grabeklis, S.; Goriainov, S.V.; Chistyakov, V.V.; Sergeeva, M.G.; Reiser, G. Astrocytes synthesize primary and cyclopentenone prostaglandins that are negative regulators of their proliferation. *Biochem. Biophys. Res. Commun.* **2018**, *500*, 204–210. [CrossRef] [PubMed]
36. Bouchette, D.; Preuss, C.V. *Zileuton*; StatPearls Publishing: Treasure Island, FL, USA, 2020.
37. Rossi, A.; Pergola, C.; Koeberle, A.; Hoffmann, M.; Dehm, F.; Bramanti, P.; Cuzzocrea, S.; Werz, O.; Sautebin, L. The 5-lipoxygenase inhibitor, zileuton, suppresses prostaglandin biosynthesis by inhibition of arachidonic acid release in macrophages. *Br. J. Pharmacol.* **2010**, *161*, 555–570. [CrossRef]
38. Pelletier, J.S.; Devine, J.; Capriotti, K.; Barone, S.B.; Capriotti, J.A. Topical application of povidone-iodine/dimethylsulfoxide ophthalmic gel preparation in Dutch-Belted rabbits. *Cutan. Ocul. Toxicol.* **2019**, *38*, 221–226. [CrossRef]
39. Gordon, D.M. Dimethyl sulfoxide in ophthalmology, with special reference to possible toxic effects. *Ann. N. Y. Acad. Sci.* **1967**, *141*, 392–402. [CrossRef]
40. Maibach, H.I.; Feldmann, R.J. The effect of DMSO on percutaneous penetration of hydrocortisone and testosterone in. *Ann. N. Y. Acad. Sci.* **1967**, *141*, 423–427. [CrossRef]
41. Capriotti, K.; Capriotti, J.A. Dimethyl sulfoxide: History, chemistry, and clinical utility in dermatology. *J. Clin. Aesthet. Dermatol.* **2012**, *5*, 24–26.
42. Hanna, C.; Fraunfelder, F.T.; Meyer, S.M. Effects of dimethyl sulfoxide on ocular inflammation. *Ann. Ophthalmol.* **1977**, *9*, 61. [PubMed]
43. Zileuton: Cayman Chemical Product Information. Available online: https://www.caymanchem.com/pdfs/10006967.pdf (accessed on 1 June 2020).
44. Del Castillo, F.B.; Cantu-Dibildox, J.; Sanz-González, S.M.; Zanon-Moreno, V.C.; Pinazo-Durán, M.D. Cytokine expression in tears of patients with glaucoma or dry eye disease: A prospective, observational cohort study. *Eur. J. Ophthalmol.* **2018**, *29*, 437–443. [CrossRef]
45. Ambaw, Y.A.; Chao, C.; Ji, S.; Raida, M.; Torta, F.; Wenk, M.R.; Tong, L. Tear eicosanoids in healthy people and ocular surface disease. *Sci. Rep.* **2018**, *8*, 11296. [CrossRef] [PubMed]

46. Altinsoy, A.; Dileköz, E.; Kul, O.; Ilhan, S.Ö.; Tunccan, O.G.; Seven, I.; Bagriacik, E.U.; Sarioglu, Y.; Or, M.; Ercan, Z.S. A Cannabinoid Ligand, Anandamide, Exacerbates Endotoxin-Induced Uveitis in Rabbits. *J. Ocul. Pharmacol. Ther.* **2011**, *27*, 545–552. [CrossRef]
47. Vangaveti, V.; Baune, B.T.; Kennedy, R.L. Hydroxyoctadecadienoic acids: Novel regulators of macrophage differentiation and atherogenesis. *Ther. Adv. Endocrinol. Metab.* **2010**, *1*, 51–60. [CrossRef] [PubMed]
48. Yoshida, Y.; Umeno, A.; Ogawa, Y.; Shichiri, M.; Murotomi, K.; Horie, M. Chemistry of Lipid Peroxidation Products and Their Use as Biomarkers in Early Detection of Diseases. *J. Oleo Sci.* **2015**, *64*, 347–356. [CrossRef]
49. Sevanian, A.; Mead, J.F.; Stein, R.A. Epoxides as products of lipid autoxidation in rat lungs. *Lipids* **1979**, *14*, 634–643. [CrossRef]
50. Thompson, D.; Hammock, B.D. Dihydroxyoctadecamonoenoate esters inhibit the neutrophil respiratory burst. *J. Biosci.* **2007**, *32*, 279–291. [CrossRef]
51. Seen, S.; Tong, L. Dry eye disease and oxidative stress. *Acta Ophthalmol.* **2017**, *96*, e412–e420. [CrossRef]
52. Perez-Garmendia, R.; Rodriguez, A.L.D.E.; Ramos-Martinez, I.; Zuñiga, N.M.; Gonzalez-Salinas, R.; Quiroz-Mercado, H.; Zenteno, E.; Hernández, E.R.; Hernández-Zimbrón, L.F.; Martínez-Ramos, I. Interplay between Oxidative Stress, Inflammation, and Amyloidosis in the Anterior Segment of the Eye; Its Pathological Implications. *Oxid. Med. Cell. Longev.* **2020**, *2020*, 6286105. [CrossRef]
53. Kojima, T.; Wakamatsu, T.H.; Dogru, M.; Ogawa, Y.; Igarashi, A.; Ibrahim, O.M.A.; Inaba, T.; Shimizu, T.; Noda, S.; Obata, H.; et al. Age-Related Dysfunction of the Lacrimal Gland and Oxidative Stress: Evidence from the Cu,Zn-superoxide dismutase-1 (Sod1) knockout mice. *Am. J. Pathol.* **2012**, *180*, 1879–1896. [CrossRef] [PubMed]
54. Caligiuri, S.P.; Love, K.; Winter, T.; Gauthier, J.; Taylor, C.G.; Blydt-Hansen, T.; Zahradka, P.; Aukema, H.M. Dietary Linoleic Acid and α-Linolenic Acid Differentially Affect Renal Oxylipins and Phospholipid Fatty Acids in Diet-Induced Obese Rats. *J. Nutr.* **2013**, *143*, 1421–1431. [CrossRef] [PubMed]
55. Rao, N.L.; Dunford, P.J.; Xue, X.; Jiang, X.; Lundeen, K.A.; Coles, F.; Riley, J.P.; Williams, K.N.; Grice, C.A.; Edwards, J.P.; et al. Anti-Inflammatory Activity of a Potent, Selective Leukotriene A4 Hydrolase Inhibitor in Comparison with the 5-Lipoxygenase Inhibitor Zileuton. *J. Pharmacol. Exp. Ther.* **2007**, *321*, 1154–1160. [CrossRef] [PubMed]
56. Suh, J.H.; Yum, E.K.; Cho, Y.S. Synthesis and Biological Evaluation of N-Aryl-5-aryloxazol-2-amine Derivatives as 5-Lipoxygenase Inhibitors. *Chem. Pharm. Bull.* **2015**, *63*, 573–578. [CrossRef]
57. Altan, S.; Oğurtan, Z. Dimethyl sulfoxide but not indomethacin is efficient for healing in hydrofluoric acid eye burns. *J. Int. Soc. Burn. Inj.* **2017**, *43*, 232–244. [CrossRef]
58. Altan, S.; Sağsöz, H.; Oğurtan, Z. Topical dimethyl sulfoxide inhibits corneal neovascularization and stimulates corneal repair in rabbits following acid burn. *Biotech. Histochem.* **2017**, *92*, 619–636. [CrossRef]
59. Toczołowski, J.; Wolski, T.; Klamut-Sory, K. Effect of drugs inhibiting the formation of hydroxide radicals on healing of experimental corneal ulcer. *Klin. Ocz.* **1992**, *94*, 83.
60. Skrypuch, O.W.; Tokarewicz, A.C.; Willis, N.R. Effects of dimethyl sulfoxide on a model of corneal alkali injury. *Can. J. Ophthalmol.* **1987**, *22*, 17–20.
61. Elisia, I.; Nakamura, H.; Lam, V.; Hofs, E.; Cederberg, R.; Cait, J.; Hughes, M.R.; Lee, L.; Jia, W.; Adomat, H.H.; et al. DMSO Represses Inflammatory Cytokine Production from Human Blood Cells and Reduces Autoimmune Arthritis. *PLoS ONE* **2016**, *11*, e0152538. [CrossRef]
62. Nagy, L.; Tontonoz, P.; Alvarez, J.G.; Chen, H.; Evans, R.M. Oxidized LDL regulates macrophage gene expression through ligand activation of PPARgamma. *Cell* **1998**, *93*, 229–240. [CrossRef]
63. AlSalem, M.; Wong, A.; Millns, P.; Arya, P.H.; Chan, M.S.L.; Bennett, A.J.; Barrett, D.A.; Chapman, V.; Kendall, D.A. The contribution of the endogenous TRPV1 ligands 9-HODE and 13-HODE to nociceptive processing and their role in peripheral inflammatory pain mechanisms. *Br. J. Pharmacol.* **2013**, *168*, 1961–1974. [CrossRef] [PubMed]
64. Balicki, I. Clinical study on the application of tacrolimus and DMSO in the treatment of chronic superficial keratitis in dogs. *Pol. J. Vet. Sci.* **2012**, *15*, 667–676. [CrossRef] [PubMed]
65. Pelletier, J.S.; Stewart, K.P.; Capriotti, K.; Capriotti, J.A. Rosacea Blepharoconjunctivitis Treated with a Novel Preparation of Dilute Povidone Iodine and Dimethylsulfoxide: A Case Report and Review of the Literature. *Ophthalmol. Ther.* **2015**, *4*, 143–150. [CrossRef] [PubMed]

66. Pelletier, J.S.; Capriotti, K.; Stewart, K.S.; Capriotti, J.A. Demodex Blepharitis Treated with a Novel Dilute Povidone-Iodine and DMSO System: A Case Report. *Ophthalmol. Ther.* **2017**, *6*, 361–366. [CrossRef] [PubMed]
67. Bhalerao, H.; Koteshwara, K.; Chandran, S. Brinzolamide Dimethyl Sulfoxide in Situ Gelling Ophthalmic Solution: Formulation Optimisation and In Vitro and In Vivo Evaluation. *AAPS PharmSciTech* **2020**, *21*, 69. [CrossRef]
68. Roda, M.; Corazza, I.; Bacchi-Reggiani, M.L.; Pellegrini, M.; Taroni, L.; Giannaccare, G.; Versura, P. Dry Eye Disease and Tear Cytokine Levels—A Meta-Analysis. *Int. J. Mol. Sci.* **2020**, *21*, 3111. [CrossRef]
69. Silva, B.; De Miranda, A.; Rodrigues, F.; Silveira, A.M.; Resende, G.D.S.; Moraes, M.F.D.; De Oliveira, A.P.; Parreiras, P.; Barcelos, L.S.; Teixeira, M.; et al. The 5-lipoxygenase (5-LOX) Inhibitor Zileuton Reduces Inflammation and Infarct Size with Improvement in Neurological Outcome Following Cerebral Ischemia. *Curr. Neurovasc. Res.* **2015**, *12*, 398–403. [CrossRef]
70. Sahin, A.; Kam, W.R.; Darabad, R.R.; Topilow, K.; Sullivan, D.A. Regulation of Leukotriene B4Secretion by Human Corneal, Conjunctival, and Meibomian Gland Epithelial Cells. *Arch. Ophthalmol.* **2012**, *130*, 1013–1018. [CrossRef]
71. Masoudi, S.; Zhao, Z.; Stapleton, F.; Willcox, M.D. Contact Lens–Induced Discomfort and Inflammatory Mediator Changes in Tears. *Eye Contact Lens Sci. Clin. Pract.* **2017**, *43*, 40–45. [CrossRef]
72. Tager, A.M.; Bromley, S.K.; Medoff, B.D.; Islam, S.A.; Bercury, S.D.; Friedrich, E.B.; Carafone, A.D.; Gerszten, R.E.; Luster, A.D. Leukotriene B4 receptor BLT1 mediates early effector T cell recruitment. *Nat. Immunol.* **2003**, *4*, 982–990. [CrossRef]
73. Goodarzi, K.; Goodarzi, M.; Tager, A.M.; Luster, A.D.; Von Andrian, U.H. Leukotriene B4 and BLT1 control cytotoxic effector T cell recruitment to inflamed tissues. *Nat. Immunol.* **2003**, *4*, 965–973. [CrossRef]
74. Harauma, A.; Saito, J.; Watanabe, Y.; Moriguchi, T. Potential for daily supplementation of n-3 fatty acids to reverse symptoms of dry eye in mice. *Prostaglandins Leukot. Essent. Fat. Acids* **2014**, *90*, 207–213. [CrossRef] [PubMed]
75. Downie, L.E.; Ng, S.M.; Lindsley, K.B.; Akpek, E.K. Omega-3 and omega-6 polyunsaturated fatty acids for dry eye disease. *Cochrane Database Syst. Rev.* **2019**, *12*, CD011016. [CrossRef] [PubMed]
76. Silva, D.A.; Nai, G.; Giuffrida, R.; Sgrignoli, M.R.; Dos Santos, D.R.; Donadão, I.V.; Andrade, S.F.; DiNallo, H.R.; Andrade, S.F. Oral omega 3 in different proportions of EPA, DHA, and antioxidants as adjuvant in treatment of keratoconjunctivitis sicca in dogs. *Arq. Bras. Oftalmol.* **2018**, *81*, 421–428. [CrossRef]

biomedicines

MDPI

Article

Gender-Related Differences in Trimethylamine and Oxidative Blood Biomarkers in Cardiovascular Disease Patients

Laura Bordoni [1], Donatella Fedeli [1], Marco Piangerelli [2], Iwona Pelikant-Malecka [3,4], Adrianna Radulska [3,4], Joanna J. Samulak [5], Angelika K. Sawicka [5,6], Lukasz Lewicki [7], Leszek Kalinowski [3,4,8], Robert A. Olek [9,*] and Rosita Gabbianelli [1,*]

1 Unit of Molecular Biology, School of Pharmacy, University of Camerino, 62032 Camerino, Italy; laura.bordoni@unicam.it (L.B.); donatella.fedeli@unicam.it (D.F.)
2 Computer Science Division and Mathematics Division, School of Science and Technology, University of Camerino, 62032 Camerino, Italy; Marco.piangerelli@unicam.it
3 Department of Medical Laboratory Diagnostics, Medical University of Gdansk, 80-211 Gdansk, Poland; iwpe-ma@gumed.edu.pl (I.P.-M.); adrianna.radulska@gumed.edu.pl (A.R.); leszek.kalinowski@gumed.edu.pl (L.K.)
4 Biobanking and Biomolecular Resources Research Infrastructure Poland (BBMRI.PL), 80-211 Gdansk, Poland
5 Doctoral School for Physical Culture Sciences, 80-336 Gdansk, Poland; joanna.samulak@awf.gda.pl (J.J.S.); angelika.sawicka@awf.gda.pl (A.K.S.)
6 Department of Human Physiology, Faculty of Health Sciences, Medical University of Gdansk, 80-210 Gdansk, Poland
7 University Center for Cardiology, Gdansk, Debinki 2, 80-211 Gdansk, Poland; luklewicki@gmail.com
8 Gdansk University of Technology, Narutowicza 11/12, 80-233 Gdansk, Poland
9 Department of Athletics, Strength and Conditioning, Poznan University of Physical Education, 61-871 Poznan, Poland
* Correspondence: robert.olek@aol.com (R.A.O.); rosita.gabbianelli@unicam.it (R.G.); Tel.: +48-61-8355270 (R.A.O.); +39-0737-403208 (R.G.)

Received: 23 June 2020; Accepted: 20 July 2020; Published: 23 July 2020

Abstract: Gender differences in the burden of cardiovascular disease (CVD) have been observed worldwide. In this study, plasmatic levels of trimethylamine (TMA) and blood oxidative biomarkers have been evaluated in 358 men (89 controls and 269 CVD patients) and 189 women (64 control and 125 CVD patients). The fluorescence technique was applied to determine erythrocyte membrane fluidity using 1,6-diphenyl-1,3,5-hexatriene (DPH) and Laurdan, while lipid hydroperoxides were assessed by diphenyl−1-pyrenylphosphine (DPPP). Results show that levels of plasmatic TMA were higher in healthy men with respect to healthy women ($p = 0.0001$). Significantly lower TMA was observed in male CVD patients (0.609 ± 0.104 μM) compared to healthy male controls (0.680 ± 0.118 μM) ($p < 0.001$), while higher levels of TMA were measured in female CVD patients (0.595 ± 0.115 μM) with respect to female controls (0.529 ± 0.073 μM) ($p < 0.001$). DPPP was significantly higher in healthy control men than in women ($p < 0.001$). Male CVD patients displayed a lower value of DPPP (2777 ± 1924) compared to healthy controls (5528 ± 2222) ($p < 0.001$), while no significant changes were measured in females with or without CVD ($p > 0.05$). Membrane fluidity was significantly higher ($p < 0.001$) in the hydrophobic bilayer only in control male subjects. In conclusion, gender differences were observed in blood oxidative biomarkers, and DPPP value might be suggested as a biomarker predictive of CVD only in men.

Keywords: gender; membrane erythrocyte; hydroperoxides; biomarker; DPPP; DPH; TMA; cardiovascular disease; data analysis; precision–recall

---

1. Introduction

Cardiovascular disease (CVD) represents one of the primary causes of death worldwide. Data from the World Health Organization (WHO) identify CVD responsible for 37% of all deaths in the European Union (40% and 34% of all deaths in females and males, respectively). Ischemic heart disease accounts for 20% of CVD deaths in females and 19% in males. Stroke is the second most common cause of CVD deaths, accounting for 13% of all CVD deaths in females and 9% in males [1].

Genetics, gender, ethnicity, lifestyle, and socioeconomical position contribute to outline cardiovascular health from a prenatal period of life. Diseases like diabetes, hypertension, obesity, and unhealthy diets are major risk factors [2]. Genes on sex chromosomes can influence the genes in autosomes and sex steroids testosterone and estrogen; variations of androgen receptor, whose locus is on chromosome X, determine sex differences in cardiovascular regulatory mechanisms [3].

CVD can be influenced by early life risk factors; indeed, an association between low body weight at birth and an increased risk of developing CVD later in life has been observed in both genders [4,5]. Maternal low protein intake and/or high fat diet increase the risk of developing non-communicable diseases; time-dependent malnutrition during prenatal life modulates the epigenome differently, leading to CVD or other diseases (i.e., obesity, glucose intolerance) in adult age, according to biological sex [6,7].

During recent years, several studies have highlighted differences in the incidence of heart disease in women and men [8–14]. The prevalence of CVD is higher in males than in females [8]. Women develop CVD later in life, with a higher risk of stroke [9]. A different number of deaths due to CVD is also reported [10,11].

The increased incidence of death in women due to CVD seems to be associated with atypical symptoms [10] and different distributions of risk factors [11]. Diabetes and dyslipidemia have a higher impact in females than in males [11]. Women in their premenopausal life are more protected from CVD than men by estrogens, so their first myocardial infarction occurs when they are about ten years older than men. Epidemiological analysis in the period 1980–2010 reveals that CHD incidence was more reduced in men than in women; however, mortality due to CHD was higher in men than in women until old age [9]. A large case-control study (involving 24,767 people from 262 centers in 52 countries) on the association between modifiable risk factors (i.e., diet, alcohol intake, smoking, physical inactivity, psychosocial stress) and CHD incidence shows a higher impact of social determinants in women than in men [15]. Thus, better identification of sex differences in CVD is of crucial significance to develop additional strategies to prevent and treat more efficiently CVD in women and men.

In this context, oxidative stress represents a key process depending on several aspects (i.e., genetics, lifestyle, environment, etc.) that can affect numerous cell functions. Active metabolites are produced following redox reactions; e.g., the oxidation of trimethylamine (TMA) to trimethylamine N-oxide (TMAO) [16], which can be monitored due to its involvement in inflammation, atherosclerosis development, and impact on visceral adiposity [17–20]. Moreover, at both the plasma membrane level and lipoproteins, lipid oxidation leads to hydroperoxides production, which significantly contributes to the oxidation of TMA into TMAO, as it has been observed from in vitro and ex vivo studies [21,22]; then, since TMAO is a reactive molecule, it might promote foam cells formation [23]. The crosstalk between lipid peroxidation and TMA metabolism might include gender differences that could provide further insights on CVD; hence, the collection of evidence on this aspect could promote a gender approach to modulate CVD risk.

To identify biomarkers useful to characterizing gender differences in CVD, the present study assesses several blood biomarkers: the plasma TMA, the erythrocyte plasma membrane fluidity, and lipid hydroperoxides are measured in 358 men (89 controls and 269 CVD patients) and 189 women (64 controls and 125 CVD patients). A different profile in controls and CVD subjects has been identified according to gender; a direct correlation between plasma TMA level and erythrocyte lipid hydroperoxides measured by the DPPP probe has been measured in men, while DPH fluorescence anisotropy was inversely correlated to TMA and DPPP.

2. Experimental Section

2.1. Subjects

In total, 358 male (89 controls and 269 CVD patients) and 189 females (64 controls and 125 CVD patients) were recruited in Wejherowo Cardiovascular Center. Inclusion criteria for CVD patients were the diagnosis of elective or urgent coronary angiography, established according to the Third Universal Definition of Myocardial Infarction, and 2015 European Society of Cardiology guidelines [24,25]. The control group was recruited amongst the subjects without a self-reported medical history of CVD (Table 1). The present study was approved by the Regional Bioethical Committee in Gdansk (KB-27/16, 28 December 2016 and extended KB 32-17, 16 November 2017). Informed consent was obtained from all subjects.

Table 1. Characteristics of the Study Participants.

	Control F = 64/M = 89	CVD F = 125/M = 269
Obesity (BMI ≥ 30)	14/30	46/98
Hypertension	22/41	102/199
Hyperlipidemia	16/24	78/186
Diabetes mellitus	5/16	41/77
Current or past smokers	7/52	43/153

F—females; M—males.

2.2. Samples Collection

Blood samples were collected in EDTA-containing tubes; plasma samples obtained by centrifugation at 1300× *g* for 10 min at 18–25 °C were kept frozen at −80 °C until TMA analysis. Erythrocytes were kept frozen at −80 °C and used for membrane isolation.

2.3. Plasma TMA and TMAO

Plasma TMA and TMAO were determined by the Ultra High Performance Liquid Chromatography (UHPLC) tandem mass spectrometry method, based on methods described previously [26,27]. UHPLC separation was performed on an XBridge ® HILIC 3.5 µm (3.0 × 50 mm, Waters, MA, USA) column on a NEXERA Shimadzu UHPLC system coupled with QT4500 SCIEX. Trimethyl-d9-amine HCl (d9-TMA, C/D/N ISOTOPES INC., Quebec, Canda) was used as an internal standard. The 3 µM of d9-TMA working solution of internal standard (ISWS) was prepared in methanol/acetonitrile (15:85) and 0.1% formic acid (*v/v*) (Merck KGaA, Darmstadt, Germany). Calibration samples, QC, and plasma samples were prepared by the addition 100 µL of cold ISWS to 50 µL of each sample type. All samples were vortexed and kept on ice for 15 min for protein precipitation. Centrifuged samples (14,000 rpm, 4 °C, for 20 min.) were divided into two parts: without dilution, which were used for the analysis of TMA concentration and diluted (5:95 of ISWS) for analysis of TMAO. The mobile phase was 70% of acetonitrile with 0.1% formic acid (*v/v*) and 30% of 15 mmol/L ammonium formate with 0.1% formic acid (*v/v*) (Merck KGaA, Darmstadt, Germany) at a flow rate of 0.4/min. The mass spectrometer was operated in multiple-reaction monitoring (MRM)-positive electrospray ionization (ESI+). The mass spectrometer optimized settings were as follows: IonSpray Voltage = 5.5 kV, source temperature = 300 °C, collision gas = 8, and curtain gas = 30.0. Ion transitions used for quantitation: *m/z* 60.1 → 44.0 for TMA, *m/z* 76.1 → 59.0 for TMAO and *m/z* 69.1 → 49.1 for d9-TMA. Calibration curves ranges were from 0.1 to 30 µM and 0.3 to 30 µM for TMA and TMAO, respectively. The limits of quantification were 0.1 µM for TMA and 0.3 µM for TMAO.

2.4. Erythrocyte Plasma Membrane Preparation

Erythrocyte membranes were obtained by progressive hemolysis; cells were incubated in 5 mM Na_2HPO_4, pH 7.4 at 4 °C for 20 min and centrifuged at 9000× *g* for 15 min at 4 °C. The additional steps of incubation with 2.5 and 1.25 mM Na_2HPO_4 at pH 7.4 and centrifugation were done to obtain white membranes.

2.5. Erythrocyte Membrane Fluidity

Membrane fluidity was measured on erythrocyte membrane using 1,6-Diphenyl−1,3,5-hexatriene (DPH) (Molecular Probes, Eugene, OR, USA) and 6-lauroyl−2-dimethylaminonaphthalene (Laurdan) (Molecular Probes, Eugene, OR, USA).

A Hitachi 4500 spectrofluorometer was used for fluorescence measurements.

All samples were normalized to the final protein concentration of 0.4 mg/mL, determined using the Pierce BCA Protein Assay Kit (Thermo Scientific, Waltham, MA, USA).

Steady-state fluorescence anisotropy (r) of DPH was carried out in 1 mL of sodium phosphate buffer (2.5 mM, pH 7.4), containing 0.4 mg of the plasma membrane and DPH at the final concentration of 1 μM after 1 h of incubation at 37 °C using excitation and emission wavelengths of 360 and 430 nm, respectively, according to the equation [28]:

$$r = (I_{||} - I_{\perp} g)/(I_{||} + 2I_{\perp} g) \quad (1)$$

where g is the grating correction factor for the optical system, obtained from the ratio of the perpendicular and the parallel polarized emission components when the excitation light is polarized in the horizontal plane, and $I_{||}$ and $I_{\perp}$ are the intensities measured with the polarization plane parallel and perpendicular to that of the exciting beam.

Generalized polarization of Laurdan (GP340) was analyzed in 1 mL of sodium phosphate buffer (2.5 mM, pH 7.4), containing 0.4 mg of the plasma membrane and Laurdan at the final concentration of 1 μM after 5 min of incubation at 37 °C using an excitation wavelength of 340 and emission of 440 and 490 nm, respectively, according to Parasassi's equation [29]:

$$GP340 = (I_B - I_R)/(I_B + I_R) \quad (2)$$

where I_B and I_R are the intensities at the blue (440 nm) and red (490 nm) edges of the emission spectrum and correspond to the fluorescence emission maximum in the gel and liquid crystalline phases of the bilayer, respectively [30].

2.6. DPPP Assay

Erythrocyte membrane lipid hydroperoxides were detected using a membrane-localized fluorescent probe Diphenyl−1-pyrenylphosphine (DPPP) (Cayman Chemical Co., Ann Arbor, MI, USA), that reacts specifically with hydroperoxides and becomes highly fluorescent when oxidized [22]. Lipid hydroperoxide formation occurs considerably in plasma membranes from unsaturated fatty acids during oxidative stress [31,32]; the measure of lipid hydroperoxides represents a crucial step of the propagative lipid peroxidation, which affects membrane and protein conformation with important outcomes on their functionality [32]. DPPP represents a sensitive and reproducible quantitative method of total lipid hydroperoxide analysis [33].

Membrane samples, normalized to the final protein concentration of 0.4 mg/mL, were incubated with 1 μM DPPP in 1 mL PBS at 37 °C for 5 min in the dark. The fluorescence intensity of the samples was measured using 351 and 380 nm as excitation and emission wavelengths, respectively. Results are expressed as fluorescence intensity (arbitrary units, a.u.).

2.7. Statistical Analysis

Shapiro–Wilk was used to test the normality of data distribution. The Kruskal–Wallis test and Spearman correlation were used to determine significant differences among analyzed variables and correlations, respectively. Precision–recall curves were calculated using the Scikit-learn library for Python. They were used for testing the power of the logistic regression model based on DPPP and DPH for males and females, respectively. If not differently specified, statistical analyses were performed using the SPSS package for Windows, v.20.0 (SPSS Inc., Chicago, IL, USA).

3. Results

3.1. Descriptive Statistics

Of the 547 recruited subjects, 358 were male and 189 females. Within the male group, 89 were healthy controls, while 269 were CVD patients. The male controls' and CVD patients' mean ages were 62.6 ± 8.5 and 65.0 ± 12.0, respectively. Within the female group, 64 women were healthy controls, while 125 were CVD patients. The female controls' and CVD patients' mean ages were 66.8 ± 6.7 and 69.5 ±10.3, respectively.

3.2. Gender Differences in the Plasma TMA Level

Plasma TMA levels were significantly different in the two genders, i.e., healthy control men show higher levels of TMA (0.680 ± 0.118 μM) than women (0.529 ± 0.073) ($p = 0.0001$). Plasma TMA levels were significantly lower in male CVD patients compared to controls (Figure 1) ($p < 0.001$). At the same time, a higher TMA level in female CVD subjects with respect to healthy controls of the same gender was observed (Figure 1) ($p < 0.001$).

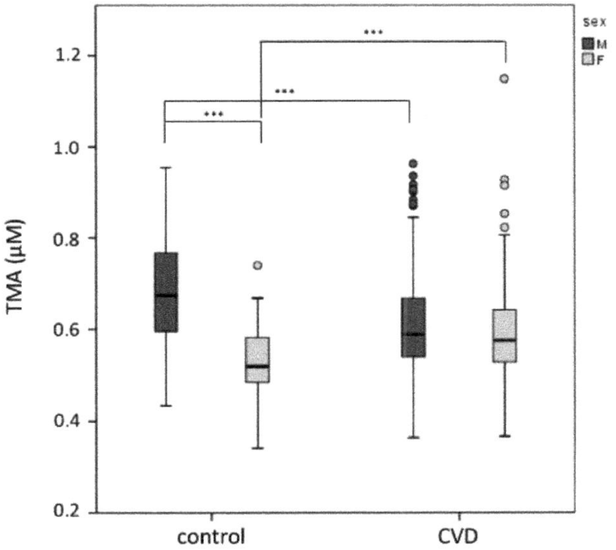

Figure 1. Plasma TMA level in males and females. The male control group displays higher plasma TMA levels compared to female controls. Male CVD patients show a lower TMA value with respect to healthy controls of the same gender, while an opposite result was observed in the female groups. Male controls ($n = 89$) and male CVD patients ($n = 269$). Female controls ($n = 64$) and female CVD patients ($n = 125$), *** $p < 0.001$.

3.3. Gender Differences in the Erythrocyte Plasma Membrane Fluidity

Erythrocyte plasma membrane fluidity was analyzed using fluorescent probes that localize at different depths of the bilayer. The analysis of the hydrophobic region of the bilayer by DPH showed significant changes in fluorescence anisotropy (r) in controls: male subjects have a lower value of anisotropy (r = 0.129 ± 0.558) compared to females (r = 0.166 ± 0.425) ($p < 0.001$). Male CVD patients present a higher value of anisotropy with respect to controls (Figure 2) ($p < 0.001$), while no changes were observed in female CVD subjects with respect to healthy controls of the same gender (Figure 2) ($p > 0.05$).

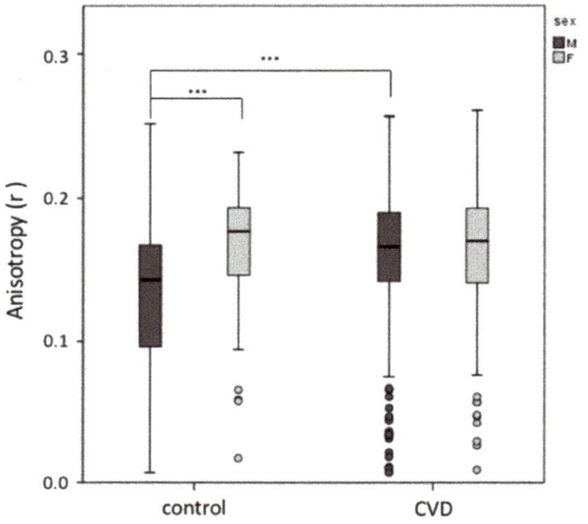

Figure 2. DPH fluorescence anisotropy (r) in plasma membrane erythrocytes from males and females. The measured membrane fluidity was higher in male controls with respect to female controls. Male CVD patients have a lower DPH membrane fluidity with respect to healthy controls of the same gender. Male controls ($n = 89$) and male CVD patients ($n = 269$), *** $p < 0.001$. Female controls ($n = 64$) and female CVD patients ($n = 125$).

The analysis of the hydrophilic–hydrophobic region by Laurdan showed no changes in generalized polarization of Laurdan between males and females, as well as in healthy/unhealthy subjects.

3.4. Gender Differences in the Erythrocyte Lipid Hydroperoxide Level (DPPP)

Lipid hydroperoxide levels were measured in erythrocyte plasma membrane using the fluorescent probe DPPP. DPPP fluorescence was significantly different between healthy males and females, with men displaying higher values (5528 ± 2222) than women (2616 ± 1065) ($p < 0.001$). Male CVD patients show lower values of DPPP compared to healthy controls of the same gender (Figure 3) ($p < 0.001$), while no changes in females with or without CVD were measured (Figure 3) ($p > 0.05$). Interestingly, the DPPP was directly related to TMA levels (Spearman correlation = 0.317; $p < 0.001$) in the male group (Figure 4), but not in the female group (Spearman correlation = 0.067; $p = 0.361$) (Figure 4). On the other hand, TMA showed a negative correlation with DPH in males ($p < 0.001$) (Figure 4), but not in females ($p > 0.05$) (Figure 4).

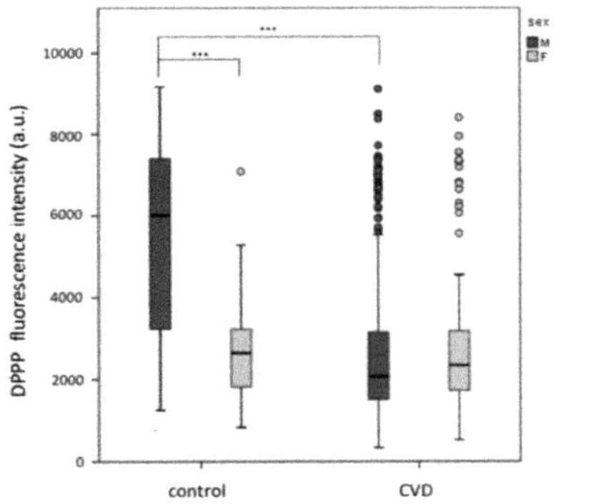

Figure 3. Lipid hydroperoxides (DPPP) in erythrocytes from male and female subjects. Lipid hydroperoxides were higher in the male control group with respect to female controls. Male CVD patients have a lower hydroperoxides level with respect to healthy controls of the same gender. Male controls ($n = 89$) and male CVD patients ($n = 269$), *** $p < 0.001$. Female controls ($n = 64$) and female CVD patients ($n = 125$). Results are expressed as fluorescence intensity (arbitrary units, a.u.).

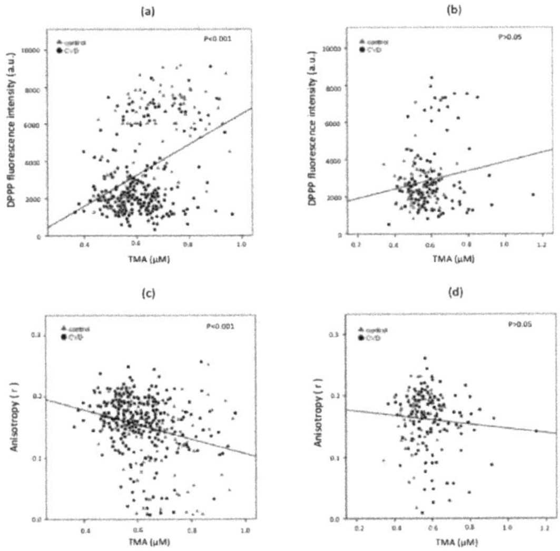

Figure 4. Correlations between plasma TMA levels and DPPP in males (**a**) or females (**b**) and DPH anisotropy (r), in the male (**c**) or female (**d**) groups. Only in the male group, erythrocyte membrane lipid hydroperoxide (DPPP fluorescence intensity, a.u.) correlates positively, and membrane fluidity (anisotropy, r) inversely with plasma TMA.

3.5. Precision–Recall Curves

Results from the precision–recall analysis, resulting by using a logistic model, show that only in this work, the precision–recall curves (or PR curves) were used because of the presence of unbalanced data. These curves were built by calculating the precision and recall as the classification threshold changes. PR curves show precision on the y-axis, against the recall on the x-axis. Those quantities are defined as follows:

$$\text{Precision} = \text{TP}/(\text{TP} + \text{FP}) \quad (3)$$

$$\text{Recall} = \text{TP}/(\text{TP} + \text{FN}) \quad (4)$$

Where true positive (TP), false positive (FP), and false negative (FN) values were applied. In order to assign a value to those parameters, a cut-off for distinguishing persons between the two classes (controls and CVD) was set. Changing the cut-off allows us to obtain different values for TP, FP, and FN, while the real number of the CVD and controls remains the same. A PR curve shows the relationship between precision and recalls for every possible cut-off value. Thus, every point on the PR curve represents the precision and recall for a chosen cut-off. The best cut-off is the one that allows us to have values of precision and recall both closer to 1. Figure 5 shows the curves for each logistic model. Greater area under the curve and better the classifier performances: this suggests that DPPP Males classifier, with an area under the PR curve of 0.941, is the best performing model among all the classifier that has been used. In this model, the cut-off value that allows to have the highest precision and recall is shown in Figure 5a. It is worth noting that 69 values of the DPH in the original dataset were missing. Those values are almost equally divided in each class (39 CVD and 30 controls). The dataset was imputed by estimating the empirical DPH distribution and using its mean for replacing the missing values.

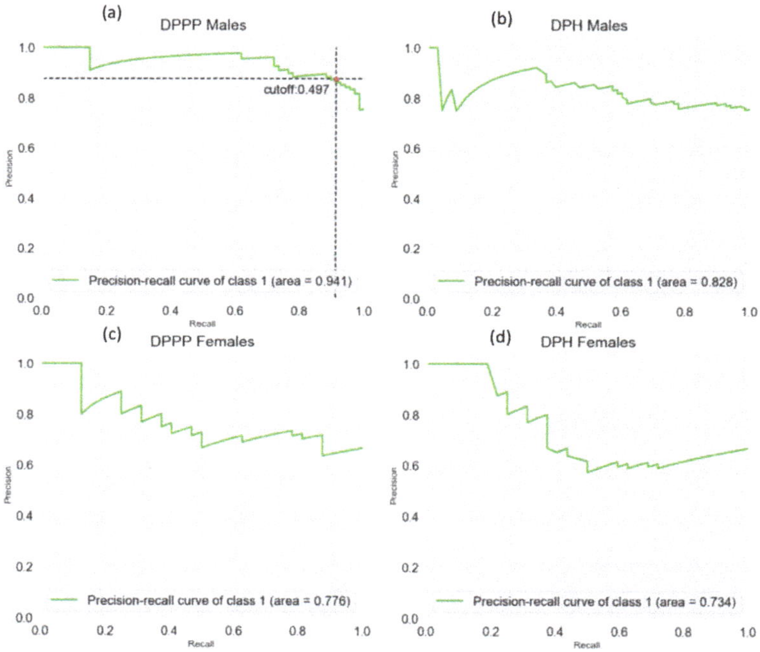

Figure 5. Precision–recall analysis. The four PR curves present the precision–recall analysis. In the insets, the values of the area under the curves are reported. In the DPPP males curve (**a**), the cut-off value of 0.497 is indicated. The precision–recall curve (**a**) highlights that erythrocyte lipid hydroperoxides, measured by DPPP, in men may suggest this parameter as a biomarker to predict CVD in men. The precision–recall curve for DPPP classifier in females (**b**), for DPH classifier in males (**c**), and for DPH classifier in females (**d**).

4. Discussion

Our study shows a direct correlation between plasma TMA and erythrocyte lipid hydroperoxides measured by DPPP in men. Plasma TMA in controls is higher in men than in women, but it decreases in male patients with CVD, while it increases in female affected by CVD. TMA production depends mainly on the activity of the gut microflora, which can metabolize dietary choline (phosphatidylcholine, phosphocholine, sphingomyelin, etc.), betaine, and L-carnitine contained in animal food (i.e., meat, fish, egg, etc.). TMA can also be achieved from the catabolism of ergothioneine contained in vegetarian food (i.e., mushrooms, beans). TMA from gut reaches the liver by portal circulation, where flavin monooxygenases (FMO3) catalyze its conversion in the TMAO. Lower expression of FMO3 has been associated with decreased plasma TMAO levels [21,34]. TMAO can also derive from the consumption of fish meals [35]; as observed in mice, it can be produced through the direct oxidation of TMA [22]. TMAO is distributed to tissues, where it works as an osmolyte or can be cleared by the kidneys. It has been suggested that TMAO is involved in the development of atherosclerosis by promoting foam cells formation and atherogenic plaques [36,37]. TMAO contributes to about 11% of the variation in atherosclerosis susceptibility in mice [21], and its level correlates with several characteristics of plaque instability, such as markers of inflammation, platelet activation, and intraplaque hemorrhage [22].

Gender differences in the level of FMO3 have been observed, and a lower TMAO production in the liver of male mice compared to females was measured [21]. The gender difference of TMAO production in mice has also been associated with testosterone level, which is able to downregulate FMO3, and to modulate estrogen-dependent upregulation of FMO3 expression; the testosterone can decrease TMAO levels, and, accordingly, this could explain the lower levels of TMAO in males than in females [38]. Furthermore, an increased excretion rate of TMAO in male mice was measured with respect to female animals when mice were treated with choline; in the same animals, TMA level was higher in male than in female mice. Comparably, in our study, TMA was significantly higher in men than in women; within the group of the same sex, the decreased level of TMA in male CVD patients might be associated with sex-hormone regulation and to its different direct oxidation to TMAO. Females with CVD show higher TMA levels than healthy females, and this might be related to gender differences in the redox system and metabolic responses [11]. Under physiological conditions, women appear to be less susceptible to oxidative stress than men, and this can impact differently on CVD development (i.e., coronary heart disease); gender differences in oxidative stress response might affect the risk of developing atherosclerosis [11]. A link between TMA oxidation and free radicals has been observed; increased TMAO levels have been associated with vascular inflammation through activation of the NLRP3 inflammasome by reactive oxygen species (ROS) due to the TMAO inhibition of the SIRT3-SOD 2-mtROS pathway [39]. ROS production increases in several inflammatory diseases and they have an active role in CVD [40]. In our study, healthy men display higher levels of TMA and lipid hydroperoxides measured by DPPP than male CVD patients. Remarkably, the lipid hydroperoxides in erythrocyte membrane might represent a biomarker of CVD. The precision–recall curves (Figure 5) demonstrate that DPPP can be used to predict CVD only in men. Since our model can discriminate between ill and healthy people, and our goal is to minimize the number of false negatives, only the PR curve of the DPPP males, with an area under the curve of 0.941, can be considered as a possible prognostic factor.

As previously reported, biomarkers of oxidative stress were lower in females than in males [11,41], and healthy women have lower DPPP levels than healthy men. However, in female CVD patients, lipid hydroperoxides increase in respect to males affected by CVD. Changes in the DPPP in men and women could be due also to the double role of ROS, which, in addition to catalyzing the oxidative process, can also have a regulatory function. Lipid hydroperoxides are involved in the stress signaling that mediates several cellular responses (i.e., induction of antioxidant enzymes, apoptotic death) and may have gender-dependent regulations. Furthermore, the different level of hydroperoxides may also be related to differences in the metabolic pathways involved in the removal of lipid hydroperoxides and in the repairing reactions; indeed, lipid hydroperoxides should be removed to avoid the propagation of lipid peroxidation [42]. The excision/reduction/repair pathway comprises the activity of several enzymes like phospholipase A2, glutathione peroxidase (GPX), and an acyltransferase, which, as reported in the kinetic models, are less involved in hydroperoxide repair with respect to the enzymes phospholipid hydroperoxide glutathione peroxidase (PHGPX), phospholipase A2, and acyltransferase, that work through reduction/excision/repair reactions. Transfected cells with PHGPX were particularly efficient in removing lipid hydroperoxides; PHGPH can interact more easily than GPX with polar (i.e., H_2O_2)

and lower polarity substrates (i.e., lipid hydroperoxides). Gender differences in glutathione peroxidase and phospholipase A2 activity have been observed, and they might contribute to partially explain the gender differences in lipid hydroperoxide levels [11,42–45].

The increased DPH fluorescence anisotropy in male CVD patients compared to controls indicates a reduced fluidity in the hydrophobic region of the membrane. The decline of membrane fluidity negatively interferes with the membrane protein dynamicity and finally, influences protein functions. Lower fluidity can depend on the fatty acid composition, the oxidative process at lipid or protein level, and metabolic regulation [30,46]. Lipid composition varies according to the diet: a diet rich in mono-polyunsaturated fatty acids (i.e., extra virgin olive oil (EVOO), seed) modulates bilayer composition toward a more fluid state of lipids, compared to a saturated fatty acid diet (i.e., meat, cheese). Oxidative processes decrease membrane fluidity due to the increased number of intermolecular interactions. In healthy subjects, DPH anisotropy was higher in women than in men, and no changes in fluidity were measured in women, even in the presence of CVD. Considering the gender difference observed in lipid hydroperoxides, fluidity changes could mainly depend on dietary lipid composition and metabolic regulation. Changes in lipid profile (i.e., triglycerides, HDL-cholesterol), smoking, and diabetes have a stronger negative impact in post-menopausal women than men, while total cholesterol and LDL have a more significant effect in men [11,47]. Besides, hyperlipidemia and diabetes can amplify oxidative stress, with substantial implications for atherosclerosis development.

The main limitation of this study is the lack of subjects' dietary habits, including alcohol consumption, to correlate the observed changes at the membrane level. Smoking habits cannot explain observed differences in DPH anisotropy, TMA, and hydroperoxide levels. On the other hand, gender differences measured in the peripheral biomarkers TMA, DPPP, and DPH represent remarkable data, which could be used to better address gender-specific therapies for CVD. Besides, weak changes in TMAO measured in our groups (Supplementary Material Table S1) could be only partially associated with plasma TMA levels. Finally, the direct correlation between plasma TMA and hydroperoxides level that emerged from this study warrants attention, and its potential use as a blood biomarker predictive of CVD in men might have relevant implications in CVD prevention.

Future studies able to correlate gender differences of other biochemical parameters associated with enzymes involved in the regulation of plasma TMA metabolism are warranted, especially considering that recently TMA, but not TMAO, has been proposed as a marker of cardiovascular risk [48,49]. Furthermore, additional studies aimed at the correlation between food components and membrane lipid redox state could be useful to investigate.

5. Conclusions

Gender differences in CVD have been identified in plasma TMA level and at the erythrocyte membrane level. Healthy females have a lower basal level of TMA and lipid hydroperoxides than males, while their membrane in the hydrophobic region results in less fluid than in healthy males. Female CVD patients are characterized by a higher plasma TMA than their healthy controls, while no differences in lipid hydroperoxides and membrane fluidity between control and CVD females were measured. Male CVD patients show a decreased fluidity in the hydrophobic region of the erythrocyte membrane. Erythrocyte lipid hydroperoxides measured by DPPP can be proposed as new biomarkers to predict CVD in men.

Supplementary Materials: Supplementary Materials can be found at http://www.mdpi.com/2227-9059/8/8/238/s1.

Author Contributions: Conceptualization, L.B., R.A.O. and R.G.; methodology, D.F., I.P.-M. and A.R.; formal analysis, L.B. and M.P.; software, M.P.; investigation, D.F., I.P.-M., A.R., J.J.S., A.K.S. and L.L.; resources, R.G. and L.L.; writing—original draft preparation, R.G.; writing—review and editing, L.B and A.K.S.; visualization, L.B. and M.P.; supervision, R.G. and R.A.O.; funding acquisition, R.G. and L.K. All authors have read and agreed to the published version of the manuscript.

Funding: This research was funded by R.G, grant no FPA000033 and Polish Ministry of Science and Higher Education Poland, grant no DIR/WK2017/01.

Acknowledgments: We thank the students Ilaria Marazzani and Valentina Marinozzi for their assistance during the fluorescence measurements performed at the Unit of Molecular Biology of the University of Camerino.

Conflicts of Interest: The authors declare no conflict of interest.

References

1. Wilkins, E.; Wilson, L.; Wickramasinghe, K.; Bhatnagar, P.; Leal, J.; Luengo-Fernandez, R.; Burns, R.; Rayner, M.; Townsend, N. *European Cardiovascular Disease Statistics 2017*. European Heart Network. Available online: http://www.ehnheart.org/images/CVD-statistics-report-August-2017.pdf (accessed on 15 February 2017).
2. Mishra, R. Monica Determinants of cardiovascular disease and sequential decision-making for treatment among women: A Heckman's approach. *SSM Popul. Health.* **2019**, *7*, 100365. [CrossRef] [PubMed]
3. Shufelt, C.L.; Pacheco, C.; Tweet, M.S.; Miller, V.M. Sex-Specific Physiology and Cardiovascular Disease. *Adv. Exp. Med. Biol.* **2018**, *1065*, 433–454. [CrossRef] [PubMed]
4. Hales, C.N.; Barker, D.J.P. The thrifty phenotype hypothesis. *Br. Med. Bull.* **2001**, *60*, 5–20. [CrossRef] [PubMed]
5. Barker, D. The Developmental Origins of Adult Disease. *J. Am. Coll. Nutr.* **2004**, *23*, 588S–595S. [CrossRef] [PubMed]
6. Calkins, K.; Devaskar, S.U. Fetal origins of adult disease. *Curr. Probl. Pediatr. Adolesc. Health Care* **2011**, *41*, 158–176. [CrossRef] [PubMed]
7. Santos, M.S.; Joles, J.A. Early determinants of cardiovascular disease. *Best Pract. Res. Clin. Endocrinol. Metab.* **2012**, *26*, 581–597. [CrossRef]
8. Virani, S.S.; Alonso, A.; Benjamin, E.J.; Bittencourt, M.S.; Callaway, C.W.; Carson, A.P.; Chamberlain, A.M.; Chang, A.R.; Cheng, S.; Delling, F.N.; et al. Heart Disease and Stroke Statistics—2020 Update: A Report From the American Heart Association. *Circulation* **2020**, *141*. [CrossRef]
9. Bots, S.H.; Peters, S.A.E.; Woodward, M. Sex differences in coronary heart disease and stroke mortality: A global assessment of the effect of ageing between 1980 and 2010. *BMJ Glob. Health* **2017**, *2*, e000298. [CrossRef]
10. Kawamoto, K.R.; Davis, M.B.; Duvernoy, C.S. Acute Coronary Syndromes: Differences in Men and Women. *Curr. Atheroscler. Rep.* **2016**, *18*, 73. [CrossRef]
11. Kander, M.C.; Cui, Y.; Liu, Z. Gender difference in oxidative stress: A new look at the mechanisms for cardiovascular diseases. *J. Cell. Mol. Med.* **2016**, *21*, 1024–1032. [CrossRef]
12. Benjamin, E.J.; Blaha, M.J.; Chiuve, S.E.; Cushman, M.; Das, S.R.; Deo, R.; De Ferranti, S.D.; Floyd, J.; Fornage, M.; Gillespie, C.; et al. Heart Disease and Stroke Statistics—2017 Update: A Report From the American Heart Association. *Circulation* **2017**, *135*. [CrossRef] [PubMed]
13. Garcia, M.; Mulvagh, S.L.; Merz, C.N.B.; Buring, J.E.; Manson, J.E. Cardiovascular Disease in Women: Clinical Perspectives. *Circ. Res.* **2016**, *118*, 1273–1293. [CrossRef]
14. Bordoni, L.; Sawicka, A.K.; Szarmach, A.; Winklewski, P.J.; Olek, R.; Gabbianelli, R. A Pilot Study on the Effects of l-Carnitine and Trimethylamine-N-Oxide on Platelet Mitochondrial DNA Methylation and CVD Biomarkers in Aged Women. *Int. J. Mol. Sci.* **2020**, *21*, 1047. [CrossRef] [PubMed]
15. Rosengren, A.; Hawken, S.; Ounpuu, S.; Sliwa, K.; Zubaid, M.; Almahmeed, W.A.; Blackett, K.N.; Sitthiamorn, C.; Sato, H.; Yusuf, S.; et al. Association of psychosocial risk factors with risk of acute myocardial infarction in 11119 cases and 13648 controls from 52 countries (the IN- TERHEART study): Case-control study. *Lancet* **2004**, *364*, 953–962. [CrossRef]
16. Winter, S.E.; A Lopez, C.; Baumler, A.J. The dynamics of gut-associated microbial communities during inflammation. *EMBO Rep.* **2013**, *14*, 319–327. [CrossRef]
17. Ding, L.; Chang, M.; Guo, Y.; Zhang, L.; Xue, C.; Yanagita, T.; Zhang, T.; Wang, Y. Trimethylamine-N-oxide (TMAO)-induced atherosclerosis is associated with bile acid metabolism. *Lipids Health Dis.* **2018**, *17*, 286. [CrossRef] [PubMed]
18. Janeiro, M.H.; Ramirez, M.J.; Milagro, F.; Martínez, J.A.; Solas, M. Implication of Trimethylamine N-Oxide (TMAO) in Disease: Potential Biomarker or New Therapeutic Target. *Nutrients* **2018**, *10*, 1398. [CrossRef] [PubMed]

19. Annunziata, G.; Maisto, M.; Schisano, C.; Ciampaglia, R.; Narciso, V.; Hassan, S.T.S.; Tenore, G.C.; Novellino, E. Effect of Grape Pomace Polyphenols With or Without Pectin on TMAO Serum Levels Assessed by LC/MS-Based Assay: A Preliminary Clinical Study on Overweight/Obese Subjects. *Front. Pharmacol.* **2019**, *10*, 575. [CrossRef]
20. Barrea, L.; Annunziata, G.; Muscogiuri, G.; Di Somma, C.; Laudisio, D.; Maisto, M.; De Alteriis, G.; Tenore, G.C.; Colao, A.; Savastano, S. Trimethylamine-N-oxide (TMAO) as Novel Potential Biomarker of Early Predictors of Metabolic Syndrome. *Nutrients* **2018**, *10*, 1971. [CrossRef]
21. Bennett, B.J.; Vallim, T.Q.D.A.; Wang, Z.; Shih, D.M.; Meng, Y.; Gregory, J.; Allayee, H.; Lee, R.; Graham, M.; Crooke, R.; et al. Trimethylamine-N-oxide, a metabolite associated with atherosclerosis, exhibits complex genetic and dietary regulation. *Cell Metab.* **2013**, *17*, 49–60. [CrossRef]
22. Koay, Y.C.; Chen, Y.-C.; Wali, A.J.; Luk, A.W.S.; Li, M.; Doma, H.; Reimark, R.; Zaldivia, M.T.K.; Habtom, H.T.; E Franks, A.; et al. Plasma levels of trimethylamine-N-oxide can be increased with 'healthy' and 'unhealthy' diets and do not correlate with the extent of atherosclerosis but with plaque instability. *Cardiovasc. Res.* **2020**. [CrossRef] [PubMed]
23. Geng, J.; Yang, C.; Wang, B.; Zhang, X.; Hu, T.; Gu, Y.; Li, J. Trimethylamine N-oxide promotes atherosclerosis via CD36-dependent MAPK/JNK pathway. *Biomed. Pharmacother.* **2018**, *97*, 941–947. [CrossRef] [PubMed]
24. Thygesen, K.; Alpert, J.; Jaffe, A.S.; Simoons, M.L.; Chaitman, B.R.; White, H.D. Third Universal Definition of Myocardial Infarction. *Glob. Hear.* **2012**, *7*, 275–295. [CrossRef] [PubMed]
25. Roffi, M.; Patrono, C.; Collet, J.-P.; Mueller, C.; Valgimigli, M.; Andreotti, F.; Bax, J.J.; Borger, M.A.; Brotons, C.; Chew, D.P.; et al. 2015 ESC Guidelines for the management of acute coronary syndromes in patients presenting without persistent ST-segment elevation: Task Force for the Management of Acute Coronary Syndromes in Patients Presenting without Persistent ST-Segment Elevation of the European Society of Cardiology (ESC). *Eur. Hear. J.* **2015**, *37*, 267–315. [CrossRef]
26. Grinberga, S.; Dambrova, M.; Latkovskis, G.; Strele, I.; Konrade, I.; Hartmane, D.; Sevostjanovs, E.; Liepinsh, E.; Pugovics, O. Determination of trimethylamine-N-oxide in combination with L-carnitine and γ-butyrobetaine in human plasma by UPLC/MS/MS. *Biomed. Chromatogr.* **2015**, *29*, 1670–1674. [CrossRef] [PubMed]
27. Awwad, H.M.; Geisel, J.; Obeid, R. Determination of trimethylamine, trimethylamine N-oxide, and taurine in human plasma and urine by UHPLC-MS/MS technique. *J. Chromatogr. B Anal. Technol. Biomed. Life Sci.* **2016**, *1038*, 12–18. [CrossRef] [PubMed]
28. Shinitzky, M.; Barenholz, Y. Fluidity parameters of lipid regions determined by fluorescence polarization. *Biochim. Biophys. Acta* **1978**, *515*, 367–394. [CrossRef]
29. Parasassi, T.; De Stasio, G.; D'Ubaldo, A.; Gratton, E. Phase fluctuation in phospholipid membranes revealed by Laurdan fluorescence. *Biophys. J.* **1990**, *57*, 1179–1186. [CrossRef]
30. Vadhana, D.; Carloni, M.; Fedeli, N.; Nasuti, C.; Gabbianelli, R. Perturbation of Rat Heart Plasma Membrane Fluidity Due to Metabolites of Permethrin Insecticide. *Cardiovasc. Toxicol.* **2011**, *11*, 226–234. [CrossRef]
31. Bordoni, L.; Fedeli, N.; Nasuti, C.; Capitani, M.; Fiorini, D.; Gabbianelli, R. Permethrin pesticide induces NURR1 up-regulation in dopaminergic cell line: Is the pro-oxidant effect involved in toxicant-neuronal damage? *Comp. Biochem. Physiol. C Toxicol. Pharmacol.* **2017**, *201*, 51–57. [CrossRef]
32. Girotti, A.W. Lipid hydroperoxide generation, turnover, and effector action in biological systems. *J. Lipid Res.* **1998**, *39*, 1529–1542. [PubMed]
33. Sohn, J.-H.; Taki, Y.; Ushio, H.; Ohshima, T. Quantitative determination of total lipid hydroperoxides by a flow injection analysis system. *Lipids* **2005**, *40*, 203–209. [CrossRef] [PubMed]
34. Shih, D.M.; Zhu, W.; Schugar, R.C.; Meng, Y.; Jia, X.; Miikeda, A.; Wang, Z.; Zieger, M.; Lee, R.; Graham, M.; et al. Genetic Deficiency of Flavin-Containing Monooxygenase 3 (Fmo3) Protects Against Thrombosis but Has Only a Minor Effect on Plasma Lipid Levels—Brief Report. *Arter. Thromb. Vasc. Boil.* **2019**, *39*, 1045–1054. [CrossRef] [PubMed]
35. Cho, C.E.; Taesuwan, S.; Malysheva, O.V.; Bender, E.; Tulchinsky, N.F.; Yan, J.; Sutter, J.L.; Caudill, M.A.; Espin, J.C. Back cover: Trimethylamine-N-oxide (TMAO) response to animal source foods varies among healthy young men and is influenced by their gut microbiota composition: A randomized controlled trial. *Mol. Nutr. Food Res.* **2017**, *61*, 1770016. [CrossRef]
36. Wang, Z.; Klipfell, E.; Bennett, B.J.; Koeth, R.; Levison, B.S.; Dugar, B.; Feldstein, A.E.; Britt, E.B.; Fu, X.; Chung, Y.-M.; et al. Gut flora metabolism of phosphatidylcholine promotes cardiovascular disease. *Nature* **2011**, *472*, 57–63. [CrossRef]

37. Roncal, C.; Martínez-Aguilar, E.; Orbe, J.; Ravassa, S.; Fernández-Montero, A.; Saenz-Pipaon, G.; Ugarte, A.; De Mendoza, A.E.-H.; Rodríguez, J.A.; Fernández-Alonso, S.; et al. Trimethylamine-N-Oxide (TMAO) Predicts Cardiovascular Mortality in Peripheral Artery Disease. *Sci. Rep.* **2019**, *9*, 15580–15588. [CrossRef]
38. Falls, J.G.; Ryu, D.-Y.; Cao, Y.; Levi, P.E.; Hodgson, E. Regulation of Mouse Liver Flavin-Containing Monooxygenases 1 and 3 by Sex Steroids. *Arch. Biochem. Biophys.* **1997**, *342*, 212–223. [CrossRef]
39. Chen, M.; Zhu, X.; Ran, L.; Lang, H.; Yi, L.; Mi, M. Trimethylamine-N-Oxide Induces Vascular Inflammation by Activating the NLRP3 Inflammasome Through the SIRT3-SOD2-mtROS Signaling Pathway. *J. Am. Hear. Assoc.* **2017**, *6*. [CrossRef]
40. Panth, N.; Paudel, K.R.; Parajuli, K. Reactive Oxygen Species: A Key Hallmark of Cardiovascular Disease. *Adv. Med.* **2016**. [CrossRef]
41. Ide, T.; Tsutsui, H.; Ohashi, N.; Hayashidani, S.; Suematsu, N.; Tsuchihashi, M.; Tamai, H.; Takeshita, A. Greater oxidative stress in healthy young men compared with premenopausal women. *Arter. Thromb. Vasc. Boil.* **2002**, *22*, 438–442. [CrossRef]
42. Félix, R.; Valentão, P.; Andrade, P.B.; Félix, C.; Novais, S.C.; Lemos, M.F. Evaluating the In Vitro Potential of Natural Extracts to Protect Lipids from Oxidative Damage. *Antioxidants* **2020**, *9*, 231. [CrossRef] [PubMed]
43. Hamon, I.; Valdès, V.; Franck, P.; Buchweiller, M.-C.; Fresson, J.; Hascoët, J.M. Différences liées au sexe dans le métabolisme du glutathion (GSH) du grand prématuré. *Archives de Pédiatrie* **2011**, *18*, 247–252. [CrossRef] [PubMed]
44. Brilakis, E.S.; Khera, A.; McGuire, D.K.; See, R.; Banerjee, S.; Murphy, S.A.; De Lemos, J.A. Influence of race and sex on lipoprotein-associated phospholipase A2 levels: Observations from the Dallas Heart Study. *Atherosclerosis* **2008**, *199*, 110–115. [CrossRef]
45. Kuslys, T.; Vishwanath, B.S.; Frey, F.J.; Frey, B.M. Differences in phospholipase A 2 activity between males and females and Asian Indians and Caucasians. *Eur. J. Clin. Investig.* **1996**, *26*, 310–315. [CrossRef] [PubMed]
46. Bordoni, L.; Fedeli, D.; Fiorini, D.; Gabbianelli, R. Extra Virgin Olive Oil and Nigella sativa Oil Produced in Central Italy: A Comparison of the Nutrigenomic Effects of Two Mediterranean Oils in a Low-Grade Inflammation Model. *Antioxidants* **2019**, *9*, 20. [CrossRef]
47. Gao, Z.; Chen, Z.; Sun, A.; Deng, X. Gender differences in cardiovascular disease. *Med. Nov. Technol. Devices* **2019**, *4*, 100025. [CrossRef]
48. Jaworska, K.; Hering, D.; Mosieniak, G.; Bielak-Zmijewska, A.; Pilz, M.; Konwerski, M.; Gasecka, A.; Kapłon-Cieślicka, A.; Filipiak, K.; Sikora, E.; et al. TMA, A Forgotten Uremic Toxin, but Not TMAO, Is Involved in Cardiovascular Pathology. *Toxins* **2019**, *11*, 490. [CrossRef]
49. Jaworska, K.; Konop, M.; Hutsch, T.; Perlejewski, K.; Radkowski, M.; Grochowska, M.; Bielak-Zmijewska, A.; Mosieniak, G.; Sikora, E.; Ufnal, M. Trimethylamine But Not Trimethylamine Oxide Increases With Age in Rat Plasma and Affects Smooth Muscle Cells Viability. *J. Gerontol. Ser. A Boil. Sci. Med Sci.* **2019**, *75*, 1276–1283. [CrossRef]

biomedicines

MDPI

Article

Effects of an 8-Week Protein Supplementation Regimen with Hyperimmunized Cow Milk on Exercise-Induced Organ Damage and Inflammation in Male Runners: A Randomized, Placebo Controlled, Cross-Over Study

Sihui Ma [1,†], Takaki Tominaga [2,†], Kazue Kanda [3], Kaoru Sugama [3], Chiaki Omae [2], Shunsuke Hashimoto [4], Katsuhiko Aoyama [4], Yasunobu Yoshikai [5] and Katsuhiko Suzuki [1,*]

1 Faculty of Sport Sciences, Waseda University, Tokorozawa 359-1192, Japan; masihui@toki.waseda.jp
2 Graduate School of Sport Sciences, Waseda University, Tokorozawa 359-1192, Japan; t.tominaga7713@gmail.com (T.T.); chappy-ld312@moegi.waseda.jp (C.O.)
3 Research Institute for Life Support Innovation, Waseda University, Shinjuku 162-0041, Japan; rurishijimikanda@gmail.com (K.K.); k.sugama@kurenai.waseda.jp (K.S.)
4 Ortho Corporation, Shibuya 150-0002, Japan; hashimoto@kenko.co.jp (S.H.); aoyama@kenko.co.jp (K.A.)
5 Division of Host Defense, Medical Institute of Bioregulation, Kyushu University, Fukuoka 812-8582, Japan; yoshikai@bioreg.kyushu-u.ac.jp
* Correspondence: katsu.suzu@waseda.jp; Tel.: +81-04-2947-6898
† These authors contributed equally to this article.

Received: 10 February 2020; Accepted: 2 March 2020; Published: 4 March 2020

Abstract: Prolonged strenuous exercise may induce inflammation, cause changes in gastrointestinal permeability, and lead to other unfavorable biological changes and diseases. Nutritional approaches have been used to prevent exercise-induced inflammatory responses and gastrointestinal disorders. Hyperimmunized milk, obtained by immunizing cows against specific antigens, promotes the development of immunity against pathogens, promotes anti-inflammatory effects, and protects intestinal function. Immune protein (IMP) is a concentrated product of hyperimmunized milk and is a more promising means of supplementation to protect against acute infections and inflammation. To determine whether IMP has protective properties against exercise-induced gastrointestinal dysfunction and inflammation, we examined biochemical markers, intestinal damage markers, and pro-/anti-inflammatory profiles of young male runners using a randomized, placebo controlled, cross-over design. Urine samples were collected and used for measurements of creatinine, *N*-acetyl-β-D-glucosaminidase, osmotic pressure, and specific gravity. Titin was measured as a muscle damage marker. Further, urine concentrations of complement 5a, calprotectin, fractalkine, myeloperoxidase, macrophage colony-stimulating factor, monocyte chemotactic protein-1, intestinal fatty acid binding protein (I-FABP), interferon (IFN)-γ, interleukin (IL)-1β, IL-1 receptor antagonist, IL-2, IL-4, IL-6, IL-8, IL-10, IL-12p40, and tumor necrosis factor (TNF)-α were measured by enzyme-linked immunosorbent assays. We demonstrated that urine osmotic pressure, urine specific gravity, I-FABP, IFN-γ, IL-1β, and TNF-α were reduced by 8 weeks of IMP supplementation, indicating that IMP may have potential in preventing strenuous exercise-induced renal dysfunction, increased intestinal permeability, and inflammation. Thus, IMP supplementation may be a feasible nutritional approach for the prevention of unfavorable exercise-induced symptoms.

Keywords: hyperimmunized milk; exercise; inflammation; intestinal permeability; cytokine

---

1. Introduction

Prolonged strenuous exercise may induce unfavorable biological changes and symptoms, including inflammatory responses, such as leukocyte infiltration [1–3]; gastrointestinal (GI) incidents, such as diarrhea, nausea, and gastric pain [4–6]; delayed-onset muscle soreness; muscle and internal organ injury; and immune suppression [7–11].

Strenuous exercise can also induce intestinal barrier dysfunction. The GI mucosa serves as the first line of defense against invasion from non-self antigens [12]. Functional loss of the GI barrier, consisting of the enterocyte membranes, tight junctions, mucous, and localized macrophages, may bring unwanted biological and pathological consequences by allowing harmful substances (e.g., bacteria, xenobiotics, hydrolytic enzymes, and so forth) to enter into the circulation [13].

Many athletes use aspirin, ibuprofen, and other non-steroidal anti-inflammatory drugs (NSAIDs) to treat inflammation-induced algesthesia [14]. However, NSAIDs inhibit cyclooxygenase (COX) in the GI mucosa, aggravating the GI symptoms and harming athletes' performance and wellbeing. Therefore, supplementation for protecting the GI barrier merits consideration [15].

Hyperimmunized milk is obtained by immunizing cows against specific antigens. This technique results in the enrichment of various immunoglobulins in the milk product [16]. In 1957, Stolle first produced hyperimmunized milk by injecting cows with various bacteria pathogenic to humans (26 kinds of antigens, including *Escherichia coli*, *Salmonella typhimurium*, *Shigella dysenteriae*, *Staphylococcus pyogenes*, *Proteus vulgaris*, and others) [16]. Hyperimmunized milk is reported to possess health-promoting effects, including immunoregulatory, performance-enhancing effects, and NSAID-induced GI damage-preventing effects [17–20]. For instance, oral administration of milk from cows hyperimmunized against pathogenic bacteria is reported to down-regulate inflammatory responses in the gut, and may reduce allergic disease [21], protect against radiation-induced opportunistic infection and lethality [22,23], alleviate inflammatory responses to carrageenin [24], abrogate the lymphocyte response to concanavalin A [25], and prevent or treat neonatal bacterial infection [26].

Hyperimmunized protein, also known as "immune protein (IMP)", is a concentrated product of hyperimmunized milk, and therefore provides more promise as a supplement to protect individuals from acute inflammation. Wang et al. reported that oral administration of bovine milk from hyperimmunized cows down-regulated Th17 and Th2 responses and reduced interleukin (IL)-17A in the gut [21]. Additionally, IL-1β, IL-2, IL-6, and tumor necrosis factor (TNF)-α production were reduced, and collagen-induced arthritis was reported as being alleviated with 49 days of administration of hyperimmune colostrum [27]. When injected with a novel anti-inflammatory factor isolated from milk from hyperimmunized cows, a mastitis mouse model showed less mammary inflammation, and edema was suppressed by as much as 80% in carrageenin-challenged rats [24]. However, to the best of our knowledge, the protective effect of neither hyperimmunized milk nor IMP on exercise-induced inflammation and other adverse events have been reported to date. Therefore, we sought to test the potential benefits of IMP supplementation on prolonged strenuous exercise.

In order to determine whether IMP has protective properties on exercise-induced organ damage and inflammation, we examined biochemical markers, cytokine excretion profiles, and organ damage markers in young male runners undergoing a 3000 m full-speed running test (3000 m time trial (3000 m TT)) with or without 8-week IMP supplementation.

2. Materials and Methods

2.1. Experimental Design

We designed a double-blind randomized cross-over placebo-controlled study. The participants were recruited to participate in two separate experimental trials with a 1 month wash out period: supplementation of either (1) immune protein (IMP trial) or (2) placebo protein (PLA trial). All of the participants were asked to complete three separate 3000 m TT at three time points in each trial (first race: before supplementation, M0; second race: 1 month after supplementation, M1; third race: 2 months after supplementation, M2) (Figure 1). The experimental protocols were approved by the Ethics Committee of Waseda University (2017-319, date of approval: 11 April 2018). Written informed consent was obtained from all the participants prior to their enrollment in the study. The experiments were carried out from April 2018 to January 2019.

2.2. Participants

Seven young men participated in this study. The participants were recreationally active and had no chronic diseases. The characteristics of the participants were as follows: age, 18.7 ± 1.5 (mean ± standard deviation, SD) years; height, 171.8 ± 7.7 cm; body mass, 60.4 ± 3.1 kg. Participants read and signed an informed consent form prior to engaging in the study. Inclusion criteria were as follows: (a) participants had to be male long-distance runners from Waseda University between the ages of 18 and 30 years old; (b) participants had to be healthy and free of any known disease, determined by a medical history questionnaire; (c) participants had to be individuals who do not change training loads and diet content/amount during the experimental period; and (d) participants had to abstain from supplemental protein or amino acids for 3 months prior to participating. A physical activity questionnaire and medical history form were filled out prior to participation to establish that physical activity requirements were met and to identify potential risk factors that could be aggravated by participation in the study.

2.3. Immune Protein Supplementation

Following an initial baseline 3000 m TT, subjects were asked to take IMP powder (IMP trial) or a matched placebo (normal protein powder, PLA trial) two times a day for 8 weeks. IMP and placebo were provided in packaged, single doses (10 g), and were obtained from Ortho Inc. (Ortho Incorporation, Tokyo, Japan). IMP and placebo are administrated by mixing with water.

2.4. Experimental Protocol

After recruitment, the subjects were counter-balanced on the basis of body weight and 3000 m TT into a PLA or IMP trial. There were no significant differences between groups for any of these variables.

The subjects carried out 3000 m TTs at time point of M0, M1, and M2. The time trials were carried out on an athletic field. The food and fluid intake of subjects was not restricted on the days of the races (Figure 1). IMP or PLA were consumed over 2 months, separated by a 1-month wash-out period, according to previous studies [28–30]. Ratings of perceived exertion (RPE) were obtained using the Borg scale. Body composition and body fat percentage were obtained using an InBody 720 Body Composition Analyzer (Inbody Japan Inc., Tokyo, Japan). Participants were asked to self-report if they experienced discomfort during the experiment period.

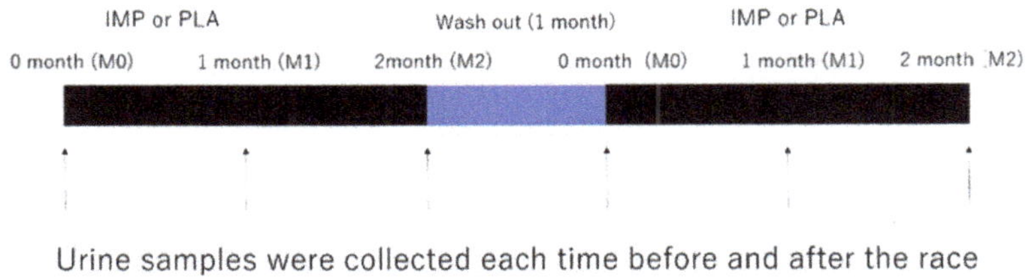

Figure 1. Experimental design. Immune protein powder (IMP) or a matched placebo (normal protein powder, PLA) were administered for 2 months in a cross-over randomized controlled trial (RCT). Arrows indicate the times at which 3000 m time trials were performed.

2.5. Urine Sampling and Analysis

Pre-exercise urine samples (Pre) were collected 30–60 min before each 3000 m TT. After the pre-sampling, participants were allowed to perform warm-up exercises ad libitum prior to the 3000 m TT. Post-exercise urine samples (Post) were collected within 30 min after completion of the time trial. The urinary excretion of participants was not restricted before exercise. The collected urine samples were centrifuged at 1000× *g* for 10 min to remove sediments. The supernatants were stored at −80°C until analysis.

2.6. Assays for Urine Biochemistry, Inflammatory Substances, and Organ Damage Markers

Urine creatinine, *N*-acetyl-β-D-glucosaminidase (NAG), osmotic pressure, and specific gravity were measured by Koutou-Biken Co. (Koutou-Biken Co., Tsukuba, Japan).

IL-1β, IL-6, and TNF-α concentrations were measured with Quantikine high sensitivity (HS) enzyme-linked immunosorbent assay (ELISA) kits (R&D Systems Inc., Minneapolis, MN, USA). IL-1 receptor antagonist (ra), monocyte chemotactic protein (MCP)-1, and macrophage colony-stimulating factor (M-CSF) concentrations were also measured with Quantikine ELISA kits (R&D Systems Inc., Minneapolis, MN, USA). Intestinal fatty acid binding protein (I-FABP) and fractalkine concentrations were measured with Duoset ELISA kits (R&D Systems Inc., Minneapolis, MN, USA). IL-2, IL-4, IL-8, IL-10, IL-12p40, complement 5a (C5a), and interferon (IFN)-γ concentrations were measured with OptEIA ELISA kits (Becton Dickinson Biosciences, San Diego, CA, USA). Calprotectin and myeloperoxidase (MPO) concentrations were measured with ELISA kits (Hycult biotechnology Inc, Uden, The Netherlands). Titin concentration was measured by ELISA as previously described [31]. The absorbance was measured spectrophotometrically on a VersaMax Microplate Reader (Molecular Devices Inc., San Jose, CA, USA) according to the manufacturer's instructions. The concentration of each protein was calculated by comparison with a calibration curve established in the same measurement.

2.7. Statistical Analysis

The sample size was calculated using the program G*Power [32]. Six subjects were required to detect an effect size of $f = 0.5$ for the within-between interaction, with a power of 0.8 and a significance level of 0.05 under the assumption of a correlation coefficient among repeated measures $r = 0.7$ and a nonsphericity correction of $\varepsilon = 0.5$. Data are presented as means ± SD. A two-way analysis of variance (ANOVA) was performed to determine the main effects of protein (IMP or PLA) or time points for 3000 m race time, body composition, ΔRPE, and body fat percentage. A three-way ANOVA with mixed-effects analysis was performed to determine the main effects of protein (IMP or PLA), time points (M0, M1, and M2), and exercise. Urine creatinine was used for urinary parameters' correction. Statistical significance was defined as $p < 0.05$. Statistical analysis was performed using GraphPad 8.0 (Graphpad, Ltd., La Jolla, CA, USA).

3. Results

3.1. Body Composition, RPE, and 3000 m Time Trial Results

No significant interaction was observed between IMP and PLA in race time (Figure 2). Body weight, body fat percentage, and RPE were not different between participants in the IMP trial and PLA trial (Figure 3). No adverse events were self-reported or observed during the study period.

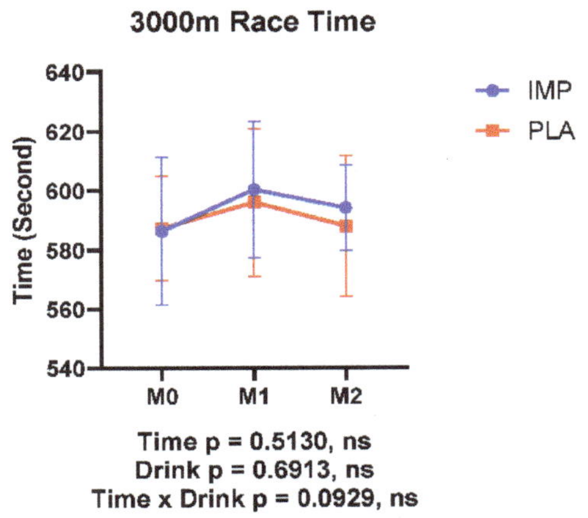

Figure 2. Results of 3000 m time trials. The data are presented as means ± SD.

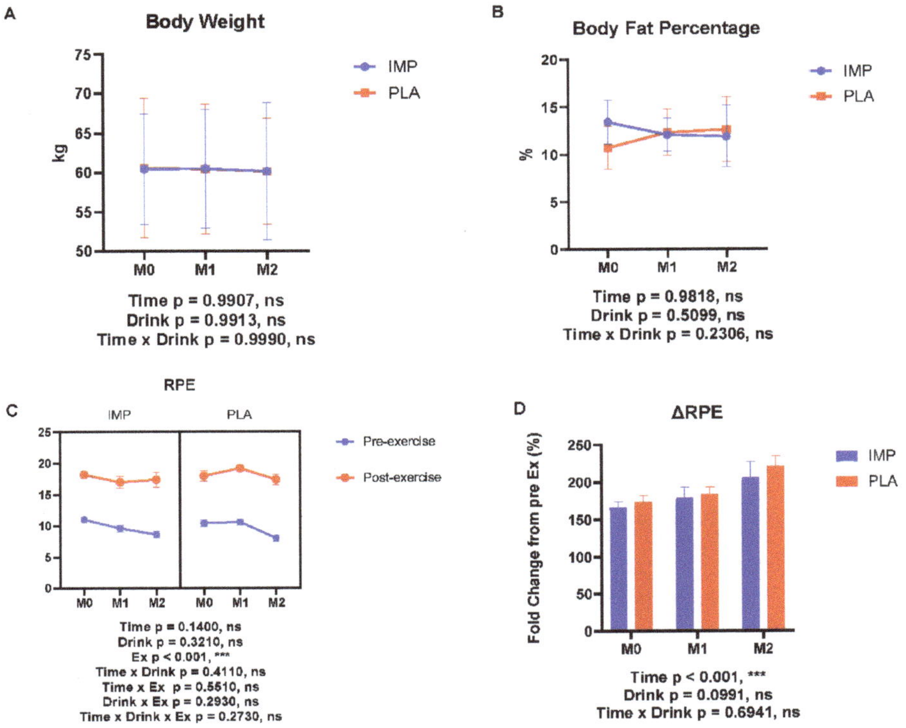

Figure 3. Body composition, body fat percentage, and ratings of perceived exertion (RPE) results. (**A**) Body weight change, (**B**) change in body fat percentage, (**C**) RPE at each time point, and (**D**) RPE change between IMP and PLA. The data are presented as means ± SD. *** $p < 0.001$.

3.2. Renal Function Markers

NAG, urine osmotic pressure, and specific gravity were measured as indicators of renal function. The right side of each figure in Figure 3 shows the data of the PLA supplementation period and the left side shows the data of the IMP supplementation period. Urine NAG was increased by exercise, indicating renal damage occurred after 3000 m TT (Figure 4A). However, in the IMP period, significant interaction effects on urine osmotic pressure changed and specific gravity change were observed (Figure 4B,C). Summary data are available in Table 1.

Table 1. Summary of data from Figures 4–10.

Name	Trial	M0		M1		M2	
		IMP	PLA	IMP	PLA	IMP	PLA
NAG> (IU/L)	Pre Post	2.729 ± 1.438 8.543 ± 2.540	1.714 ± 1.182 7.257 ± 4.712	2.729 ± 0.991 10.457 ± 5.369	2.943 ± 1.258 5.629 ± 1.847	2.500 ± 1.956 11.971 ± 8.136	2.471 ± 1.423 9.029 ± 7.692
UOP mOSm/L	Pre Post	878.7 ± 205.1 785.8 ± 130.2	642.5 ± 275.9 580.3 ± 179.7	869.4 ± 284.2 867.3 ± 86.36	906.2 ± 193.6 676.0 ± 169.4	672.7 ± 205.5 729.0 ± 63.38	879.7 ± 188.6 670.7 ± 211.8
SPG	Pre Post	1.026 ± 0.006 1.024 ± 0.003	1.019 ± 0.008 1.018 ± 0.006	1.025 ± 0.008 1.027 ± 0.004	1.025 ± 0.006 1.018 ± 0.009	1.019 ± 0.004 1.022 ± 0.003	1.024 ± 0.006 1.020 ± 0.006
I-FABP (pg/mgCr)	Pre Post	196.8 ± 52.90 4783 ± 2491	354.0 ± 473.5 6335 ± 2411	183.7 ± 195.1 3635 ± 1249	232.0 ± 283.4 5139 ± 2331	370.0 ± 450.9 4845 ± 2402	205.9 ± 206.8 7609 ± 4507
Titin (pg/mgCr)	Pre Post	912.0 ± 613.6 978.1 ± 637.1	1329 ± 1147 1466 ± 846.7	1050 ± 1146 802.1 ± 400.1	968.5 ± 849.9 11901 ± 720.4	828.6 ± 561.3 848.5 ± 586.2	838.8 ± 621.9 1355 ± 1238
IFN-γ (pg/mgCr)	Pre Post	2.030 ± 1.089 1.716 ± 0.710	3.694 ± 2.713 2.273 ± 1.261	2.351 ± 0.998 1.488 ± 0.206	2.004 ± 0.971 2.273 ± 1.261	2.801 ± 0.908 1.821 ± 0.797	1.990 ± 0.785 2.834 ± 1.665
IL-1β (pg/mgCr)	Pre Post	0.132 ± 0.073 0.272 ± 0.089	0.285 ± 0.292 0.462 ± 0.355	0.152 ± 0.107 0.210 ± 0.088	0.189 ± 0.153 0.496 ± 0.559	0.251 ± 0.148 0.235 ± 0.169	0.150 ± 0.084 0.297 ± 0.161
TNF-α (pg/mgCr)	Pre Post	0.139 ± 0.123 0.121 ± 0.104	0.073 ± 0.051 0.153 ± 0.132	0.153 ± 0.098 0.082 ± 0.053	0.107 ± 0.170 0.091 ± 0.087	0.124 ± 0.074 0.069 ± 0.074	0.096 ± 0.127 0/231 ± 0.240
C5a (ng/mgCr)	Pre Post	0.991 ± 1.998 4.726 ± 4.349	0.232 ± 0.219 5.362 ± 7.272	0.181 ± 0.079 2.992 ± 2.598	0.125 ± 0.068 3.766 ± 5.757	0.125 ± 0.058 2.967 ± 2.559	0.125 ± 0.057 1.782 ± 1.073
Calprotectin (ng/mgCr)	Pre Post	21.18 ± 22.26 27.31 ± 21.49	12.25 ± 11.94 29.43 ± 27.06	15.47 ± 14.25 25.68 ± 19.60	17.19 ± 26.81 31.23 ± 34.14	10.40 ± 9.010 23.56 ± 21.63	13.30 ± 11.63 26.53 ± 29.17
Fractalkine (pg/mgCr)	Pre Post	0.241 ± 0.251 0.104 ± 0.200	0.398 ± 0.200 0.276 ± 0.357	0.329 ± 0.488 0.295 ± 0.484	0.385 ± 0.274 2.276 ± 0.357	0.323 ± 0.214 0.252 ± 0.380	0.579 ± 0.422 0.356 ± 0.507
MCP-1 (pg/mgCr)	Pre Post	175.6 ± 96.93 341.7 ± 238.7	166.4 ± 75.83 364.7 ± 241.2	151.8 ± 40.74 257.2 ± 97.94	208.3 ± 60.27 294.3 ± 58.86	183.8 ± 75.61 320.48 ± 195.4	202.8 ± 139.8 325.4 ± 113.7
MPO (ng/mgCr)	Pre Post	0.181 ± 0.090 0.202 ± 0.076	0.535 ± 0.620 0.384 ± 0.224	0.234 ± 0.126 0.377 ± 0.216	0.199 ± 0.063 0.254 ± 0.102	0.256 ± 0.109 0.219 ± 0.075	0.432 ± 0.500 0.436 ± 0.354
M-CSF (pg/mgCr)	Pre Post	1206 ± 501.5 3904 ± 1550	831.9 ± 596.4 3766 ± 2213	706.1 ± 395.9 3100 ± 1563	875.2 ± 311.3 2987 ± 688.3	714.5 ± 324.1 3274 ± 977.6	714.8 ± 389.8 3375 ± 1041
IL-4 (pg/mgCr)	Pre Post	12.76 ± 17.64 14.78 ± 15.49	5.900 ± 3.816 21.63 ± 24.64	20.34 ± 18.00 10.50 ± 9.960	24.65 ± 26.71 23.54 ± 32.92	17.95 ± 19.85 10.87 ± 14.31	30.44 ± 39.17 36.49 ± 44.67
IL-10 (pg/mgCr)	Pre Post	7.875 ± 5.324 6.883 ± 3.913	18.55 ± 13.73 13.31 ± 6.581	11.12 ± 6.290 8.265 ± 3.075	11.46 ± 5.722 9.332 ± 6.126	12.88 ± 1.372 7.371 ± 5.916	9.478 ± 2.233 12.28 ± 5.593
IL-2 (pg/mgCr)	Pre Post	9.136 ± 2.035 9.079 ± 2.721	21.94 ± 7.037 23.51 ± 15.03	11.34 ± 8.41 16.08 ± 13.32	9.022 ± 3.647 19.07 ± 15.58	7.782 ± 3.061 11.80 ± 8.148	10.49 ± 5.818 12.74 ± 4.582
IL-12p40 (pg/mgCr)	Pre Post	72.08 ± 92.78 41.16 ± 27.32	82.30 ± 69.99 66.71 ± 47.09	61.79 ± 26.67 24.63 ± 13.15	64.49 ± 56.61 53.56 ± 55.21	56.42 ± 31.53 35.61 ± 33.74	49.23 ± 33.20 59.48 ± 48.20
IL-1ra (pg/mgCr)	Pre Post	2660 ± 1798 4340 ± 3328	3221 ± 2392 5053 ± 4958	2382 ± 1412 4522 ± 3244	3314 ± 2953 4690 ± 2889	2501 ± 1237 4172 ± 2276	2262 ± 1490 4211 ± 2819
IL-6 (pg/mgCr)	Pre Post	0.445 ± 0.392 0.798 ± 0.530	0.527 ± 0.267 0.780 ± 0.557	0.397 ± 0.212 1.418 ± 1.423	0.676 ± 0.302 1.021 ± 0.861	0.484 ± 0.359 0.907 ± 0.579	0.794 ± 0.619 1.839 ± 1.897
IL-8 (pg/mgCr)	Pre Post	9.168 ± 7.782 3.786 ± 1.791	6.491 ± 5.077 4.969 ± 1.629	5.460 ± 4.316 8.400 ± 5.455	5.112 ± 2.853 8.615 ± 6.825	4.541 ± 3.988 7.604 ± 6.530	3.935 ± 2.887 9.366 ± 7.042

IMP: results of immune protein trial, PLA: results of placebo trial, UOP: urinary osmotic pressure, and SPG: urine-specific gravity. The data are presented as means ± SD.

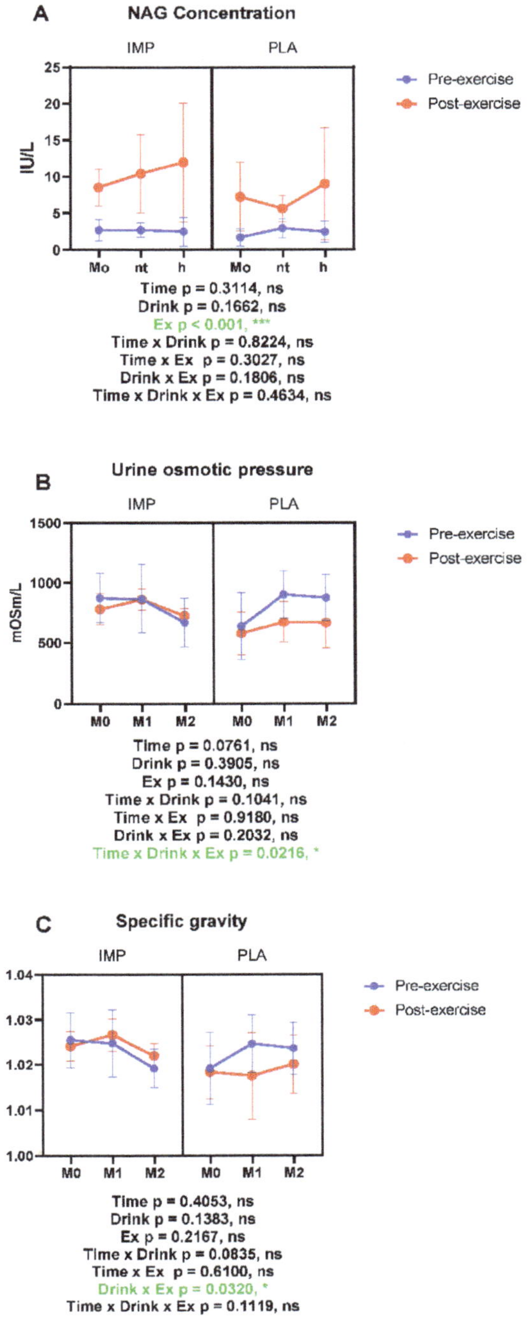

Figure 4. Results of renal function. (**A**) *N*-acetyl-β-D-glucosaminidase (NAG) concentration, (**B**) urine osmotic pressure, and (**C**) urine-specific gravity. The data are presented as means ± SD. * $p < 0.05$, and *** $p < 0.001$. Green text indicates a significance <0.05

3.3. Intestine Damage Marker

I-FABP was measured as an intestinal damage marker. According to our results, I-FABP was increased significantly after 3000 m TTs, indicating intestinal damage. When I-FABP concentration was corrected with creatinine, it indicated that IMP supplementation attenuated the exercise-induced increase of I-FABP significantly (Figure 5). Summary data are available in Table 1.

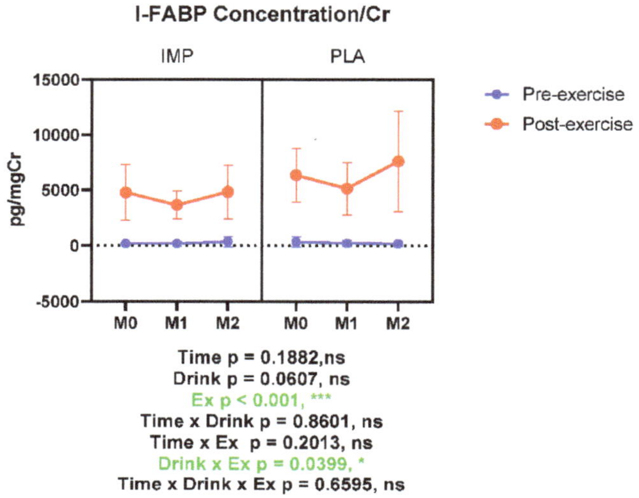

Figure 5. Urine intestinal fatty acid binding protein (I-FABP) concentration corrected with creatinine. The data are presented as means ± SD. * $p < 0.05$ and *** $p < 0.001$. Green text indicates a significance <0.05.

3.4. Muscle Damage Marker

Titin was measured as a muscle damage marker, which was not altered by 3000 m TTs. IMP did not alter titin concentration (Figure 6). Summary data are available in Table 1.

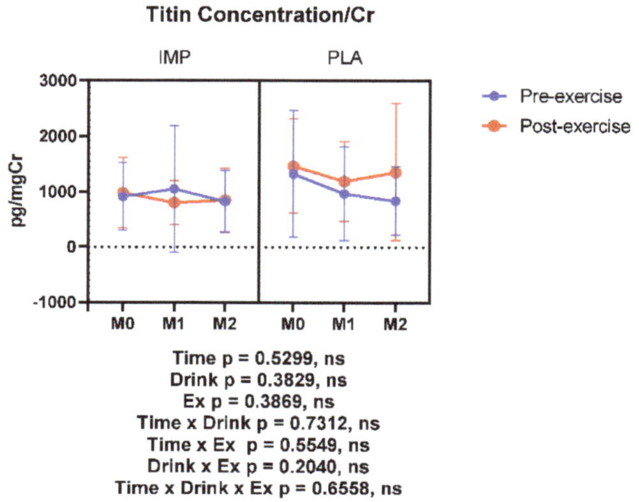

Figure 6. Urine titin concentration corrected with creatinine. The data are presented as means ± SD.

3.5. Inflammatory Substance Profile

The inflammatory markers IFN-γ, IL-1β, TNF-α, C5a, calprotectin, fractalkine, MCP-1, MPO, and M-CSF were measured in subjects' urine. In the placebo period, IFN-γ, IL-1β, and TNF-α tended to increase after exercise. However, in the IMP supplementation period, the exercise-induced increase of the above cytokines was inhibited (IFN-γ and TNF-α), or trended towards being inhibited (IL-1β), according to interactions between drink and exercise (Figure 7). Summary data are available in Table 1.

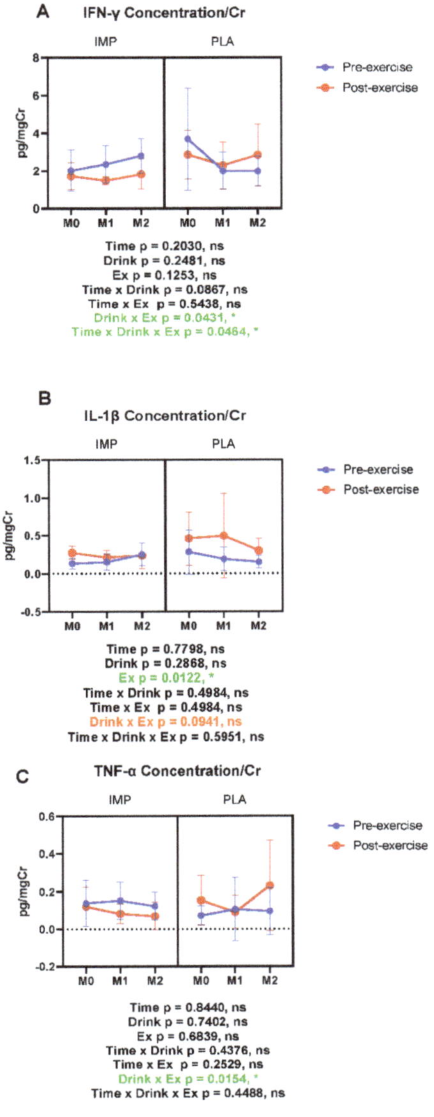

Figure 7. Urine interferon (IFN)-γ (**A**), interleukin (IL)-1β (**B**), and tumor necrosis factor (TNF)-α (C) concentrations corrected with creatinine. The data are presented as means ± SD. * p <0.05. Green text indicates a significance <0.05 and orange text indicates a significance <0.10.

C5a, calprotectin, MCP-1, and M-CSF were increased by 3000 m TTs. Fractalkine showed a trend of being decreased with 3000 m TTs, whereas urine MPO was not altered. IMP did not alter the above inflammatory substances (Figure 8). Summary data are available in Table 1.

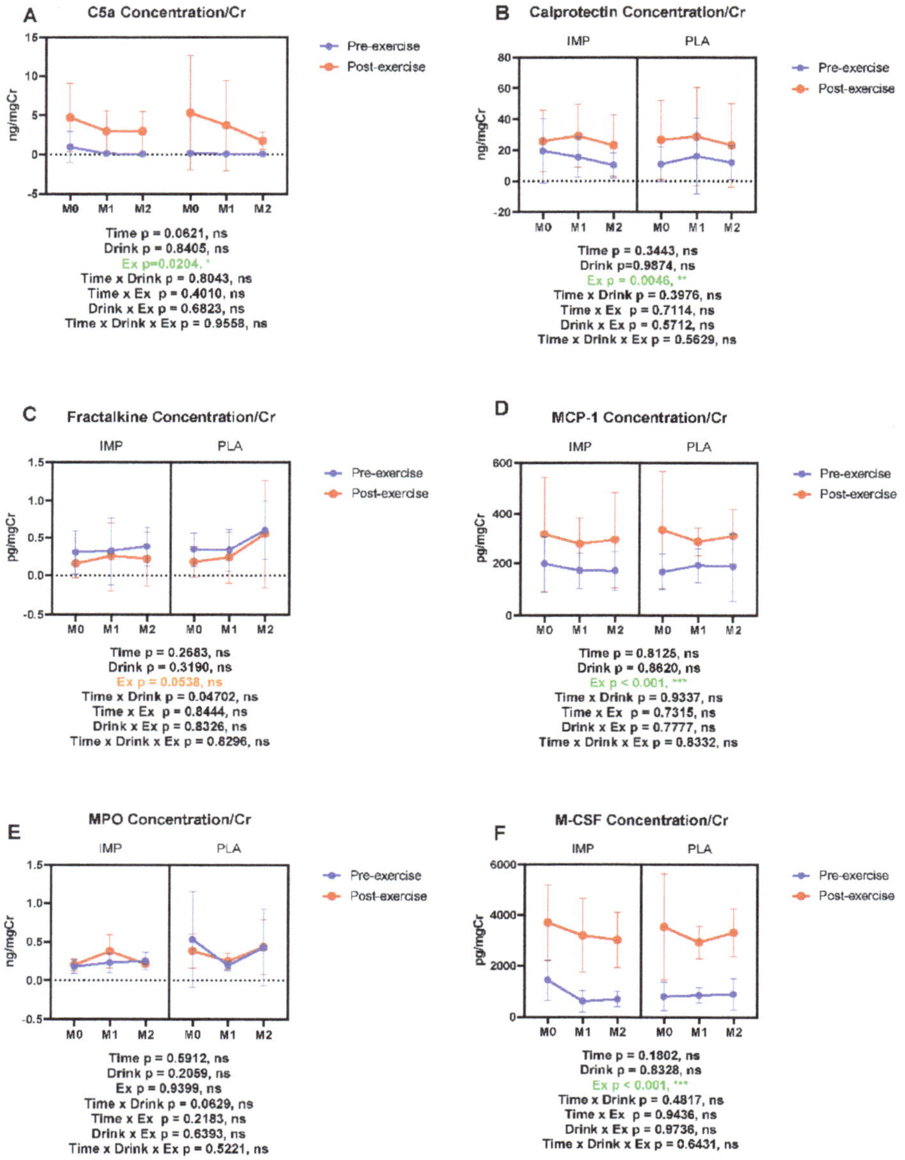

Figure 8. Urine complement 5a (C5a) (**A**), calprotectin (**B**), fractalkine (**C**), monocyte chemotactic protein (MCP)-1 (**D**), myeloperoxidase (MPO) (**E**), and macrophage colony-stimulating factor (M-CSF) (**F**) concentrations corrected with creatinine. The data are presented as means ± SD. * $p < 0.05$ and *** $p < 0.001$. Green text indicates a significance <0.05 and orange text indicates a significance <0.10.

The concentrations of immunoregulatory cytokines, IL-2, IL-4, IL-10, and IL-12p40 were measured. Urine IL-4 was not altered by 3000 m TTs (Figure 9A). Urine IL-10 and IL-12p40 were decreased by 3000 m TTs (Figure 9B,D). Urine IL-2 showed a trend of being decreased by 3000 m TTs (Figure 9C). IMP did not alter the concentrations of the above immunoregulatory cytokines (Figure 9). Summary data are available in Table 1.

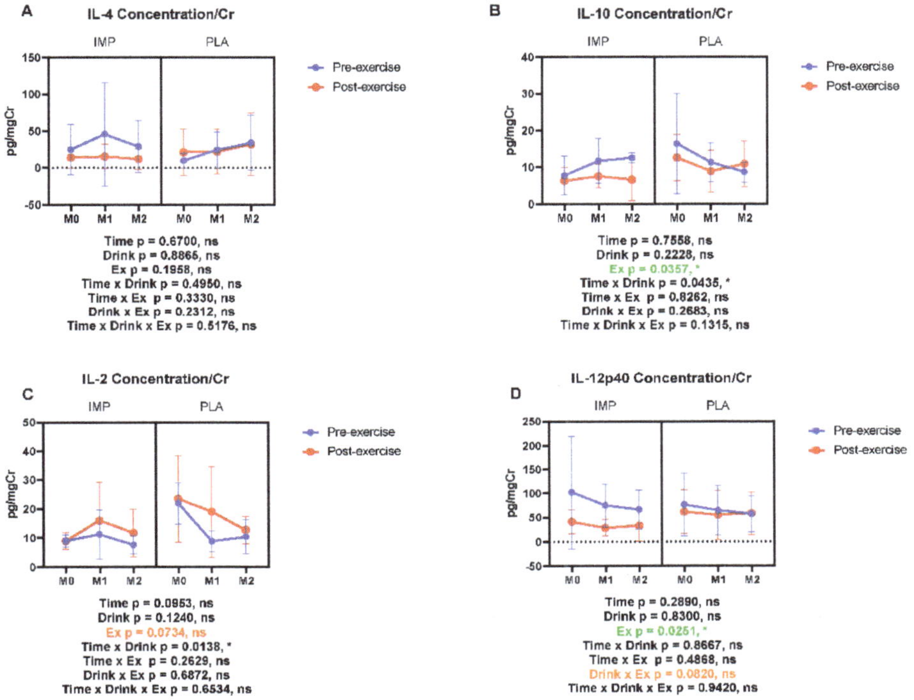

Figure 9. Urine IL-4 (**A**), IL-10 (**B**), IL-2 (**C**), and IL-12p40 (**D**) concentrations corrected with creatinine. The data are presented as means ± SD. * $p < 0.05$. Green text indicates a significance < 0.05 and orange text indicates a significance <0.10.

The concentrations of IL-1ra and IL-6, anti-inflammatory and multi-functional cytokines respectively, and IL-8, a neutrophil-activating cytokine, were measured. IL-1ra and IL-6 were increased by 3000 m TTs (Figure 10A,B). IL-8 was not altered by 3000 m TTs. IMP did not alter the concentrations of these cytokines (Figure 10). Summary data are available in Table 1.

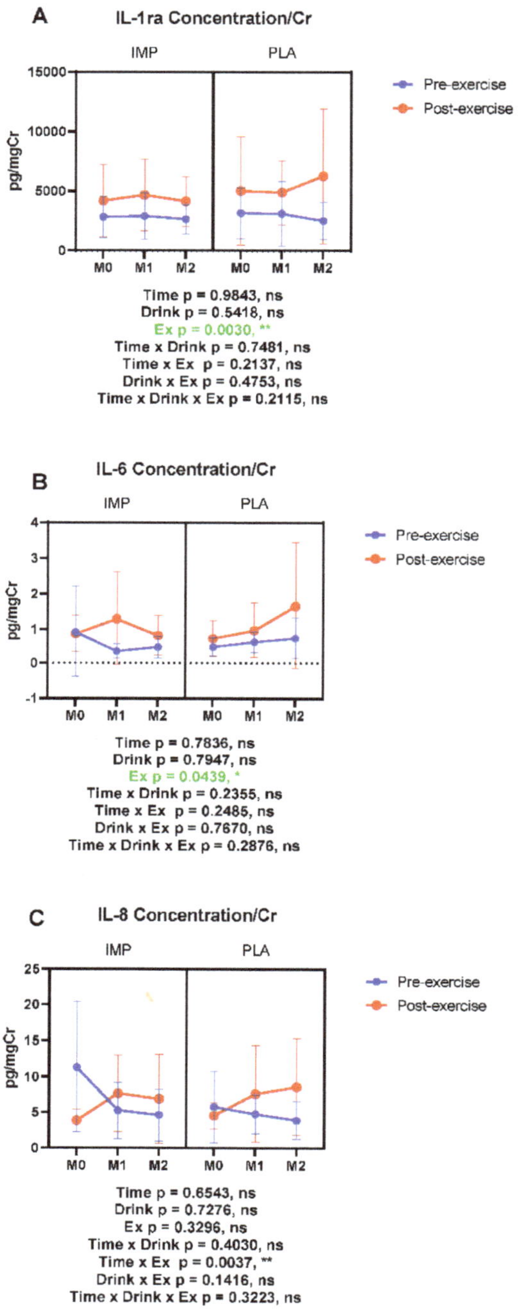

Figure 10. Urine IL-1 receptor antagonist (ra) (**A**), IL-6 (**B**), and IL-8 (**C**) concentrations corrected with creatinine. The data are presented as means ± SD. * $p < 0.05$ and ** $p < 0.01$. Green text indicates a significance < 0.05.

4. Discussion

In the present study, we used urine samples, rather than plasma or serum samples, as a non-invasive way to evaluate exercise-induced biomarker kinetics. In urine, the concentrations of C5a, calprotectin, MCP-1, M-CSF, IL-1ra, IL-6, IL-10, and IL-12p40 showed significant changes with a 3000 m TT, whereas the concentrations of fractalkine and IL-2 showed marginally significant changes. However, MPO, IL-4, IL-8, and titin were not altered in urine samples with a 3000 m TT.

Strenuous exercise may induce renal dysfunction, or even acute renal failure [33]. In the present study, an increase in the concentration of NAG indicated that a 3000 m TT induced renal tubular damage. Though IMP did not affect NAG, with 8 weeks of IMP supplementation, urine osmotic pressure and specific gravity were not significantly affected by exercise, indicating that IMP may have protective effects on renal condensing function.

Cytokine kinetics are well documented for their quick responses to strenuous exercise, reflecting a transient perturbation to the immune system [1–3]. We demonstrated that IFN-γ, IL-13, and TNF-α were reduced by an 8-week IMP supplementation regimen, indicating that IMP may have potential in preventing strenuous exercise-induced inflammation. A great body of literature has demonstrated that strenuous exercise causes an inflammatory response and structural damage to the body, and that nutritional approaches have been used to prevent exercise-induced inflammatory response [1–3]. For example, supplementation with polyphenols and flavonoids has been used to prevent inflammation in exercise [34,35]. The potential mechanisms of this protection are thought to be related to classical inflammation pathways and the Toll-like receptor 4-mediated pathway by down-regulating down-stream protein and cytokine production [36]. Additionally, a low carbohydrate, high fat ketogenic diet has also been reported to have the potential to prevent exercise-induced inflammation [37]. Volunteers consuming a proprietary milk protein supplement for 8 weeks reported significant alleviation in joint pain and walked a significantly longer distance during a 6-min walking test [38]. Therefore, nutritional intervention may be a feasible method of protecting athletes from exercise-induced inflammation and muscle or organ damage.

Athletes report GI symptoms during training and competition frequently [39]. I-FABP is reported to reflect functional changes in exercise-induced intestinal permeability. Although the mechanism of exercise-induced GI symptoms is not fully understood, 90 min of running at a challenging pace may induce significant elevation of serum I-FABP concentrations, and symptomatic athletes have been reported to exhibit higher lipopolysaccharide (LPS) activity, indicating intestinal damage and increased intestinal permeability [39]. Although LPS from the portal circulation will be scavenged and removed from the body by Kupffer cells, LPS clearance might be overwhelmed during prolonged intense exercise, leading to the leakage of LPS from the liver into the central circulation, therefore leading to endotoxemia and exercise-induced heat stroke [40]. Several supplementation methods, including the administration of probiotics, have been considered for GI treatment in athletes. It has been reported that a carbohydrate (CHO)-containing beverage has protective effects on gastroduodenal function but showed no protective effects on intestinal function [41]. Acute oral glutamine supplementation prior to exercise prevented the rise of plasma endotoxin and nuclear factor-κB (NF-κB) activation in peripheral blood mononuclear cells [42]. However, adding glutamine to a CHO-containing beverage has no additional protective effects [43]. Fish protein hydrolysates, combined with indomethacin supplementation, reduced intestinal permeability by 62% [44]. Additionally, 4 weeks of supplementation with a multi-strain probiotic was reported to provide a small reduction ($d = 0.25$) in symptoms of gastrointestinal discomfort and increase running time to exhaustion, but failed to adjust exercise-induced plasma IL-1ra, IL-6, and IL-10 alternation [45]. According to our results, IMP supplementation significantly alleviated the elevation of I-FABP, which is a biomarker of GI permeability, benefitting GI integrity and potentially contributing to the prevention of exercise-induced endotoxemia and heat stroke.

Exhaustive exercise elicits systematic inflammatory responses and hypercytokinemia (also known as "cytokine storm") [46]. In fact, many studies have consistently shown that interleukins, such as IL-1β,

IL-1ra, and IL-6, and cytokines from the interferon family and tumor necrosis factor family increase markedly after endurance exercise [47–50]. In the present study, a 2-month IMP supplementation effectively inhibited the elevation of IFN-γ, IL-1β, and TNF-α. These preventive effects may be attributed to the protective role of IMP on LPS leakage by improving GI integrity.

Products from hyperimmunized animals have been reported for their properties in treating endogenous infections, including intestinal bacteria stimulation and rotavirus diarrhea [51]. The anti-inflammatory properties of these products have also been reported [21,24,25]. After administration of 10 g of bovine hyperimmune colostrum immunoglobulin three times a day for 5 days, healthy male volunteers showed a trend toward less diarrhea after being challenged with *Cryptosporidium parvum* [52]. The mechanism of how products from hyperimmunized animals protect individuals from endogenous infection is unknown; however, results of the present study indicate that these mechanisms may be related to the retention of GI integrity and the improvement of LPS-induced endogenous inflammation.

Similar to IMP, bovine colostrum, the "early milk," is abundant in bioactive components, including immune, growth, and antimicrobial factors [53,54]. In a cross-over study, after 2 weeks of daily supplementation with bovine colostrum, treadmill running-induced intestinal permeability was reduced by 80% [55]. Moreover, Playford et al. reported that bovine colostrum supplementation may have the potential to reduce NSAID-induced increases in intestinal permeability [55]. The mechanisms for this action have been demonstrated as being improved maintenance of tight junctions under thermal, and possibly oxidative, stresses [52–55]. An et al. showed that bovine colostrum significantly inhibited IL-1β-induced IL-8 and intracellular adhesion molecule-1 mRNA expression, suppressed IL-1β-induced NF-κB activation and cyclooxygenase-2 protein expression levels, and blocked translocation of p65 into the nucleus in HT29 cells [56]. Bovine colostrum has been also evaluated for its antibacterial activity against *Escherichia coli*, *Staphylococcus aureus*, *Proteus vulgaris*, *Enterobacter aerogenes*, and *Salmonella typhi* [57]. Due to its similarities to colostrum, IMP might function through similar mechanisms. However, the mechanisms underlying the beneficial effects of IMP should be investigated in further studies.

In the present study, we used a 1-month wash-out period to avoid carry-over effects. This period was chosen on the basis of subjects' activity levels and according to previous studies [28–30]. However, a longer wash-out period may better prevent carry-over effects. Another limitation in the present study is the lack of exercise-induced symptoms observed and reported by the participants according to the self-report questionnaires, though biochemical changes were seen with urine analyses. Whether IMP will contribute its benefits to more strenuous exercise requires validation, and further studies are encouraged.

5. Conclusions

We demonstrated that urine osmotic pressure, urine specific gravity, I-FABP, IFN-γ, IL-1β, and TNF-α were reduced in runners provided an 8-week IMP supplementation regimen, indicating that IMP may have the potential to prevent strenuous exercise-induced renal dysfunction, increased intestinal permeability, and inflammation. Thus, IMP supplementation may provide a feasible nutritional approach for the prevention of unfavorable exercise-induced disorders.

Author Contributions: Conceptualization, K.S. (Katsuhiko Suzuki); investigation, S.M., T.T., K.K., K.S. (Kaoru Sugama) and C.O.; resources, S.H. and K.A.; supervision, K.S. (Katsuhiko Suzuki) and Y.Y.; writing—original draft, S.M.; writing—review and editing, T.T., K.S. (Kaoru Sugama), and K.S. (Katsuhiko Suzuki). All authors have read and agreed to the published version of the manuscript.

Funding: This work was supported by research funds endowed to K.S. (Katsuhiko Suzuki) from Ortho Corporation, Japan.

Conflicts of Interest: The authors declare no conflict of interest. The funders (Ortho Corporation) had no role in study design, data collection and analysis, decision to publish, or preparation of the manuscript.

References

1. Suzuki, K. Chronic Inflammation as an Immunological Abnormality and Effectiveness of Exercise. *Biomolecules* **2019**, *9*, 223. [CrossRef] [PubMed]
2. Suzuki, K. Cytokine Response to Exercise and Its Modulation. *Antioxidants* **2018**, *7*, 17. [CrossRef]
3. Goh, J.; Lim, C.L.; Suzuki, K. Effects of Endurance-, Strength-, and Concurrent Training on Cytokines and Inflammation. In *Concurrent Aerobic and Strength Training: Scientific Basics and Practical Applications*; Schumann, M., Rønnestad, B.R., Eds.; Springer International Publishing: Cham, Switzerland, 2019; pp. 125–138. ISBN 978-3-319-75547-2.
4. van Wijck, K.; Lenaerts, K.; van Loon, L.J.C.; Peters, W.H.M.; Buurman, W.A.; Dejong, C.H.C. Exercise-Induced Splanchnic Hypoperfusion Results in Gut Dysfunction in Healthy Men. *PLoS ONE* **2011**, *6*, e22366. [CrossRef] [PubMed]
5. Lis, D.; Ahuja, K.D.; Stellingwerff, T.; Kitic, C.M.; Fell, J. Case study: Utilizing a low FODMAP diet to combat exercise-induced gastrointestinal symptoms. *Int. J. Sport Nutr. Exerc. Metab.* **2016**, *26*, 481–487. [CrossRef] [PubMed]
6. Costa, R.J.S.; Snipe, R.M.J.; Kitic, C.M.; Gibson, P.R. Systematic review: Exercise-induced gastrointestinal syndrome—Implications for health and intestinal disease. *Aliment. Pharmacol. Ther.* **2017**, *46*, 246–265. [CrossRef] [PubMed]
7. Kawamura, T.; Suzuki, K.; Takahashi, M.; Tomari, M.; Hara, R.; Gando, Y.; Muraoka, I. Involvement of Neutrophil Dynamics and Function in Exercise-Induced Muscle Damage and Delayed-Onset Muscle Soreness: Effect of Hydrogen Bath. *Antioxidants* **2018**, *7*, 127. [CrossRef]
8. Ma, S.; Suzuki, K. Keto-Adaptation and Endurance Exercise Capacity, Fatigue Recovery, and Exercise-Induced Muscle and Organ Damage Prevention: A Narrative Review. *Sports* **2019**, *7*, 40. [CrossRef]
9. Peake, J.; Suzuki, K. Neutrophil activation, antioxidant supplements and exercise-induced oxidative stress. *Exerc. Immunol. Rev.* **2004**, *10*, 129–141.
10. Peake, J.; Neubauer, O.; Walsh, N.P.; Simpson, R.J. Recovery of the immune system after exercise. *J. Appl. Physiol.* **2017**, *122*, 1077–1087. [CrossRef]
11. Campbell, J.P.; Turner, J.E. Debunking the Myth of Exercise-Induced Immune Suppression: Redefining the Impact of Exercise on Immunological Health Across the Lifespan. *Front. Immunol.* **2018**, *9*, 648. [CrossRef]
12. Tokuhara, D.; Kurashima, Y.; Kamioka, M.; Nakayama, T.; Ernst, P.; Kiyono, H. A comprehensive understanding of the gut mucosal immune system in allergic inflammation. *Allergol. Int.* **2019**, *68*, 17–25. [CrossRef] [PubMed]
13. Lin, L.; Zhang, J. Role of intestinal microbiota and metabolites on gut homeostasis and human diseases. *BMC Immunol.* **2017**, *18*, 2. [CrossRef] [PubMed]
14. Donnelly, A.E.; Maughan, R.J.; Whiting, P.H. Effects of ibuprofen on exercise-induced muscle soreness and indices of muscle damage. *Br. J. Sports Med.* **1990**, *24*, 191–195. [CrossRef] [PubMed]
15. Lambert, G.P.; Boylan, M.; Laventure, J.P.; Bull, A.; Lanspa, S. Effect of aspirin and ibuprofen on GI permeability during exercise. *Int. J. Sports Med.* **2007**, *28*, 722–726. [CrossRef] [PubMed]
16. Brunser, O.; Espinoza, J.; Figueroa, G.; Araya, M.; Spencer, E.; Hilpert, H.; Link-Amster, H.; Brüssow, H. Field trial of an infant formula containing anti-rotavirus and anti-Escherichia coli milk antibodies from hyperimmunized cows. *J. Pediatr. Gastroenterol. Nutr.* **1992**, *15*, 63–72. [CrossRef]
17. Ormrod, D.J.; Miller, T.E. Milk from hyperimmunized dairy cows as a source of a novel biological response modifier. *Agents Actions* **1993**, *38*, C146–C149. [CrossRef]
18. Cordle, C.T.; Duska-McEwen, G.; Janas, L.M.; Malone, W.T.; Hirsch, M.A. Evaluation of the immunogenicity of protein hydrolysate formulas using laboratory animal hyperimmunization. *Pediatr. Allergy Immunol.* **1994**, *5*, 14–19. [CrossRef]
19. Greenblatt, H.C.; Adalsteinsson, O.; Brodie, D.A.; Fitzpatrick-McElligott, S.G. Method of Preventing, Countering, or Reducing NSAID-Induced Gastrointestinal Damage by Administering Milk or Egg Products from Hyperimmunized Animals 1998. U.S. Patent No. 5,772,999, 30 June 1998.
20. Kisic, J.A.; Shipp, T.E. Combination of Plasma and Hyperimmunized Products for Increased Performance 2003. U.S. Patent No. 6,569,447, 27 May 2003.

21. Wang, Y.; Lin, L.; Yin, C.; Othtani, S.; Aoyama, K.; Lu, C.; Sun, X.; Yoshikai, Y. Oral administration of bovine milk from cows hyperimmunized with intestinal bacterin stimulates lamina propria T lymphocytes to produce Th1-biased cytokines in mice. *Int. J. Mol. Sci.* **2014**, *15*, 5458–5471. [CrossRef]
22. Ishida, A.; Yoshikai, Y.; Murosaki, S.; Hidaka, Y.; Nomoto, K. Administration of milk from cows immunized with intestinal bacteria protects mice from radiation-induced lethality. *Biotherapy* **1992**, *5*, 215–225. [CrossRef]
23. Kobayashi, T.; Ohmori, T.; Yanai, M.; Kawanishi, G.; Yoshikai, Y.; Nomoto, K. Protective Effect of Orally Administering Immune Milk on Endogenous Infection in X-Irradiated Mice. *Agric. Biol. Chem.* **1991**, *55*, 2265–2272.
24. Kravets, S.; Kravets, A.; Jacobson, M. Medical Food Composition and Methods Management of Inflammatory Processes in Mammals 2011. U.S. Patent Application No. 12,885,530, 11 April 2011.
25. Owens, W.E.; Nickerson, S.C. Evaluation of an Anti-Inflammatory Factor Derived from Hyperimmunized Cows. *Proc. Soc. Exp. Biol. Med.* **1989**, *190*, 79–86. [CrossRef] [PubMed]
26. Fayer, R.; Andrews, C.; Ungar, B.L.P.; Blagburn, B. Efficacy of hyperimmune bovine colostrum for prophylaxis of cryptosporidiosis in neonatal calves. *J. Parasitol.* **1989**, *75*, 393–397. [CrossRef]
27. Hung, L.H.; Wu, C.H.; Lin, B.F.; Hwang, L.S. Hyperimmune colostrum alleviates rheumatoid arthritis in a collagen-induced arthritis murine model. *J. Dairy Sci.* **2018**, *101*, 3778–3787. [CrossRef] [PubMed]
28. Bähr, M.; Fechner, A.; Krämer, J.; Kiehntopf, M.; Jahreis, G. Lupin protein positively affects plasma LDL cholesterol and LDL: HDL cholesterol ratio in hypercholesterolemic adults after four weeks of supplementation: A randomized, controlled crossover study. *Nutr. J.* **2013**, *12*, 107. [CrossRef] [PubMed]
29. Jenkins, D.J.; Kendall, C.W.; Garsetti, M.; Rosenberg-Zand, R.S.; Jackson, C.J.; Agarwal, S.; Rao, A.V.; Diamandis, E.P.; Parker, T.; Faulkner, D.; et al. Effect of soy protein foods on low-density lipoprotein oxidation and ex vivo sex hormone receptor activity—A controlled crossover trial. *Metab. Clin. Exp.* **2000**, *49*, 537–543. [CrossRef]
30. Spence, L.A.; Lipscomb, E.R.; Cadogan, J.; Martin, B.; Wastney, M.E.; Peacock, M.; Weaver, C.M. The effect of soy protein and soy isoflavones on calcium metabolism in postmenopausal women: A randomized crossover study. *Am. J. Clin. Nutr.* **2005**, *81*, 916–922. [CrossRef]
31. Kanda, K.; Sakuma, J.; Akimoto, T.; Kawakami, Y.; Suzuki, K. Detection of titin fragments in urine in response to exercise-induced muscle damage. *PLoS ONE* **2017**, *12*, e0181623. [CrossRef]
32. Faul, F.; Erdfelder, E.; Lang, A.G.; Buchner, A. G*power 3: A flexible statistical power analysis program for the social, behavioral, and biomedical sciences. *Behav. Res. Methods* **2007**, *39*, 175–191. [CrossRef]
33. Sinert, R.; Kohl, L.; Rainone, T.; Scalea, T. Exercise-Induced Rhabdomyolysis. *Ann. Emerg. Med.* **1994**, *23*, 1301–1306. [CrossRef]
34. Yada, K.; Suzuki, K.; Oginome, N.; Ma, S.; Fukuda, Y.; Iida, A.; Radak, Z. Single Dose Administration of Taheebo Polyphenol Enhances Endurance Capacity in Mice. *Sci. Rep.* **2018**, *8*, 14625. [CrossRef]
35. Konrad, M.; Nieman, D.C.; Henson, D.A.; Kennerly, K.M.; Jin, F.; Wallner-Liebmann, S.J. The Acute Effect of Ingesting a Quercetin-Based Supplement on Exercise-Induced Inflammation and Immune Changes in Runners. *Int. J. Sport Nutr. Exerc. Metab.* **2011**, *21*, 338–346. [CrossRef] [PubMed]
36. Ma, S.; Suzuki, K. Toll-like Receptor 4: Target of Lipotoxicity and Exercise-Induced Anti-inflammatory Effect? *Annu. Nutr. Food Sci.* **2018**, *2*, 1027.
37. Ma, S.; Huang, Q.; Yada, K.; Liu, C.; Suzuki, K. An 8-Week Ketogenic Low Carbohydrate, High Fat Diet Enhanced Exhaustive Exercise Capacity in Mice. *Nutrients* **2018**, *10*, 673. [CrossRef]
38. Ziegenfuss, T.N.; Kerksick, C.M.; Kedia, A.W.; Sandrock, J.; Raub, B.; Lopez, H.L. Proprietary Milk Protein Concentrate Reduces Joint Discomfort While Improving Exercise Performance in Non-Osteoarthritic Individuals. *Nutrients* **2019**, *11*, 283. [CrossRef]
39. Pugh, J.N.; Impey, S.G.; Doran, D.A.; Fleming, S.C.; Morton, J.P.; Close, G.L. Acute high-intensity interval running increases markers of gastrointestinal damage and permeability but not gastrointestinal symptoms. *Appl. Physiol. Nutr. Metab.* **2017**, *42*, 941–947. [CrossRef] [PubMed]
40. Lim, C.L.; Suzuki, K. Systemic inflammation mediates the effects of endotoxemia in the mechanisms of heat stroke. *Biol. Med.* **2017**, *9*, 376–378. [CrossRef]
41. Lambert, G.P.; Broussard, L.J.; Mason, B.L.; Mauermann, W.J.; Gisolfi, C.V. Gastrointestinal permeability during exercise: Effects of aspirin and energy-containing beverages. *J. Appl. Physiol.* **2001**, *90*, 2075–2080. [CrossRef] [PubMed]

42. Zuhl, M.; Dokladny, K.; Mermier, C.; Schneider, S.; Salgado, R.; Moseley, P. The effects of acute oral glutamine supplementation on exercise-induced gastrointestinal permeability and heat shock protein expression in peripheral blood mononuclear cells. *Cell Stress Chaperones* **2015**, *20*, 85–93. [CrossRef] [PubMed]
43. Marchbank, T.; Limdi, J.K.; Mahmood, A.; Elia, G.; Playford, R.J. Clinical trial: Protective effect of a commercial fish protein hydrolysate against indomethacin (NSAID)-induced small intestinal injury. *Aliment. Pharmacol. Ther.* **2008**, *28*, 799–804. [CrossRef]
44. Shing, C.M.; Peake, J.M.; Lim, C.L.; Briskey, D.; Walsh, N.P.; Fortes, M.B.; Ahuja, K.D.K.; Vitetta, L. Effects of probiotics supplementation on gastrointestinal permeability, inflammation and exercise performance in the heat. *Eur. J. Appl. Physiol.* **2014**, *114*, 93–103. [CrossRef]
45. Sarker, S.A.; Casswall, T.H.; Juneja, L.R.; Hoq, E.; Hossain, I.; Fuchs, G.J.; Hammarström, L. Randomized, placebo-controlled, clinical trial of hyperimmunized chicken egg yolk immunoglobulin in children with rotavirus diarrhea. *J. Pediatr. Gastroenterol. Nutr.* **2001**, *32*, 19–25. [CrossRef] [PubMed]
46. Suzuki, K. Inflammatory responses to exercise and its prevention. *Curr. Top. Biochem. Res.* **2018**, *19*, 37–42.
47. Sugama, K.; Suzuki, K.; Yoshitani, K.; Shiraishi, K.; Kometani, T. Urinary excretion of cytokines versus their plasma levels after endurance exercise. *Exerc. Immunol. Rev.* **2013**, *19*, 29–48. [PubMed]
48. Sugama, K.; Suzuki, K.; Yoshitani, K.; Shiraishi, K.; Kometani, T. IL-17, neutrophil activation and muscle damage following endurance exercise. *Exerc. Immunol. Rev.* **2012**, *18*, 116–127.
49. Sugama, K.; Suzuki, K.; Yoshitani, K.; Shiraishi, K.; Miura, S.; Yoshioka, H.; Mori, Y.; Kometani, T. Changes of thioredoxin, oxidative stress markers, inflammation and muscle/renal damage following intensive endurance exercise. *Exerc. Immunol. Rev.* **2015**, *21*, 130–142.
50. Peake, J.; Della Gatta, P.; Suzuki, K.; Nieman, D. Cytokine expression and secretion by skeletal muscle cells: Regulatory mechanisms and exercise effects. *Exerc. Immunol. Rev.* **2015**, *21*, 8–25.
51. Okhuysen, P.C.; Chappell, C.L.; Crabb, J.; Valdez, L.M.; Douglass, E.T.; DuPont, H.L. Prophylactic Effect of Bovine Anti-Cryptosporidium Hyperimmune Colostrum Immunoglobulin in Healthy Volunteers Challenged with Cryptosporidium parvum. *Clin. Infect. Dis.* **1998**, *26*, 1324–1329. [CrossRef]
52. Shing, C.M.; Peake, J.M.; Suzuki, K.; Jenkins, D.G.; Coombes, J.S. Bovine Colostrum Modulates Cytokine Production in Human Peripheral Blood Mononuclear Cells Stimulated with Lipopolysaccharide and Phytohemagglutinin. *J. Interferon Cytokine Res.* **2009**, *29*, 37–44. [CrossRef]
53. Shing, C.M.; Peake, J.M.; Suzuki, K.; Okutsu, M.; Pereira, R.; Stevenson, L.; Jenkins, D.G.; Coombes, J. Effects of bovine colostrum supplementation on immune variables in highly trained cyclists. *J. Appl. Physiol.* **2007**, *102*, 1113–1122. [CrossRef]
54. Davison, G.; Marchbank, T.; March, D.S.; Thatcher, R.; Playford, R.J. Zinc carnosine works with bovine colostrum in truncating heavy exercise–induced increase in gut permeability in healthy volunteers. *Am. J. Clin. Nutr.* **2016**, *104*, 526–536. [CrossRef]
55. Playford, R.J.; Macdonald, C.E.; Calnan, D.P.; Floyd, D.N.; Podas, T.; Johnson, W.; Wicks, A.C.; Bashir, O.; Marchbank, T. Co-administration of the health food supplement, bovine colostrum, reduces the acute non-steroidal anti-inflammatory drug-induced increase in intestinal permeability. *Clin. Sci.* **2001**, *100*, 627–633. [CrossRef] [PubMed]
56. An, M.J.; Cheon, J.H.; Kim, S.W.; Park, J.J.; Moon, C.M.; Han, S.Y.; Kim, E.S.; Kim, T.I.; Kim, W.H. Bovine colostrum inhibits nuclear factor κB–mediated proinflammatory cytokine expression in intestinal epithelial cells. *Nutr. Res.* **2009**, *29*, 275–280. [CrossRef] [PubMed]
57. Yadav, R.; Angolkar, T.; Kaur, G.; S Buttar, H. Antibacterial and Anti-inflammatory Properties of Bovine Colostrum. *Recent Pat. Inflamm. Allergy Drug Discov.* **2016**, *10*, 49–53. [CrossRef] [PubMed]

biomedicines

MDPI

Article

The Use of Natural Agents to Counteract Telomere Shortening: Effects of a Multi-Component Extract of *Astragalus mongholicus* Bunge and Danazol

Isabelle Guinobert [1], Claude Blondeau [1], Bruno Colicchio [2], Noufissa Oudrhiri [3], Alain Dieterlen [2], Eric Jeandidier [4], Georges Deschenes [5], Valérie Bardot [1], César Cotte [1], Isabelle Ripoche [6], Patrice Carde [7], Lucile Berthomier [6] and Radhia M'Kacher [8,*]

1 Groupe PiLeJe, 37 Quai de Grenelle, 75015 Paris Cedex 15, Naturopôle, Les Tiolans, 03800 Saint-Bonnet de Rochefort, France; i.guinobert@pileje.com (I.G.); c.blondeau@pileje.com (C.B.); v.bardot@pileje.com (V.B.); c.cotte@pileje-industrie.com (C.C.)

2 IRIMAS, Institut de Recherche en Informatique, Mathématiques, Automatique et Signal, Université de Haute-Alsace, 68093 Mulhouse, France; bruno.colicchio@uha.fr (B.C.); alain.dieterlen@uha.fr (A.D.)

3 Service d'Hématologie Moléculaire et Cytogénétique Paul Brousse CHU Paris Sud, Université Paris Sud, Inserm UMRS935, 94800 Villejuif, France; noufissa.oudrhiri@aphp.fr

4 Service de Génétique Médicale, Groupe Hospitalier de la Région de Mulhouse et Sud-Alsace, 68070 Mulhouse, France; jeandidiere@ghrmsa.fr

5 Service de Néphrologie, APHP-Hôpital Robert Debré, 75019 Paris, France; georges.deschenes@aphp.fr

6 Institut de Chimie de Clermont-Ferrand, Université Clermont Auvergne, CNRS, SIGMA Clermont, BP 10448, 63000 Clermont-Ferrand, France; isabelle.ripoche@sigma-clermont.fr (I.R.); lucile.berthomier@sigma-clermont.fr (L.B.)

7 Département d'hématologie, Gustave Roussy Cancer Campus, université Paris Saclay, 94803 Villejuif, France; dr.pcarde@gmail.com

8 Cell Environment, DNA damage R&D, 75020 Paris, France

* Correspondence: radhia.mkacher@cell-environment.com; Tel.: +33-01-48-81-30-38

Received: 19 December 2019; Accepted: 7 February 2020; Published: 12 February 2020

Abstract: A link between telomere shortening and oxidative stress was found in aging people and patients with cancer or inflammatory diseases. Extracts of *Astragalus* spp. are known to stimulate telomerase activity, thereby compensating telomere shortening. We characterized a multi-component hydroethanolic root extract (HRE) of *Astragalus mongholicus* Bunge and assessed its effects on telomeres compared to those of danazol. Astragalosides I to IV, flavonoids, amino acids and sugars were detected in the HRE. Samples of peripheral blood lymphocytes with short telomeres from 18 healthy donors (mean age 63.5 years; range 32–86 years) were exposed to a single dose of 1 μg/mL HRE or danazol for three days. Telomere length and telomerase expression were then measured. Significant elongation of telomeres associated to a less toxicity was observed in lymphocytes from 13/18 donors following HRE treatment (0.54 kb (0.15–2.06 kb)) and in those from 9/18 donors after danazol treatment (0.95 kb (0.06–2.06 kb)). The rate of cells with short telomeres (<3 kb) decreased in lymphocytes from all donors after exposure to either HRE or danazol, telomere elongation being telomerase-dependent. These findings suggest that the HRE could be used for the management of age-related diseases.

Keywords: *Astragalus mongholicus* Bunge; danazol; telomere; telomerase; aging

1. Introduction

The age structure of human populations is changing, with an increase in the proportion of elderly individuals [1]. Age-related diseases are currently the most important causes of morbidity and mortality worldwide [2,3]. There is consequently an urgent need to develop approaches conducive to better health in the elderly [4], thereby improving their quality of life and reducing medical costs [5,6].

Telomeres are dynamic nucleoprotein structures that protect the ends of chromosomes from degradation and activation of the DNA damage response. Telomeres are considered to be a biological clock, playing a major role in aging and genome stability [7]. It is now well-documented that telomere dysfunction is a potential biomarker for age-related diseases and can contribute to the prognosis of several diseases [8–12]. Telomere sensitivity to inflammation and oxidative stress such as ionizing radiation has been previously demonstrated [13]. This sensitivity promotes telomere shortening and replicative senescence [14] leading to chromosomal instability [15]. This phenomenon was found to occur in both proliferative and nonproliferative tissues [16]. To overcome telomere dysfunction, activation of a telomere maintenance mechanism is required to support cell proliferation and immortalization. In most cases, telomeres are elongated by telomerase, a cellular reverse transcriptase capable of compensating telomere shortening through de novo addition of (T2AG3)n [17]. However, telomerase activity can decline with age [18]. Telomerase reactivation approaches have been investigated to counteract telomere shortening and its consequences and have consequently been proposed for the treatment of age-related diseases and telomeropathies [19]. It was shown that antioxidant and anti-inflammatory agents can be used to slow the loss of telomere length [20]. Furthermore, several studies have reported telomere elongation by androgens such as danazol [7,21] and by herbal products [22–27].

In traditional Chinese medicine, *Astragali Radix* (known as Huang Qi), the dried root of *Astragalus membranaceus* (Fisch.) Bunge or *Astragalus mongholicus* Bunge, is an herbal medicine that has been used to counteract oxidative stress, inflammation and aging since ancient times [28,29]. Pharmacological studies have shown that *Astragalus* spp. extracts and their principal components (saponins, flavonoids and polysaccharides) act on aging via several mechanisms [23,30]. In addition to their antioxidant, anti-inflammatory, immunoregulatory and anticancer effects, extracts of *Astragalus* spp. have been shown to exert beneficial effects on telomeres and to stimulate telomerase activity in various models [22,23,31]. Most studies investigated cycloastragenol (TA-65), a single chemical entity isolated by a proprietary purification process from a root extract of *Astragalus membranaceus* [22,24,25,31,32].

The objective of this study was to determine the phytochemical composition of a multicomponent hydroethanolic root extract (HRE) of *Astragalus mongholicus* Bunge and to assess its effects on telomere length and telomerase expression in lymphocytes from healthy donors with short telomeres, per comparison with those of danazol, no such comparison having been made up to now within the same cohort. We demonstrated significant telomere elongation in lymphocytes exposed to HRE, associated with less toxicity than that induced by danazol treatment. This telomere elongation could be related to telomerase activation. The proportion of lymphocytes with short telomeres decreased significantly after exposure to either HRE or danazol in samples from all donors.

2. Materials and Methods

2.1. Preparation of the Hydroethanolic Root Extract of Astragalus mongholicus Bunge

Roots of *A. mongholicus* Bunge were collected in China in October 2015 and identified by Gilles Thébaud from the UniVegE service of the University of Clermont-Ferrand (France) in which a voucher specimen was deposited (CLF110821). CLF is registered in the Index Herbariorum of the New York Botanical Garden.

The liquid HRE of *A. mongholicus* Bunge evaluated in this study was produced by PiLeJe Industrie (France) according to the patented process WO2001056584A1. The batch used in this study (no. C-16K404) contained 30.7% of dry material containing 0.05% formononetin and 0.16% of astragaloside IV. The drug extract ratio (DER) of HRE, expressed as the ratio of the dry weight of the original fresh plant material to that of the resulting extract, was 3:1. After addition of glycerol, the *A. mongholicus* Bunge HRE corresponds to a formononetin-standardized extract of *A. mongholicus* Bunge (EPS Astragale, PiLeJe Laboratoire, France).

2.2. High-Performance Thin-Layer Chromatography (HPTLC) Analysis of *A. mongholicus* Bunge HRE

Standards were diluted in methanol at a concentration of 0.1 mg/mL for formononetin (Extrasynthèse, Genay, France) and 0.51 mg/mL for astragaloside IV (European Directorate for the Quality of Medicines & HealthCare, Strasbourg, France). *A. mongholicus* Bunge HRE without glycerol (4 mL) was diluted in 16 mL of a mixture of ethanol and water (50/50:*v*/*v*). The resultant solution was shaken and centrifuged for 3 min at 4400 rpm. The supernatant solution was transferred into individual vials and then subjected to HPTLC analysis.

HPTLC analysis was performed on 100.0 × 100.0 mm silica gel 60 F 254 HPTLC glass plates (Merck, Germany). Standard solutions and samples were applied to the plates in bands 8.0 mm wide using a CAMAG Automatic TLC sampler (ATS 4). The plates were developed in a CAMAG Automatic developing chamber (ADC2), derivatization being accomplished using a TLC plate heater and a CAMAG Chromatogram Immersion Device. The chromatograms were recorded by a CAMAG Visualizer with WinCATS software. The specific chromatographic conditions used for the three types of compounds analyzed are presented in Supplementary Table S1.

2.3. Liquid Chromatography/Mass Spectrometry (LC/MS) Analysis of *A. mongholicus* Bunge HRE

Ultra-high performance liquid chromatography (UHPLC) analyses were performed on an Ultimate 3000 RSLC UHPLC system (Thermo Fisher Scientific Inc., Waltham, MA, USA) coupled with a binary pump (U3000 HPG-3400RS) and a diode array detector. Compounds were separated on an Uptisphere Strategy C18 column (25 × 4.6 mm, 5 µm; Interchim, Montluçon, France) and maintained at 40 °C. The flow rate was 0.8 mL/min, and the injection volume was 5 µL. Mobile phases were phase A, 0.1% (*v*/*v*) formic acid in water and phase B, 0.1% (*v*/*v*) formic acid in acetonitrile with the linear gradient: 0–25 min, 100%–0% of phase A. The UHPLC system was connected to a Q-Exactive Orbitrap (Thermo Fisher Scientific Inc.) mass spectrometer operated in negative and positive electrospray ionization modes. Source operating conditions were: 3 kV spray voltage for the negative mode and 3.5 kV spray voltage for the positive mode; 320 °C heated capillary temperature; 475 °C auxiliary gas temperature; sheath, sweep and auxiliary gas (nitrogen) flow rate 60, 18 and 4 arbitrary units, respectively, and collision cell voltage between 20 and 50 eV. Full-scan data were obtained at a resolution of 35,000, whereas tandem mass spectrometry (MS^2) data were obtained at a resolution of 17,500. Data were processed using Xcalibur software (Thermo Fisher Scientific Inc.).

The components of the HRE were characterized according to their retention times, mass spectral data and comparison with authentic standards, when available, or otherwise with published data.

2.4. In Vitro Exposure of Cell Lines And Cytotoxicity Approach

Lymphoblastoid cells from two human cell lines (BJAB and DG-75) were treated with increasing doses of HRE (0.01, 0.1, 1 and 10 µg/mL) dissolved in ethanol 30% for 72 h at 37°C. For the controls, the same procedure was followed with ethanol alone (negative control) and with danazol (Sigma, Saint Quentin Fallavier, France; dissolved in DMSO to concentrations of 0.01, 0.1, 1 and 10 µg/mL; positive control). Survival was assessed using trypan blue, cell proliferation being evaluated on the basis of the mitotic index after cell arrest. The number of cells in metaphase and interphase were scored. The mitotic index was the ratio between the number of cells in metaphase to the total number of scored cells.

2.5. Peripheral Blood Lymphocyte In Vitro Exposure and Culture Conditions

Peripheral blood lymphocytes from 18 healthy donors (15 men and 3 women) with a mean age of 63.5 years (range 32–86 years) were used in this study. A large cohort of 150 healthy donors was used as a control. The use of samples from healthy donors has been approved by the Ethic Committee of Gustave Roussy Cancer Campus University Paris Saclay (ethical approval code: Comités de protection des personnes CPP 97/06, and Ile-de-France/ Nephrovir/ 2010). Informed consent was obtained from all donors included in this study.

Blood lymphocytes were exposed to 1 µg/mL HRE or danazol and cultured in RPMI 1640 medium (Gibco-BRL, Grand Island, NY, USA) supplemented with Glutamax, 10% fetal bovine serum (Eurobio, Courtaboeuf, France) and antibiotics (penicillin and streptomycin; Gibco-BRL) for 72 h (3 days) at 37 °C. The effects of *A. mongholicus* Bunge HRE and danazol on lymphocyte proliferation and telomere length were assessed.

2.6. Telomere Quantification

Telomeres were quantified in interphase cells using the quantitative fluorescence in situ hybridization (Q-FISH) technique with a Cy-3-labelled PNA probe specific for TTAGGG (Eurogenetec, Liège, Belgium), permitting investigation of intercellular variation in a large number of scored cells. The detailed procedure was described previously [11,12]. Quantitative image acquisition and analysis were performed using Metacyte software (Metasystem, version 3.9.1; Altlussheim, Germany). The mean fluorescence intensity (FI) of telomeres was automatically quantified in 10,000 nuclei on each slide. Settings for exposure and gain remained constant between captures. The experiments were performed in triplicate. Internal (cell line) and external (fluorescence beads) controls of the fluorescence intensity were used in each experiment. Telomere length, measured as mean FI, was also translated into the mean telomere length in kilobases (kb) using a standard curve performed in cancer patients, as well as in human cell lines using the telomeric restriction fragment (TRF) [11] (Supplementary Figure S1). Mean telomere length was expressed in kb.

2.7. Telomerase Expression Using Immunofluorescence

To quantify telomerase expression, peripheral blood lymphocytes of 6 donors were isolated in Ficoll medium (Ficoll, Biochrom AG, Berlin, Germany) and then cultured in RPMI medium (Gibco-BRL) supplemented with 10% fetal bovine serum (Eurobio, Courtaboeuf, France) and antibiotics (penicillin and streptomycin; Gibco-BRL) at 37 °C for 72 h. The detailed procedure was published previously [33].

2.8. Statistical Analysis

All data were analyzed using R software version 3.5.3 and libraries. Mean comparisons were computed using the two-sample Wilcoxon test. The following convention for symbols indicating statistical significance were used: ns for $p > 0.05$, * for $p \leq 0.05$, ** for $p \leq 0.01$, *** for $p \leq 0.001$ and **** for $p \leq 0.0001$. The regression curve presented was computed on the mean telomere length previously determined in a cohort of 150 healthy donors [34] using a linear regression model (lm).

3. Results

3.1. Characteristics of A. mongholicus Bunge HRE

HPTLC analysis revealed the presence of astragalosides, including astragaloside IV, flavonoids, including formononetin, and amino acids in the *A. mongholicus* Bunge HRE (Figure 1). Analysis by UHPLC-MS confirmed the presence of astragaloside IV and formononetin, additionally revealing the presence of astragalosides I, II and III (Supplementary Figure S2 and Tables S2 and S3). Isoflavones, including calycosin, ononin and calycosin-7-o-β-D-glucoside, were also detected. Various amino acids were identified, including L-canavanine, asparagine, aspartic acid, glutamic acid, leucine and phenylalanine.

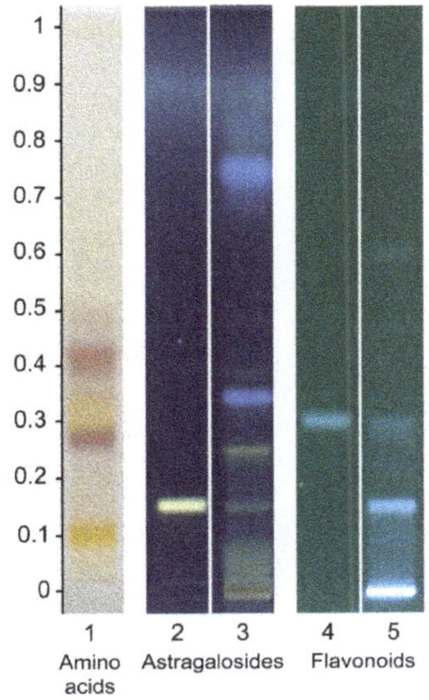

Figure 1. High-performance thin-layer chromatography (HPTLC) plate for amino acids, astragalosides and flavonoids. Track 1: *A. mongholicus* Bunge HRE (0.2 µL), Track 2: astragaloside IV (2 µL), Track 3: *A. mongholicus* Bunge HRE (1 µL), Track 4: formononetin (4 µL) and Track 5: *A. mongholicus* Bunge HRE (3.4 µL).

3.2. HRE Cytotoxicity

The cytotoxicity of HRE and danazol were assessed on the basis of cell viability and mitotic index on two human cell lines (BJAB and DG-75) and human peripheral blood lymphocytes.

The choice of these cell lines was based on their telomere status, the BJAB cell line being characterized by drastically short telomeres compared to the DG-75 cell line (Figure 2A). Cell viability following exposure to each of the four HRE and danazol doses was assessed by manual cell counting using trypan blue to stain dead cells (Figure 2B). No significant difference in cell viability was observed between cells treated with HRE at 1 µg/mL and those treated with the vehicle (control). Interestingly, BJAB cell viability was significantly higher after treatment with HRE at 0.01 µg/mL than in the controls ($p < 0.01$). In contrast, danazol 1 µg/mL induced more toxicity in BJAB cells than in DG75 cells, showing that BJAB cells are more sensitive to danazol than DG75 cells.

Similarly, the mitotic index was evaluated after the HRE and danazol treatments and compared to the control value in the cell lines (Figure 2C). With regard to the BJAB cell line, the mitotic index after HRE treatment was higher than that in the controls (more than 10.3%), confirming the high cell viability results obtained after HRE treatment. In contrast, the mitotic index was reduced in BJAB cells treated with danazol and confirmed the higher sensitivity of these cells to danazol. The results of these experiments permitted selection of an optimal dose for human lymphocyte exposure that did not induce increased toxicity, namely 1 µg/mL for both the HRE and danazol.

Mitotic index was also evaluated in peripheral blood lymphocytes from 18 healthy donors before and after exposure to 1 µg/mL of HRE or danazol during three days. Figure 3 shows the relative change in the mitotic index after HRE and danazol treatments compared to the control. A higher mitotic index was observed in 15 donors after HRE treatment versus 11 donors after danazol treatment.

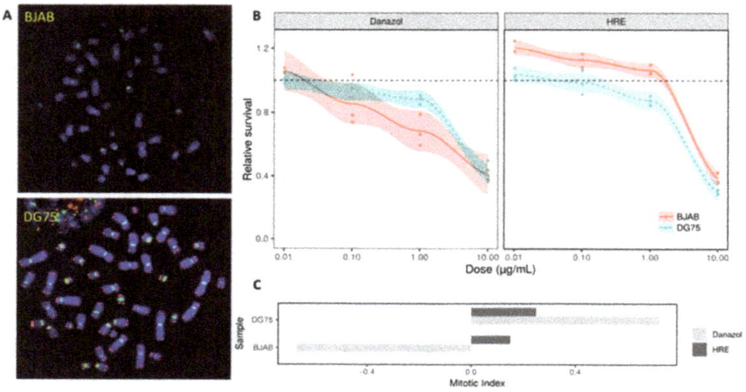

Figure 2. Toxicity of hydroethanolic root extract (HRE) and danazol. BJAB and DG-75 cells were incubated with increasing doses of the HRE or danazol for 3 days. (**A**) Metaphases from BJAB and DG75 cell lines stained with a Cy3 telomere probe (red) and FITC centromere probe (green) showing drastically short telomeres in BJAB cells. (**B**) Cell viability determined by manual cell counting after staining with trypan blue. Relative survival was calculated after in vitro exposure to the HRE or danazol. The data are representative of three independent experiments and expressed as the mean ratio ± standard error of the mean. The experiments were performed in triplicate. (**C**) Mitotic index variation after exposure to HRE and danazol for 3 days following a single dose of 1 µg/mL. Two slides were used for each condition.

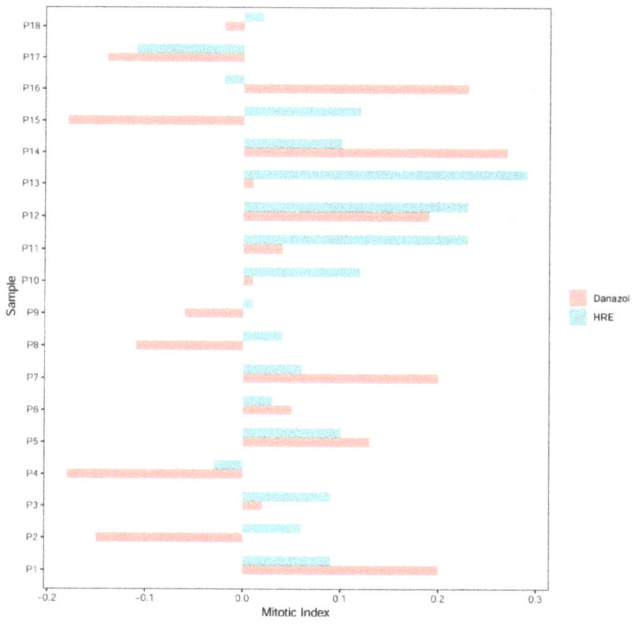

Figure 3. Toxicity of HRE and danazol treatment on circulating lymphocytes from healthy donors based on the relative change in the mitotic index after HRE and danazol treatment (1 µg/mL) compared to control values. Two slides were used to establish the mitotic index for each condition.

3.3. *In Vitro Exposure of Peripheral Blood Lymphocytes to HRE Induced Telomere Elongation and Decreased the Proportion of Cells with Short Telomeres*

Telomere length was measured using the quantitative fluorescence in situ hybridization (Q-FISH) technique in interphase cells, permitting the investigation of intercellular variation in a large number of scored cells. The mean telomere length in peripheral lymphocytes from each donor was based on the quantification of telomere signal intensity performed in triplicate. We first analyzed telomere length in a large cohort of healthy donors spanning a large age range (150 healthy donors; 2–76 years). The rate of telomere loss was calculated from the decrease in telomere length as a function of donor age. Telomere length declined at a rate of 79 pb/year ($p < 10^{-6}$, R2 = 0.29; Figure 4).

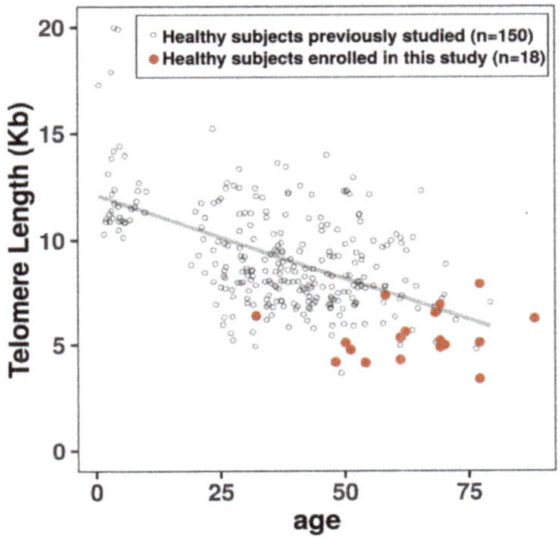

Figure 4. Telomere length in peripheral blood lymphocytes as a function of age. The healthy blood donors enrolled in this study presented very short telomeres in their peripheral blood lymphocytes compared to those of a previously studied cohort of 150 blood donors [34]. The regression line indicates natural telomere shortening with age (79 pb per year; Y = 12.1–0.79 and R2 = 0.29). Telomere length was measured by Q-FISH. Fluorescence intensity was transformed to kilobases according to the correlation between Q-FISH and Southern Blot results.

To assess the effect of HRE and danazol on telomere length, 18 healthy donors (mean age 63.5 years; range 32–86 years) with short telomeres were selected. These donors had a mean telomere length of 5.97 kb (3.47–7.94 kb; Figure 4). Telomere length in peripheral blood lymphocytes from 15 of these donors was lower than the median age-dependent telomere length (Figure 4).

After exposure to HRE, significant telomere elongation was observed in blood lymphocytes from 13 of the 18 donors (72%, 0.54 kb (0.15–2.06 kb); p < 0.001; Figure 5).

The increase in telomere length compared to that measured before treatment varied from 5% to 27% (Figure 6A). No significant change in telomere length was observed in lymphocytes from one donor, and moderate toxicity following exposure to HRE was seen in lymphocytes from four donors (Figures 5 and 6A). We have also analyzed the rate of cells with very short telomeres, less than 3kb [35]. The choice of this telomere length was based on both the telomere length observed in patients with genetic disorders related to telomere mutations, such as dyskeratosis congenita and aplastic anemia [36], and the telomere length in the cohort used in our study (mean telomere length: 5.97 kb). After HRE exposure, a decrease in the proportion of cells with very short telomeres (less than 3 kb) was observed in lymphocytes from all donors (Figure 6B and Supplementary Figure S3).

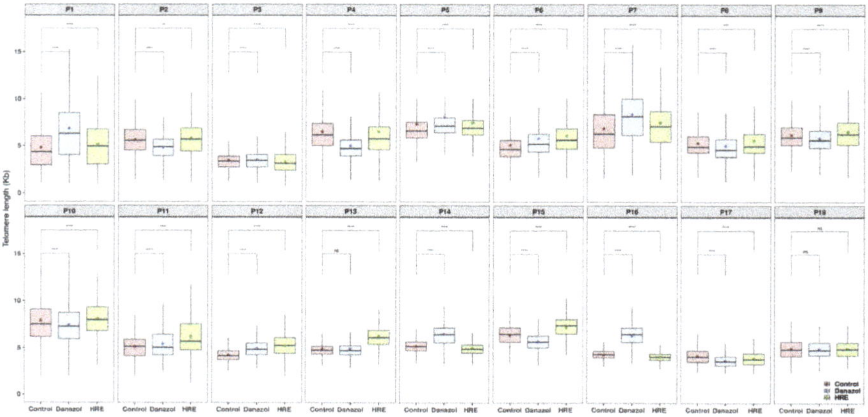

Figure 5. Box plots of telomere length in circulating lymphocytes from healthy donors determined by Q-FISH. Mean values are shown by diamond-shaped points. The middle line reflects the median, the box length reflects the interquartile range (interquartile range, 75th–25th percentiles) and the whiskers reflect the 5th and 95th percentiles. Statistical significance of the difference between telomere length of circulating lymphocytes before and after treatment with HRE and danazol (1 µg/mL) (one-way analysis of means ANOVA): **** $p < 0.0001$. NS: not significant.

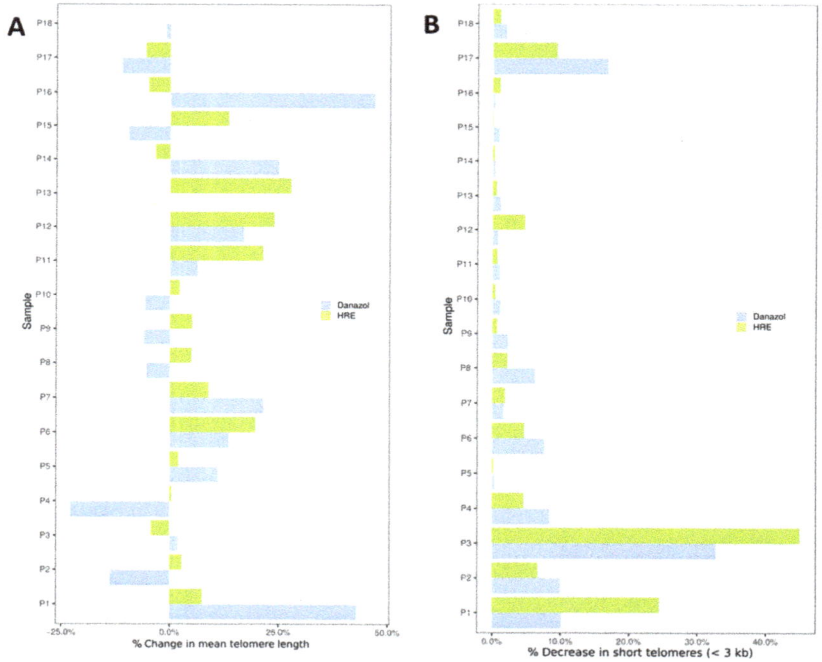

Figure 6. Changes in telomere length in circulating lymphocytes from each healthy donor after exposure to HRE and to danazol (1 µg/mL). (**A**) Change in mean telomere length and (**B**) decrease in the proportion of lymphocytes showing drastic telomere shortening (<3 kb).

After danazol exposure, significant telomere elongation was observed in cultured circulating lymphocytes from 9 of the 18 donors (50%, 0.95 kb (0.06–2.06 kb); $p < 0.001$; Figure 5). The increase in telomere length varied from 2% to 42% (Figure 6A). No significant change was observed in lymphocytes from two donors, and toxicity following exposure to danazol was seen in lymphocytes from seven donors (Figures 5 and 6A). As seen with HRE, a decrease in the rate of cells with very short telomeres (less than 3 kb) was observed in lymphocytes from all donors (Figure 6B and Supplementary Figure S3). Comparison of the effects of HRE and danazol on telomere elongation showed less toxicity and a positive response in lymphocytes from more donors following exposure to HRE (13/18) than after exposure to danazol (9/18). In a large cohort of 150 healthy donors, we determined the natural shortening of telomeres related to natural aging to be 79 pb/year [33]. The mean telomere elongation corresponded to a gain of 6.77 years of age (0.54 kb) after HRE and 12.08 years (0.95 kb) after danazol treatment.

3.4. The HRE Induced Telomerase Expression and Led to Telomerase-Dependent Elongation

Previously, we demonstrated that telomerase reverse transcriptase (hTERT) expression, assessed by immunofluorescence, was strongly correlated with telomerase activity measured by the telomeric repeat amplification protocol (TRAP) assay [33]. In this study, hTERT expression was assessed using immunofluorescence staining in six donors. A significant increase in hTERT expression was observed after exposure to HRE (0.6- to 14.4-fold relative to control) or to danazol (7.8- to 22.2-fold relative to control; Figure 7). The increase in hTERT expression observed after exposure to HRE was lower than that observed after exposure to danazol.

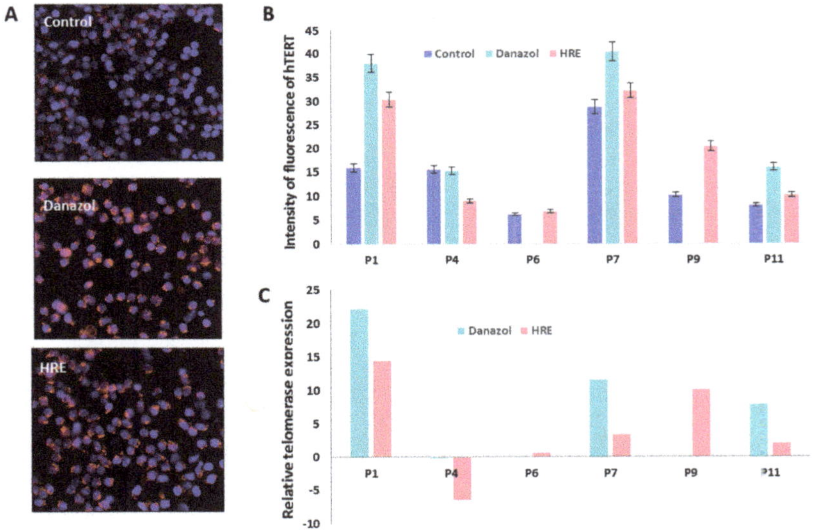

Figure 7. Telomerase expression after exposure to HRE and to danazol. (**A**) Representative image of telomerase reverse transcriptase (hTERT) expression (red) after in vitro treatment of circulating lymphocytes from healthy donors using immunofluorescence staining. Cells were counterstained with DAPI (blue) (**B**) Quantification of the intensity of fluorescence of hTERT protein; 10,000 cells were scored. All data are representative of three independent experiments and are expressed as the mean ± standard error of the mean. The experiments were performed in triplicate. (**C**) Histogram displaying the change in telomerase expression in circulating lymphocytes from healthy donors after exposure to HRE and danazol as a multiple of telomerase expression before exposure to these agents. The absence of hTERT expression for P6 and P9 after danazol treatment was due to a technical issue.

4. Discussion

Aging is a complex and multifactorial process. Telomere shortening and dysfunction, with other factors such as oxidative stress and replicative senescence, play a major role in natural aging and age-related diseases [1]. The implication of telomere dysfunction related to genetic susceptibility and/or environmental factors in genomic instability and age-related diseases has been clearly demonstrated [11,12,37]. The development of novel specific and effective agents devoid of major systemic side effects is a new challenge in the battle against aging. Telomere shortening, the relevant marker of aging, is also responsible for cellular and organismal aging. Counteracting telomere attrition and its consequences has been a main target for research during the last decade [7,22]. Regenerative medicine has also focused on strategies to maintain telomere length [31]. Androgens, such as danazol, have been used to promote telomere elongation in patients with telomeropathies or telomere syndromes [21]. Danazol has also been used to treat bone marrow syndromes for decades with mixed responses and without knowledge of the underlying mechanisms. Recently, several studies have demonstrated that danazol regulates expression of the telomerase gene in both in vitro and in animal models [38,39]. However, the results concerning telomere elongation after in vivo treatment with danazol have been inconsistent, with substantial variation between patients and evidence of poor tolerance [40]. In addition to androgens, several herbal products have been tested for their effects on telomeres [23,25,26,28]. Cycloastragenol (TA-65), a bioactive compound isolated from *Astragalus membranaceus*, has been shown to increase telomere length and activate telomerase in both preclinical and clinical studies [22,24,25,31,32,41,42].

In our laboratory, telomere length has already been evaluated in large cohorts of healthy donors and cancer patients [11,33–35]. In a large cohort of healthy donors, telomere length decreased at a rate of 79 pb per year, which is in line with the rate published by other authors [43–45]. In this study, we assessed the effects of a multi-component extract of *Astragalus mongholicus* Bunge on telomere elongation and telomerase activity in comparison to those of danazol. Up to now, no such comparison had been performed within the same cohort.

The first step in this study consisted to assess the toxicity of HRE using human cell lines. Less toxicity was observed with HRE than with danazol in terms of cellular viability and proliferation (mitotic index). These data confirmed the toxicity of danazol, which had been described previously, mainly apparent in the context of drastically short telomeres [21]. The BJAB cell line, characterized by very short telomeres, showed higher proliferation after exposure to low doses of HRE. In contrast, there was a significant decrease in cellular proliferation and the mitotic index in BJAB cells after danazol treatment. This discrepancy in the response of BJAB cells to danazol and HRE treatment could be due to the telomere shortening in these cells [46]. Additional investigations are needed to elucidate the mechanisms underlying the sensitivity of BJAB cells to treatment.

The effects of HRE and danazol on telomere elongation and telomerase expression in cultured lymphocytes were evaluated using a specific cohort of healthy blood donors presenting short telomeres essentially related to their age. We clearly demonstrated that exposure to HRE induced significant telomere elongation in lymphocytes from more than 70% of the donors and reduced the proportion of lymphocytes with short telomeres (below 3 kb) from all donors, with very moderate toxicity. This telomere elongation was related to an increase in telomerase activity. These data are in line with those of previously published studies on cycloastragenol [32,41,42].

We also showed that exposure to HRE not only achieved a telomere elongation corresponding to 6.8 years of natural aging but also decreased the proportion of cells with very short telomeres (less than 3 kb) from all the donors. These cells with drastically short telomeres are those that could be at the origin of a number of malignancies and age-related diseases [8]. The results obtained with danazol are in line with those obtained in patients with bone marrow syndromes [21], as well as in those with telomeropathies [40]. In addition, a broader heterogeneity in the responses and a higher rate of toxicity in lymphocytes of 39% (7/18) of the donors has been observed with danazol as compared to that seen with HRE. Similarly a broad heterogeneity of clinical responses has been observed in aplastic anemia in terms of response to danazol [47].

The extract tested in this work was obtained from roots of *Astragalus mongholicus* Bunge according to a patented process preserving the integrity and diversity of the plant totum, defined as the entire set of compounds contained in the part of the plant used for extraction. Phytochemical analysis of the *A. mongholicus* Bunge HRE tested revealed the presence of formononetin and astragaloside IV. Isoflavones, including calycosin, ononin and calycosin-7-o-β-D-glucoside, were also detected. In a study performed with a multi-component extract of *Astragalus membranaceus* roots [31], mild increases in telomerase were observed in a few donor T cell cultures compared to cycloastragenol, which significantly increased telomerase activity. In this study, the extract tested was "an extract of the root of *Astragalus membranaceus* but not a single purified compound entity". No other information on the composition of the extract is provided. In another study, an *Astragalus* extract (also without further specifications) was reported to induce significant telomerase activity in primary human IMR90 cells [25]. Astragaloside IV identified in our extract is most certainly responsible for at least some of the effects observed in our study. To our knowledge, no studies have been carried out with astragaloside IV alone. Cycloastragenol, with which most studies have been conducted and the effects observed, is a derivative of astragaloside IV. No data exist on the other compounds identified in our extract regarding a possible effect on telomeres and telomerase. However, it cannot be excluded that some of them are active. This remains to be investigated. In addition, compounds that were not detected in the HRE in the analyses performed, but that could still be present, could also be involved. For example, two isomers of 4-hydroxy-5-hydroxymethyl-(1,3)dioxolan-2,60-spirane-50,60,70,80-tetrahydro-indolizine-30-carbaldehyde (HDTIC), HDTIC-1 and HDTIC-2, extracted from *Astragalus membranaceus* slowed down the telomere shortening rate of 2BS cells [44].

5. Conclusions

Using a cohort of healthy elderly donors with telomere shortening related to natural aging, we demonstrated that *A. mongholicus* Bunge HRE in vitro exposure could induce telomere elongation in circulating lymphocytes. This elongation was associated with less toxicity than danazol. This data could help define potential therapeutic strategies based on the use of this natural agent in populations with drastically short telomeres. It will be important to investigate the in vivo effects of the HRE in an elderly population with and without age-related diseases. The use of a specific model involving telomeropathy (such as TERT gene mutations, for example) could increase our knowledge relevant to the introduction of the tested HRE as a possible agent for counteracting telomere shortening and its consequences.

Association of this treatment with regular physical exercise, a healthy lifestyle, diet and lower exposure to stress could be a first step in slowing the natural aging process and combatting age-related diseases. A multidisciplinary approach and the definition of adequate experimental in vivo models are needed to win the battle against premature aging.

6. Patents

The patented process number is WO2001056584A1.

Supplementary Materials: The following are available online at http://www.mdpi.com/2227-9059/8/2/31/s1. References [48–54] were cited in supplementary material.

Author Contributions: Conceived and designed the experiments: R.M. and I.G.; performed the experiments: R.M., V.B., I.R. and L.B.; analyzed the data: B.C., E.J. and A.D.; contributed reagents/materials/analysis tools: P.C., G.D., N.O., V.B. and C.C. and wrote the paper: C.B. and R.M. All authors have read and agreed to the published version of the manuscript.

Funding: This work was supported by a grant from Groupe PiLeJe to Cell Environment.

Acknowledgments: We are indebted to Annelise Bennaceur-Griscelli (Hopital Paul Brousse, Laboratoire de cytogénétique) for her help and support. We also thank Wala Najar for technical help and Vivien Paula Harry (independent medical writer) for writing and editorial assistance.

Conflicts of Interest: I.G., C.B., V.B. and C.C. are employees of Groupe PiLeJe.

References

1. Shetty, A.K.; Kodali, M.; Upadhya, R.; Madhu, L.N. Emerging anti-aging strategies-scientific basis and efficacy. *Aging Dis.* **2018**, *9*, 1165–1184. [CrossRef] [PubMed]
2. Xu, Z.; Feng, W.; Shen, Q.; Yu, N.; Yu, K.; Wang, S.; Chen, Z.; Shioda, S.; Guo, Y. Rhizoma coptidis and berberine as a natural drug to combat aging and aging-related diseases via anti-oxidation and ampk activation. *Aging Dis.* **2017**, *8*, 760–777. [CrossRef] [PubMed]
3. Aunan, J.R.; Cho, W.C.; Søreide, K. The biology of aging and cancer: A brief overview of shared and divergent molecular hallmarks. *Aging Dis.* **2017**, *8*, 628–642. [CrossRef] [PubMed]
4. Stambler, I. Recognizing degenerative aging as a treatable medical condition: Methodology and policy. *Aging Dis.* **2017**, *8*, 583–589. [CrossRef]
5. Chakrabarti, S.; Mohanakumar, K.P. Aging and neurodegeneration: A tangle of models and mechanisms. *Aging Dis.* **2016**, *7*, 111–113. [CrossRef]
6. Konar, A.; Singh, P.; Thakur, M.K. Age-associated cognitive decline: Insights into molecular switches and recovery avenues. *Aging Dis.* **2016**, *7*, 121–129. [CrossRef]
7. Martínez, P.; Blasco, M.A. Telomere-driven diseases and telomere-targeting therapies. *J. Cell Biol.* **2017**, *216*, 875–887. [CrossRef]
8. Blasco, M.A. Telomeres and human disease: Ageing, cancer and beyond. *Nat. Rev. Genet.* **2005**, *6*, 611–622. [CrossRef]
9. Vasko, T.; Hoffmann, J.; Gostek, S.; Schettgen, T.; Quinete, N.; Preisinger, C.; Kraus, T.; Ziegler, P. Telomerase gene expression bioassays indicate metabolic activation of genotoxic lower chlorinated polychlorinated biphenyls. *Sci. Rep.* **2018**, *8*, 16903. [CrossRef]
10. Kaifie, A.; Schikowsky, C.; Vasko, T.; Kraus, T.; Brümmendorf, T.H.; Ziegler, P. Additional benefits of telomere length (TL) measurements in chronic lymphocytic leukemia. *Leuk Lymphoma* **2019**, *60*, 541–543. [CrossRef]
11. M'kacher, R.; Bennaceur-Griscelli, A.; Girinsky, T.; Koscielny, S.; Delhommeau, F.; Dossou, J.; Violot, D.; Leclercq, E.; Courtier, M.H.; Béron-Gaillard, N.; et al. Telomere shortening and associated chromosomal instability in peripheral blood lymphocytes of patients with Hodgkin's lymphoma prior to any treatment are predictive of second cancers. *Int. J. Radiat. Oncol. Biol. Phys.* **2007**, *68*, 465–471. [CrossRef] [PubMed]
12. M'kacher, R.; Girinsky, T.; Colicchio, B.; Ricoul, M.; Dieterlen, A.; Jeandidier, E.; Heidingsfelder, L.; Cuceu, C.; Shim, G.; Frenze, M.; et al. Telomere shortening: A new prognostic factor for cardiovascular disease post-radiation exposure. *Radiat. Prot. Dosim.* **2015**, *164*, 134–137. [CrossRef] [PubMed]
13. Muraki, K.; Han, L.; Miller, D.; Murnane, J.P. Processing by MRE11 is involved in the sensitivity of subtelomeric regions to DNA double-strand breaks. *Nucleic Acids Res.* **2015**, *43*, 7911–7930. [CrossRef] [PubMed]
14. Hewitt, G.; Jurk, D.; Marques, F.D.; Correia-Melo, C.; Hardy, T.; Gackowska, A.; Anderson, R.; Taschuk, M.; Mann, J.; Passos, J.F. Telomeres are favoured targets of a persistent DNA damage response in ageing and stress-induced senescence. *Nat. Commun.* **2012**, *3*, 708. [CrossRef] [PubMed]
15. Murnane, J.P. Telomere loss as a mechanism for chromosome instability in human cancer. *Cancer Res.* **2010**, *70*, 4255–4259. [CrossRef] [PubMed]
16. Epel, E.S.; Blackburn, E.H.; Lin, J.; Dhabhar, F.S.; Adler, N.E.; Morrow, J.D.; Cawthon, R.M. Accelerated telomere shortening in response to life stress. *Proc. Natl. Acad. Sci. USA* **2004**, *101*, 17312–17315. [CrossRef]
17. Martínez, P.; Blasco, M.A. Telomeric and extra-telomeric roles for telomerase and the telomere-binding proteins. *Nat. Rev. Cancer* **2011**, *11*, 161–176. [CrossRef]
18. de Jesus, B.B.; Blasco, M.A. Potential of telomerase activation in extending health span and longevity. *Curr. Opin. Cell Biol.* **2012**, *24*, 739–743. [CrossRef]
19. Kannengiesser, C.; Borie, R.; Renzoni, E.A. Pulmonary fibrosis: Genetic analysis of telomere-related genes, telomere length measurement-or both? *Respirology* **2019**, *24*, 97–98. [CrossRef]

20. Prasad, K.N.; Wu, M.; Bondy, S.C. Telomere shortening during aging: Attenuation by antioxidants and anti-inflammatory agents. *Mech. Ageing Dev.* **2017**, *164*, 61–66. [CrossRef]
21. Townsley, D.M.; Dumitriu, B.; Liu, D.; Biancotto, A.; Weinstein, B.; Chen, C.; Hardy, N.; Mihalek, A.D.; Lingala, S.; Kim, Y.J.; et al. Danazol treatment for telomere diseases. *N. Engl. J. Med.* **2016**, *374*, 1922–1931. [CrossRef]
22. Jäger, K.; Walter, M. Therapeutic targeting of telomerase. *Genes* **2016**, *7*, 39. [CrossRef]
23. Liu, P.; Zhao, H.; Luo, Y. Anti-aging implications of *Astragalus membranaceus* (huangqi): A well-known chinese tonic. *Aging Dis.* **2017**, *8*, 868–886. [CrossRef]
24. Yu, Y.; Zhou, L.; Yang, Y.; Liu, Y. Cycloastragenol: An exciting novel candidate for age-associated diseases. *Exp. Ther. Med.* **2018**, *16*, 2175–2182. [CrossRef] [PubMed]
25. Ait-Ghezala, G.; Hassan, S.; Tweed, M.; Paris, D.; Crynen, G.; Zakirova, Z.; Crynen, S.; Crawford, F. Identification of telomerase-activating blends from naturally occurring compounds. *Altern. Ther. Health Med.* **2016**, *22*, 6–14. [PubMed]
26. Plant, J. Effects of essential oils on telomere length in human cells. *Med Aromat Plants* **2016**, *5*, 2. [CrossRef]
27. Yang, F.; Zhao, P.-W.; Sun, P.; Ma, L.J.; Zhao, P.W. Effect of Cynomorium songaricum polysaccharide on telomere of lung cancer A549 cells. *Zhongguo Zhong Zazhi* **2016**, *41*, 917–921. [CrossRef]
28. Yang, F.; Yan, G.; Li, Y.; Han, Z.; Zhang, L.; Chen, S.; Feng, C.; Huang, Q.; Ding, F.; Yu, Y.; et al. Astragalus polysaccharide attenuated iron overload-induced dysfunction of mesenchymal stem cells via suppressing mitochondrial ros. *Cell Physiol. Biochem.* **2016**, *39*, 1369–1379. [CrossRef]
29. Fu, J.; Wang, Z.; Huang, L.; Zheng, S.; Wang, D.; Chen, S.; Zhang, H.; Yang, S. Review of the botanical characteristics, phytochemistry, and pharmacology of *Astragalus membranaceus* (Huangqi). *Phytother. Res.* **2014**, *28*, 1275–1283. [CrossRef]
30. Li, X.; Qu, L.; Dong, Y.; Han, L.; Liu, E.; Fang, S.; Zhang, Y.; Wang, T. A review of recent research progress on the *Astragalus* genus. *Molecules* **2014**, *19*, 18850–18880. [CrossRef]
31. Molgora, B.; Bateman, R.; Sweeney, G.; Finger, D.; Dimler, T.; Effors, R.B.; Valenzuela, H.F. Functional assessment of pharmacological telomerase activators in human T cells. *Cells* **2013**, *2*, 57–66. [CrossRef]
32. Salvador, L.; Singaravelu, G.; Harley, C.B.; Flom, P.; Suram, A.; Raffaele, J.M. A natural product telomerase activator lengthens telomeres in humans: A randomized, double blind, and placebo controlled study. *Rejuvenation Res.* **2016**, *19*, 478–484. [CrossRef]
33. M'kacher, R.; Cuceu, C.; Al Jawhari, M.; Morat, L.; Frenzel, M.; Shim, G.; Lenain, A.; Hempel, W.M.; Junker, S.; Girinsky, T.; et al. The transition between telomerase and alt mechanisms in Hodgkin lymphoma and its predictive value in clinical outcomes. *Cancers* **2018**, *10*, 169. [CrossRef] [PubMed]
34. Cuceu, C.; Colicchio, B.; Jeandidier, E.; Junker, S.; Plassa, F.; Shim, G.; Mika, J.; Frenzel, M.; Al Jawhari, M.; Hempel, W.M.; et al. Independent mechanisms lead to genomic instability in hodgkin lymphoma: Microsatellite or chromosomal instability. *Cancers* **2018**, *10*, 233. [CrossRef] [PubMed]
35. Quintela-Fandino, M.; Soberon, N.; Lluch, A.; Manso, L.; Calvo, I.; Cortes, J.; Moreno-Antón, F.; Gil-Gil, M.; Martinez-Jánez, N.; Gonzalez-Martin, A.; et al. Critically short telomeres and toxicity of chemotherapy in early breast cancer. *Oncotarget* **2017**, *8*, 21472–21482. [CrossRef]
36. Savage, S.A. Beginning at the ends: Telomeres and human disease. *F1000Research* **2018**, *7*, F1000. [CrossRef]
37. Girinsky, T.; M'kacher, R.; Lessard, N.; Koscielny, S.; Elfassy, E.; Raoux, F.; Carde, P.; Santos, M.D.; Margainaud, J.P.; Sabatier, L.; et al. Prospective coronary heart disease screening in asymptomatic Hodgkin lymphoma patients using coronary computed tomography angiography: Results and risk factor analysis. *Int. J. Radiat. Oncol. Biol. Phys.* **2014**, *89*, 59–66. [CrossRef]
38. Calado, R.T.; Yewdell, W.T.; Wilkerson, K.L.; Regal, J.A.; Kajigaya, S.; Stratakis, C.A.; Young, N.S. Sex hormones, acting on the TERT gene, increase telomerase activity in human primary hematopoietic cells. *Blood* **2009**, *114*, 2236–2243. [CrossRef]
39. Bär, C.; Huber, N.; Beier, F.; Blasco, M.A. Therapeutic effect of androgen therapy in a mouse model of aplastic anemia produced by short telomeres. *Haematologica* **2015**, *100*, 1267–1274. [CrossRef]
40. Khincha, P.P.; Bertuch, A.A.; Gadalla, S.M.; GIRI, N.; Alter, B.P.; Savage, S.A. Similar telomere attrition rates in androgen-treated and untreated patients with dyskeratosis congenita. *Blood Adv.* **2018**, *2*, 1243–1249. [CrossRef]

41. Harley, C.B.; Liu, W.; Blasco, M.; Vera, E.; Andrews, W.H.; Briggs, L.A.; Raffaele, J.M. A natural product telomerase activator as part of a health maintenance program. *Rejuvenation Res.* **2011**, *14*, 45–56. [CrossRef] [PubMed]
42. de Jesus, B.B.; Schneeberger, K.; Vera, E.; Tejera, A.; Harley, C.B.; Blasco, M.A. The telomerase activator TA-65 elongates short telomeres and increases health span of adult/old mice without increasing cancer incidence. *Aging Cell* **2011**, *10*, 604–621. [CrossRef] [PubMed]
43. Vera, E.; Bernardes de Jesus, B.; Foronda, M.; Flores, J.M.; Blasco, M.A. The rate of increase of short telomeres predicts longevity in mammals. *Cell Rep.* **2012**, *2*, 732–737. [CrossRef] [PubMed]
44. Ehrlenbach, S.; Willeit, P.; Kiechl, S.; Willeit, J.; Reindl, M.; Schanda, K.; Kronenberg, F.; Brandstätter, A. Influences on the reduction of relative telomere length over 10 years in the population-based Bruneck Study: Introduction of a well-controlled high-throughput assay. *Int. J. Epidemiol.* **2009**, *38*, 1725–1734. [CrossRef] [PubMed]
45. Whittemore, K.; Vera, E.; Martínez-Nevado, E.; Sanpera, C.; Blasco, M.A. Telomere shortening rate predicts species life span. *Proc. Natl. Acad. Sci. USA* **2019**, *116*, 15122–15127. [CrossRef] [PubMed]
46. Lajoie, V.; Lemieux, B.; Sawan, B.; Lichtensztejn, D.; Lichtensztejn, Z.; Wellinger, R.; Mai, S.; Knecht, H. LMP1 mediates multinuclearity through downregulation of shelterin proteins and formation of telomeric aggregates. *Blood* **2015**, *125*, 2101–2110. [CrossRef]
47. Camitta, B.M.; Thomas, E.D.; Nathan, D.G.; Gale, R.P.; Kopecky, K.J.; Rappeport, J.M.; Santos, G.; Gordon-Smith, E.C.; Storb, R. A prospective study of androgens and bone marrow transplantation for treatment of severe aplastic anemia. *Blood* **1979**, *53*, 504–514. [CrossRef]
48. Wang, P.; Zhang, Z.; Sun, Y.; Liu, X.; Tong, T. The two isomers of HDTIC compounds from *Astragali Radix* slow down telomere shortening rate via attenuating oxidative stress and increasing DNA repair ability in human fetal lung diploid fibroblast cells. *DNA Cell Biol.* **2010**, *29*, 33–39. [CrossRef]
49. Le, A.; Ng, A.; Kwan, T.; Cusmano-Ozog, K.; Cowan, T.M. A rapid, sensitive method for quantitative analysis of underivatized amino acids by liquid chromatography-tandem mass spectrometry (LC-MS/MS). *J. Chromatogr. B Anal. Technol. Biomed. Life Sci.* **2014**, *944*, 166–174. [CrossRef]
50. MassBank of North America Spectrum KO002593 for Canavanine. 2019. Available online: http://mona.fiehnlab.ucdavis.edu/spectra/browse?query=&text=KO002593&size=10 (accessed on 25 July 2019).
51. MassBank of North America Spectrum PB000459 for Asparagine. 2019. Available online: http://mona.fiehnlab.ucdavis.edu/spectra/display/PB000459 (accessed on 25 July 2019).
52. MassBank of North America Spectrum CCMSLIB00003740029 for Glutamic Acid. 2019. Available online: http://mona.fiehnlab.ucdavis.edu/spectra/display/CCMSLIB00003740029 (accessed on 25 July 2019).
53. MassBank of North America Spectrum PR100500 for Sucrose. 2019. Available online: http://mona.fiehnlab.ucdavis.edu/spectra/display/PR100500 (accessed on 25 July 2019).
54. Jiao, J.; Gai, Q.-Y.; Luo, M.; Peng, X.; Zhao, C.J.; Fu, Y.J.; Ma, W. Direct determination of astragalosides and isoflavonoids from fresh *Astragalus membranaceus* hairy root cultures by high speed homogenization coupled with cavitation-accelerated extraction followed by liquid chromatography-tandem mass spectrometry. *RSC Adv.* **2015**, *5*, 34672–34681. [CrossRef]

biomedicines

MDPI

Article

Anti-Inflammatory Effects of Diospyrin on Lipopolysaccharide-Induced Inflammation Using RAW 264.7 Mouse Macrophages

Adnan Shahidullah [1], Ji-Young Lee [2], Young-Jin Kim [2], Syed Muhammad Ashhad Halimi [1], Abdur Rauf [3], Hyun-Ju Kim [2], Bong-Youn Kim [2] and Wansu Park [2,*]

1 Department of Pharmacy, University of Peshawar, Peshawar 25120, Pakistan; adnansuk1@gmail.com (A.S.); ashhad92@gmail.com (S.M.A.H.)

2 College of Korean Medicine, Gachon University, Seong-nam 13120, Korea; oxygen1119@naver.com (J.-Y.L.); godsentry@naver.com (Y.-J.K.); eternity0304@daum.net (H.-J.K.); famous008@daum.net (B.-Y.K.)

3 Department of Chemistry, University of Swabi, Anbar 23561, KPK, Pakistan; mashaljcs@yahoo.com

* Correspondence: pws98@gachon.ac.kr; Tel.: +82-31-750-8821

Received: 24 November 2019; Accepted: 7 January 2020; Published: 11 January 2020

Abstract: Diospyrin is a bisnaphthoquinonoid medicinal compound derived from *Diospyros lotus*, with known anti-cancer, anti-tubercular, and anti-leishmanial activities against *Leishmania donovani*. However, the effects of diospyrin on lipopolysaccharide (LPS)-induced macrophage activation and inflammation are not fully reported. In this study, the anti-inflammatory effects of diospyrin on LPS-induced macrophages were examined. Diospyrin showed no toxicity in RAW 264.7 at concentrations of up to 10 μM. Diospyrin moderated the production of nitric oxide (NO), monocyte chemotactic protein-1, macrophage inflammatory protein-1β, interleukin (IL)-6, IL-10, granulocyte colony-stimulating factor, granulocyte macrophage colony-stimulating factor, vascular endothelial growth factor, leukemia inhibitory factor, and RANTES/CCL5, as well as calcium release in LPS-induced RAW 264.7, at concentrations of up to 10 μM significantly ($p < 0.05$). Diospyrin also significantly inhibited the phosphorylation of p38 mitogen-activated protein kinase (MAPK) and mRNA expression of C/EBP homologous protein (CHOP), as well as tumor necrosis factor receptor superfamily member 6 (Fas), in LPS-induced RAW 264.7 cells at concentrations of up to 10 μM ($p < 0.05$). Diospyrin exhibits anti-inflammatory properties mediated via inhibition of NO, and cytokines in LPS-induced mouse macrophages via the ER-stressed calcium-p38 MAPK/CHOP/Fas pathway.

Keywords: diospyrin; lipopolysaccharide; anti-inflammation; macrophages; nitric oxide; cytokine; calcium; CHOP; Fas; p38 MAPK

---

1. Introduction

Immunity is essential for life. Innate immunity is important in protecting the host against the invasion of pathogenic microorganisms, including viruses, bacteria, fungi, and parasitic protozoa, as well as preventing tumor occurrence. Capone et al. reported that inflammation is an immune and physiological event in response to infection and/or several types of trauma [1]. Warnatsch et al. reported that inflammation is critical against infection, but must be regulated to prevent inflammatory disease [2].

Macrophage is a representative phagocyte. Macrophages are important inflammatory cells implicated in the initiation of inflammatory responses. They play a critical role in the pathogenesis of numerous inflammatory diseases by secreting various pro-inflammatory mediators and pro-inflammatory cytokines [3].

Zhang et al. reported that lipopolysaccharide (LPS) is regarded to be a key factor in the pathogenesis of bacterial sepsis [4].

Cytokine storm is thought to be important in the uncontrolled inflammation, which could be provoked by serious bacterial infections. Till now, treatments for cytokine storm are insufficient in spite of various antibiotics and many new vaccines. Natural compounds sometimes receive attention owing to their nontoxicity and anti-inflammatory activities. With anti-inflammatory effects, the signaling pathway of natural compounds for infections deserves careful study.

Diospyrin (Figure 1), the bisnaphthoquinonoid product derived from the medicinal plant *Diospyros lotus*, is known to exhibit anti-cancer, anti-tubercular, and anti-leishmanial activity against *Leishmania donovani* [5]. However, the effects of diospyrin on LPS-induced macrophages are not fully reported.

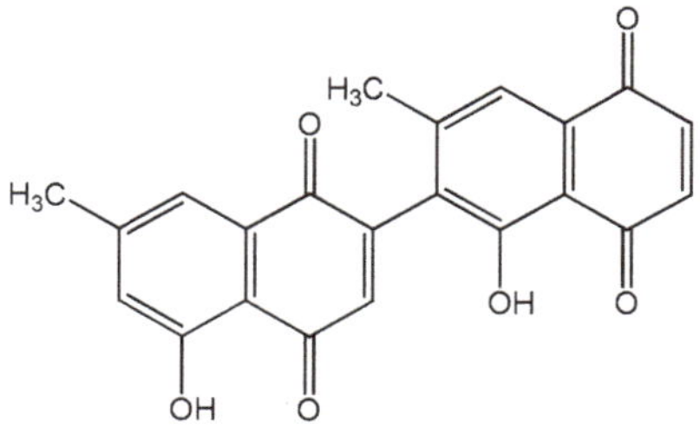

Figure 1. Chemical structure of diospyrin.

In the present study, we investigated the inhibitory effects of diospyrin on LPS-induced inflammation using RAW 264.7 mouse macrophages. Treatment with diospyrin concentrations up to 10 μM significantly modulated the excessive production of inflammatory mediators such as nitric oxide (NO), cytokines, chemokines, and growth factors. It also inhibited calcium release, phosphorylation of p38 mitogen-activated protein kinase (MAPK), and mRNA expression of C/EBP homologous protein (CHOP) and tumor necrosis factor receptor superfamily member 6 (Fas) in LPS-induced RAW 264.7 cells.

2. Materials and Methods

2.1. Materials

Dulbecco's modified Eagle's medium (DMEM), FBS, penicillin, streptomycin, PBS, and other cell culture reagents were purchased from Millipore (Billerica, MA, USA). Diospyrin was isolated from *Diospyros lotus* by Dr. Inamullah Khan. Multiplex cytokine assay kits were purchased from Millipore. The Fluo-4 calcium assay kit was supplied by Molecular Probes (Eugene, OR, USA). Real-time RT-PCR kits were ordered from Bio-Rad (Hercules, CA, USA). Phospho-p38 MAPK Antibody (T180/Y182) (eBioscience 17-9078-42) and Mouse IgG2b kappa Isotype Control (eBioscience 12-4732-81) were obtained from Life Technologies Corporation (Carlsbad, CA, USA). All other solutions for flow cytometric analysis were purchased from Thermo Fisher Scientific (Waltham, MA, USA).

2.2. Cell Viability Assay

RAW 264.7 cell line were obtained from Korea Cell Line Bank (Seoul, Korea). The modified MTT assay was used to evaluate the effect of diospyrin on viability of RAW 264.7 [6].

2.3. Quantification of NO Production

Cell were incubated with compounds for 24 h in 96-well plates and NO level in each well was evaluated using the Griess reagent assay kit (Millipore) according the manufacturer's protocol at 540 nm with a microplate reader (Bio-Rad) [6]. Indomethacin (0.5 μM) was used as a positive control.

2.4. Intracellular Calcium Assay

Cell were incubated with compounds for 18 h in 96-well plates and the intracellular calcium signaling from each well was evaluated using Fluo-4 NW Calcium Assay Kits (Thermo Fisher Scientific) according the manufacturer's protocol by a spectrofluorometer (Dynex, West Sussex, UK), with excitation and emission filters of 485 nm and 535 nm [7]. Indomethacin (0.5 μM) was used as a positive control.

2.5. Cytokines Production

Cell were incubated with materials for 24 h in 96-well plates and productions of various cytokines from each well were evaluated using Multiplex cytokine assay kits (Millipore) and Bio-Plex 200 suspension array system (Bio-Rad) according the manufacturer's protocols [7,8].

2.6. RNA Isolation and Real Time RT-PCR Analysis

Cell were incubated with materials for 18 h in six-well plates and RNA quantity was evaluated with real time RT-PCR analysis using NucleoSpin RNA kit (Macherey-Nagel, Duren, Germany), iScript cDNA Synthesis kit (Bio-Rad), the Experion RNA StdSens Analysis kit (Bio-Rad), iQ SYBR Green Supermix (Bio-Rad), and Experion Automatic Electrophoresis System (Bio-Rad) [8,9]. The target genes are listed in Table 1. The β-actin was used as a reference.

Table 1. Primers used for RT-PCR analysis.

Name [1]	Forward Primer (5′–3′)	Reverse Primer (5′–3′)
CHOP	CCACCACACCTGAAAGCAG	TCCTCATACCAGGCTTCCA
FAS	CGCTGTTTTCCCTTGCTG	CCTTGAGTATGAACTCTTAACTGTGAG
β-actin	CTAAGGCCAACCGTGAAAAG	ACCAGAGGCATACAGGGACA

[1] Primers' names; C/EBP homologous protein (CHOP), first apoptosis signal receptor (FAS), β-actin.

2.7. Flow Cytometry

After 15 min of incubation in six-well plates with compounds, cells were harvested and washed with a flow cytometry staining buffer (Thermo Fisher Scientific, Waltham, MA, USA). The cells were stained with anti-phospho-p38 MAPK antibodies according to the manufacturer's protocol. Prior to antibody staining, cells were fixed and permeabilized using Fix Buffer I (Thermo Fisher Scientific) and Perm Buffer III (Thermo Fisher Scientific), respectively. Stained cells were analyzed on the Attune NxT flow cytometer (Thermo Fisher Scientific). Unstained cells were used as negative gating control. Mouse IgG2b kappa Isotype Control was used to confirm the specificity of ohospho-p38 MAPK antibody. The raw data were analyzed using Attune NxT software (Thermo Fisher Scientific). Baicalein (25 μM) was used as a positive control. In this assay, the concentration of LPS was 0.1 μg/mL because LPS at the concentration of 1 μg/mL caused excessive effects on cellular reaction, which made the evaluation of the signaling pathway difficult.

2.8. Statistical Analysis

Data are presented as mean ± SD. All data were analyzed by one-way analysis of variance test using GraphPad Prism (ver. 4; GraphPad Software, San Diego, CA, USA).

3. Results

3.1. Effect of Diospyrin on Cell Viability

In this study, diospyrin up to a concentration of 10 μM restored the viability of RAW 264.7 cells (Figure 2A). The cell viabilities of RAW 264.7 cells, which were incubated with diospyrin at concentrations of 0.1, 1, 5, and 10 μM/mL for 24 h were 118.84% ± 11.87%, 142.4% ± 17.47%, 147.22% ± 13.28%, and 131.65% ± 8.51%, respectively, of the normal group treated with media only. On the basis of this result, diospyrin concentrations of up to 10 μM were selected for use in subsequent experiments.

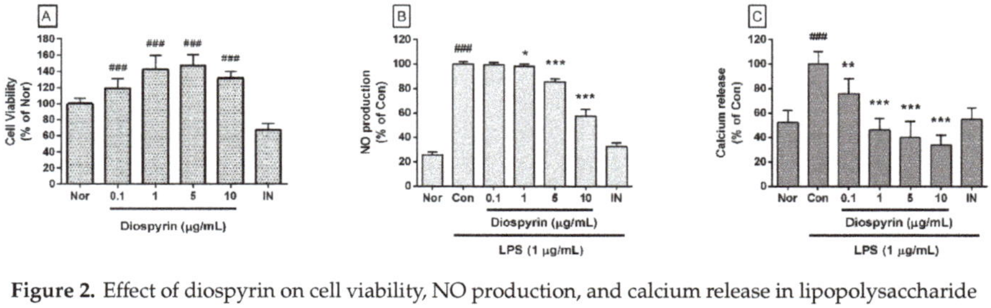

Figure 2. Effect of diospyrin on cell viability, NO production, and calcium release in lipopolysaccharide (LPS)-induced RAW 264.7 cells. After 24 h treatment, cell viability (**A**) was evaluated via a modified MTT assay and nitric oxide (NO) production (**B**) was measured using the Griess reaction assay. Calcium release (**C**) was measured with Fluo-4 calcium assay after 18 h treatment. Data are of mean ± SD and pooled from more than three independent experiments. Nor, normal group (media only); Con, control group (LPS alone); IN, indomethacin (0.5 μM). ### $p < 0.001$ vs. Nor; * $p < 0.05$ vs. Con; ** $p < 0.01$ vs. Con; *** $p < 0.001$ vs. Con.

3.2. *Effect of Diospyrin on NO Production*

Diospyrin significantly inhibited the excessive production of NO in LPS-induced RAW 264.7 cells (Figure 2B). Percentages of NO production in LPS-induced RAW 264.7 cells incubated with diospyrin at concentrations of 0.1, 1, 5, and 10 μM for 24 h were 99.15% ± 2.12%, 97.94% ± 2.11%, 85.76% ± 2.5%, and 57.35% ± 5.74%, respectively, of the control group treated with LPS only.

3.3. *Effect of Diospyrin on Intracellular Calcium Release*

In the present study, diospyrin significantly inhibited the calcium release in LPS-induced RAW 264.7 cells (Figure 2C). Percentages of calcium release in LPS-induced RAW 264.7 cells incubated with diospyrin at concentrations of 0.1, 1, 5, and 10 μM for 18 h were 75.84% ± 11.98%, 46.06% ± 9.44%, 39.5% ± 13.49%, and 33.63% ± 8.18%, respectively, of the control group treated with LPS alone.

3.4. *Effect of Diospyrin on Cytokine Production*

In the present study, diospyrin significantly reduced the excessive synthesis of monocyte chemotactic protein (MCP)-1, macrophage inflammatory protein (MIP)-1β, granulocyte colony-stimulating factor (G-CSF), granulocyte macrophage colony-stimulating factor (GM-CSF), vascular endothelial growth factor (VEGF), RANTES/CCL5, leukemia inhibitory factor (LIF; IL-6 class cytokine), interleukin (IL)-6, and IL-10 in LPS-induced RAW 264.7 cells (Figure 3). In detail, the production of MCP-1 in LPS-induced RAW 264.7 cells incubated with diospyrin at concentrations of 1, 5, and 10 μM for 24 h were 73.02% ± 13.18%, 57.02% ± 9.51%, and 61.22% ± 11.23%, respectively, of the control group treated with LPS only. The levels of MIP-1β were 97.11% ± 0.84%, 95.24% ± 1.3%, and 67.74% ± 8.73%, respectively. The levels of IL-10 following treatment with the three different concentrations of diospyrin were 78.56% ± 13.8%, 28.81% ± 10.48%, and 11.32% ± 3.87%, respectively. The levels of IL-6, G-CSF, GM-CSF, VEGF, LIF, and RANTES, following exposure to the three different concentrations of diospyrin, were as follows: 100.94% ± 1.16%, 46.37% ± 5.6%, and 4.94% ± 1.56%; 97.55% ± 1.78%, 96.19% ± 1.04%, and 43.51% ± 12.16%; 86.56% ± 8.86%, 7.15% ± 2.96%, and 1.12% ± 0.5%; 98.28% ± 3.11%, 35.78% ± 3.16%, and 21.55% ± 2.64%; 102.46% ± 4.75%, 32.2% ± 5.12%, and 4.81% ± 1.13%; and 102.55% ± 4.47%, 81.13% ± 6.81%, and 21.08% ± 5.4%, respectively.

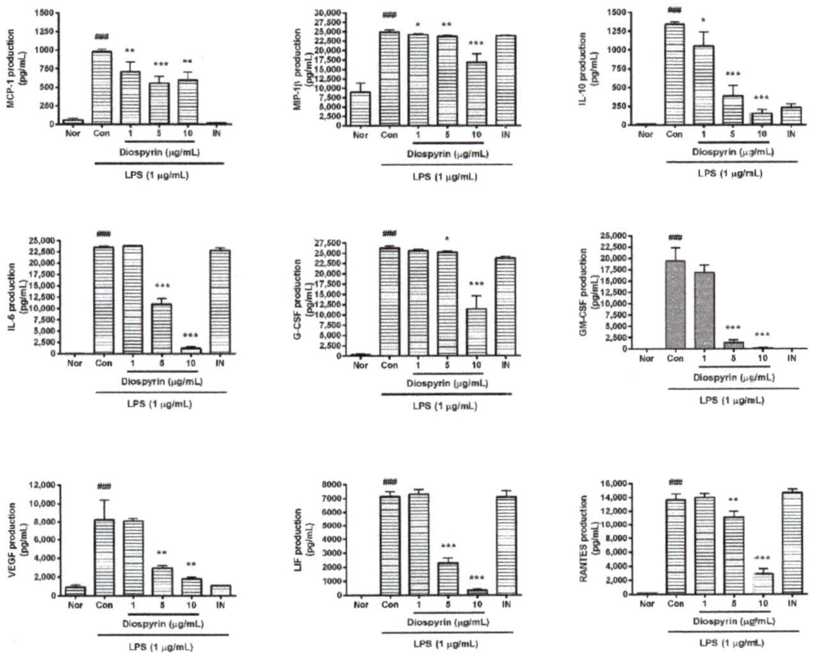

Figure 3. Effect of diospyrin on production of monocyte chemotactic protein (MCP)-1, macrophage inflammatory protein (MIP)-1β, granulocyte colony-stimulating factor (G-CSF), granulocyte macrophage colony-stimulating factor (GM-CSF), vascular endothelial growth factor (VEGF), RANTES/CCL5, leukemia inhibitory factor (LIF; IL-6 class cytokine), interleukin (IL)-6, and IL-10 in LPS-stimulated RAW 264.7. Data are of mean ± SD and pooled from more than three independent experiments. Nor, normal group (media only); Con, control group (LPS alone); IN, indomethacin (0.5 μM). ### $p < 0.001$ vs. Nor; * $p < 0.05$ vs. Con; ** $p < 0.01$ vs. Con; *** $p < 0.001$ vs. Con.

3.5. Effect of Diospyrin on mRNA Expression of CHOP and Fas

In the present study, diospyrin significantly inhibited mRNA expression of CHOP and Fas in LPS-induced RAW 264.7 cells (Figure 4). In detail, the levels of mRNA expression of CHOP in LPS-induced RAW 264.7 cells incubated with diospyrin at concentrations of 1, 5, and 10 μM for 18 h were 60.19% ± 7.79%, 3.1% ± 0.18%, and 1.71% ± 0.09%, respectively, of the control group treated with LPS only (Figure 4A), and the corresponding levels of Fas mRNA were 18.9% ± 3.54%, 12.69% ± 2.92%, and 2.86% ± 0.51%, respectively (Figure 4B). The data suggest that diospyrin inhibits calcium release from endoplasmic reticulum stores and the inflammatory reaction in LPS-induced mouse macrophages via calcium-CHOP/Fas pathway.

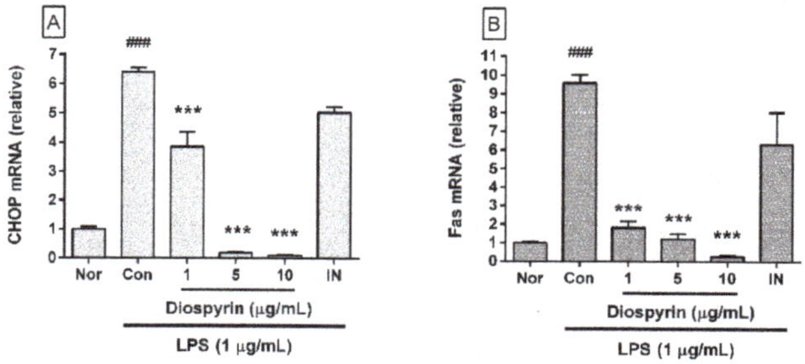

Figure 4. Effect of diospyrin on mRNA expression of C/EBP homologous protein (CHOP) (**A**) and Fas (**B**) in LPS-induced RAW 264.7 were measured with real-time RT-PCR after 18 h incubation with compounds. β-actin was used as the housekeeping gene. Nor, normal group (media only); Con, control group (LPS alone). IN denotes indomethacin (0.5 μM). Values are the mean ± SD of three independent experiments. ### $p < 0.001$ vs. Nor; *** $p < 0.001$ vs. Con.

3.6. Effect of Diospyrin on Phosphorylation of p38 MAPK

In the present study, diospyrin significantly inhibited the phosphorylation of p38 MAPK in LPS-induced RAW 264.7 cells (Figure 5). The phosphorylation of p38 MAPK in LPS-induced RAW 264.7 cells incubated with diospyrin at concentrations of 1, 5, and 10 μM for 15 min were 94.76% ± 2.14%, 84.67% ± 1.66%, and 77.77% ± 4.2%, respectively of the control group treated with LPS (0.1 μg/mL) only (Figure 5). The data suggest that diospyrin modulates the inflammatory reaction in LPS-induced mouse macrophages via p38 MAPK pathway.

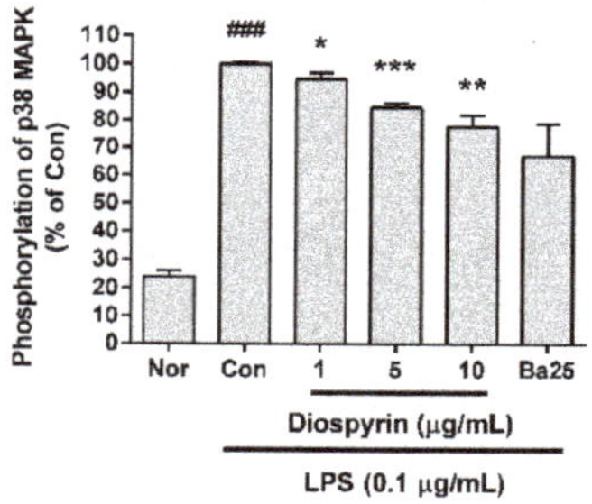

Figure 5. Effect of diospyrin on the phosphorylation of p38 MAPK in LPS-induced RAW 264.7 cells. After 15 min of treatment, the phosphorylation of p38 MAPK was measured via flow cytometry. The normal group (Nor) was treated with media only. The control group (Con) was treated with LPS (0.1 μg/mL) alone. Ba25 denotes baicalein (25 μM). Values are the mean ± SD of three independent experiments. ### $p < 0.001$ vs. Nor; * $p < 0.05$ vs. Con; ** $p < 0.01$ vs. Con; *** $p < 0.001$ vs. Con.

4. Discussion

Various bioactivities of diospyrin such as anti-cancer and anti-leishmanial effects have been reported [5]. However, the effects of diospyrin on LPS-induced macrophages have yet to be fully reported.

Macrophages and monocytes are important mediators of innate reaction and inflammation against pathogenic bacterial infection [6–10]. Ferret et al. reported that macrophages and their circulating form monocytes mediate innate immunity and inflammatory reactions by presenting foreign antigens and scavenging dead cells [11]. Medina et al. reported that macrophages produce various inflammatory mediators such as cytokines and NO in the immune activity [12].

LPS, the main component of outer membrane of Gram-negative bacteria, has been shown to induce infection, inflammation, or tissue damage, as well as mediate inflammatory responses via MAPK pathway such as p38 MAPK and extracellular signal-regulated protein kinases (ERK) [13].

Lechner et al. reported that NO plays an important role in numerous physiological and pathophysiological conditions [14]. Thiemermann et al. reported that the expression of inducible nitric-oxide synthase and the production of large quantities of NO may contribute to the pathophysiology of endotoxemia or sepsis [15]. Evans et al. reported that excessive production of NO may be responsible, at least in part, for the hypotension associated with septic shock [16]. The current data show that diospyrin exerts inhibitory effects on the production of NO in LPS-induced RAW 264.7. Thus, diospyrin might be a candidate for modulating septic shock.

Kankkunen et al. reported that inflammasome is an intracellular molecular mediator of innate immunity in inflammation [17]. Martin et al. reported that inflammasomes are multiprotein complexes that activate caspase-1 in response to infections and stress, resulting in the secretion of pro-inflammatory cytokines [18], doi et al. reported that the activated macrophages produce pro-inflammatory cytokines such as MCP-1 [19]. Pavel et al. reported that cytokines regulate the immune response to infection by binding to cytokine receptors on the plasma membrane [20]. Gadient and Patterson reported that, in addition to the systemic acute phase reaction, IL-6 and LIF are associated with several acute and chronic inflammatory diseases, including rheumatoid arthritis and bacterial meningitis [21]. Ruddy et al. reported that the levels of various cytokines such as MCP-1, G-CSF, GM-CSF, and IP-10 are increased in bronchoalveolar fluid and the lung tissue of pneumococcal pneumonia during lung inflammation [22]. Capelli et al. reported that MCP-1 and MIP-1β levels are significantly increased in patients with chronic bronchitis [23]. Zhu et al. reported that the marked upregulation of RANTES in the epithelium and subepithelium exacerbates bronchitis [24]. Coussens and Werb reported that the tumor microenvironment, which is largely orchestrated by inflammatory cells, plays an indispensable role in the neoplastic transformation, proliferation, survival, and migration of cancer cells [25]. Kyama et al. have already reported that IL-6 and VEGF induce the development of endometriosis via excessive endometrial angiogenesis [26]. Appelmann et al. have also reported that VEGF overexpression has been linked to different types of malignancies and tumors [27]. Meanwhile, Dace et al. reported that IL-10, although traditionally considered as an anti-inflammatory cytokine, also contributes to the pathobiology of autoimmune diseases [28]. Meanwhile it could be recommended to investigate levels of cytokines simultaneously using pathogen-like molecules because cytokines are various. In this study, the data represent that diospyrin moderates excessive productions of inflammatory mediators such as MCP-1, MIP-1β, IL-6, IL-10, G-CSF, GM-CSF, VEGF, LIF, and RANTES in LPS-induced RAW 264.7. This means that diospyrin could be applied to treat bacterial infectious diseases such bacterial pneumonia and bacterial meningitis. In the addition, the current results mean that diospyrin might be effective to alleviate cytokine storm caused by bacterial infection. Cytokine storm is regarded as a serious and uncontrolled increase of cytokines' level in the blood of infectious patients. Till now, treatments for cytokine storm are insufficient. Thus, diospyrin could be one of candidates for treating the uncontrolled cytokine storm revoked by bacterial infections.

Stout et al. reported that the ER calcium stores are reduced and intracellular calcium concentration is increased initially during the inflammation cascade [29]. Tabas et al. reported that the death receptor Fas is activated by CHOP, which amplifies the release of calcium from ER stores into the cytosol in ER-stressed macrophage [30]. Interestingly, Wang and Ron reported that CHOP was activated by p38 MAPK in the stressed cells [31]. Endo et al. reported that LPS triggers ER stress via overexpression of CHOP and activation of p38 MAPK, which mediates apoptosis in macrophages [32]. It is not easy to establish the MAPK signaling pathway including intracellular calcium release in inflammatory cascade. We focused on the activation of CHOP in RAW 264.7 stimulated by LPS, because CHOP is known to mediate the calcium–Fas–MAPK pathway. In the present study, diospyrin significantly inhibits the production of inflammatory cytokines, calcium release, and mRNA expression of CHOP and Fas in LPS-induced RAW 264.7 cells. Additionally, diospyrin significantly inhibited the phosphorylation of p38 MAPK in LPS-induced RAW 264.7 cells. These data suggest that diospyrin modulates LPS-induced macrophage activation via the ER-stressed calcium-p38 MAPK/CHOP/Fas pathway.

5. Conclusions

The present study demonstrates the anti-inflammatory effects of diospyrin via inhibition of NO, MCP-1, MIP-1β, IL-6, IL-10, G-CSF, GM-CSF, VEGF, LIF, and RANTES in LPS-induced macrophages mediated via the ER-stressed calcium-p38 MAPK/CHOP/Fas pathway. Further studies are needed to evaluate the medicinal benefits of diospyrin in inflammatory diseases.

Author Contributions: Conceptualization, A.S., S.M.A.H. and W.P.; methodology, A.R. and W.P.; formal analysis, J.-Y.L., Y.-J.K. and W.P.; investigation, J.-Y.L. and W.P.; resources, A.S. and A.R.; data curation, W.P.; writing—original draft preparation, W.P.; writing—review & editing, H.-J.K. and B.-Y.K.; funding acquisition, W.P. All authors have read and agreed to the published version of the manuscript.

Funding: This study was supported by the Basic Science Research Program through the National Research Foundation of Korea, funded by the Ministry of Education, Science, and Technology (2017R1A2B4004933).

Conflicts of Interest: The authors declare the absence of any conflict of interest. The funders had no role in the design of the study; in the collection, analyses, or interpretation of data; in the writing of the manuscript, or in the decision to publish the results.

References

1. Capone, F.; Guerriero, E.; Colonna, G.; Maio, P.; Mangia, A.; Castello, G.; Costantini, S. Cytokinome Profile Evaluation in Patients with Hepatitis C Virus Infection. *World J. Gastroenterol.* **2014**, *20*, 9261–9269.
2. Warnatsch, A.; Ioannou, M.; Wang, Q.; Papayannopoulos, V. Inflammation. Neutrophil Extracellular Traps License Macrophages for Cytokine Production in Atherosclerosis. *Science* **2015**, *349*, 316–320. [CrossRef]
3. O'Shea, J.J.; Ma, A.; Lipsky, P. Cytokines and Autoimmunity. *Nat. Rev. Immunol.* **2002**, *2*, 37–45. [CrossRef]
4. Zhang, F.X.; Kirschning, C.J.; Mancinelli, R.; Xu, X.P.; Jin, Y.; Faure, E.; Mantovani, A.; Rothe, M.; Muzio, M.; Arditi, M. Bacterial Lipopolysaccharide Activates Nuclear Factor-kappaB through Interleukin-1 Signaling Mediators in Cultured Human Dermal Endothelial Cells and Mononuclear Phagocytes. *J. Biol. Chem.* **1999**, *274*, 7611–7614. [CrossRef]
5. Ray, S.; Hazra, B.; Mittra, B.; Das, A.; Majumder, H.K. Diospyrin, a Bisnaphthoquinone: A Novel Inhibitor of Type I DNA Topoisomerase of Leishmania Donovani. *Mol. Pharmacol.* **1998**, *54*, 994–999. [CrossRef]
6. Yoon, S.B.; Lee, Y.J.; Park, S.K.; Kim, H.C.; Bae, H.; Kim, H.M.; Ko, S.G.; Choi, H.Y.; Oh, M.S.; Park, W. Anti-Inflammatory Effects of ScutellariaBaicalensis Water Extract on LPS-Activated RAW 264.7 Macrophages. *J. Ethnopharmacol.* **2009**, *125*, 286–290. [CrossRef]
7. Lee, J.Y.; Park, W.; Yi, D.K. Immunostimulatory Effects of Gold Nanorod and Silica-Coated Gold Nanorod on RAW 264.7 Mouse Macrophages. *Toxicol. Lett.* **2012**, *209*, 51–57. [CrossRef]
8. Kim, Y.J.; Kim, H.J.; Lee, J.Y.; Kim, D.H.; Kang, M.S.; Park, W. Anti-Inflammatory Effect of Baicalein on Polyinosinic-Polycytidylic Acid-Induced RAW 264.7 Mouse Macrophages. *Viruses* **2018**, *10*, 224. [CrossRef]
9. Kim, Y.J.; Lee, J.Y.; Kim, H.J.; Kim, D.H.; Lee, T.H.; Kang, M.S.; Park, W. Anti-Inflammatory Effects of Angelica Sinensis (Oliv.) Diels Water Extract on RAW 264.7 Induced with Lipopolysaccharide. *Nutrients* **2018**, *10*, 647. [CrossRef]
10. Lee, J.Y.; Park, W. Anti-Inflammatory Effect of Wogonin on RAW 264.7 Mouse Macrophages Induced with Polyinosinic-Polycytidylic Acid. *Molecules* **2015**, *20*, 6888–6900. [CrossRef]
11. Ferret, P.J.; Soum, E.; Negre, O.; Fradelizi, D. Auto-Protective Redox Buffering Systems in Stimulated Macrophages. *BMC Immunol.* **2002**, *3*, 3.
12. Medina, E.A.; Morris, I.R.; Berton, M.T. Phosphatidylinositol 3-Kinase Activation Attenuates the TLR2-Mediated Macrophage Proinflammatory Cytokine Response to FrancisellaTularensis Live Vaccine Strain. *J. Immunol.* **2010**, *185*, 7562–7572. [CrossRef]
13. Zong, Y.; Sun, L.; Liu, B.; Deng, Y.S.; Zhan, D.; Chen, Y.L.; He, Y.; Liu, J.; Zhang, Z.J.; Sun, J.; et al. Resveratrol Inhibits LPS-Induced MAPKs Activation Via Activation of the Phosphatidylinositol 3-Kinase Pathway in Murine RAW 264.7 Macrophage Cells. *PLoS ONE* **2012**, *7*, e44107. [CrossRef]
14. Lechner, M.; Lirk, P.; Rieder, J. Inducible Nitric Oxide Synthase (iNOS) in Tumor Biology: The Two Sides of the Same Coin. *Semin. Cancer Biol.* **2005**, *15*, 277–289. [CrossRef]

15. Thiemermann, C.; Vane, J. Inhibition of Nitric Oxide Synthesis Reduces the Hypotension Induced by Bacterial Lipopolysaccharides in the Rat in Vivo. *Eur. J. Pharmacol.* **1990**, *182*, 591–595. [CrossRef]
16. Evans, T.; Carpenter, A.; Kinderman, H.; Cohen, J. Evidence of Increased Nitric Oxide Production in Patients with the Sepsis Syndrome. *Circ. Shock* **1993**, *41*, 77–81.
17. Kankkunen, P.; Välimäki, E.; Rintahaka, J.; Palomäki, J.; Nyman, T.; Alenius, H.; Wolff, H.; Matikainen, S. TrichotheceneMycotoxins Activate NLRP3 Inflammasome through a P2X 7 Receptor and Src Tyrosine Kinase Dependent Pathway. *Hum. Immunol.* **2014**, *75*, 134–140. [CrossRef]
18. Martin, B.N.; Wang, C.; Willette-Brown, J.; Herjan, T.; Gulen, M.F.; Zhou, H.; Bulek, K.; Franchi, L.; Sato, T.; Alnemri, E.S. IKKα Negatively Regulates ASC-Dependent Inflammasome Activation. *Nat. Commun.* **2014**, *5*, 4977. [CrossRef]
19. Doi, T.; Doi, S.; Nakashima, A.; Ueno, T.; Yokoyama, Y.; Kohno, N.; Masaki, T. Mizoribine Ameliorates Renal Injury and Hypertension Along with the Attenuation of Renal Caspase-1 Expression in Aldosterone-Salt-Treated Rats. *PLoS ONE* **2014**, *9*, e93513. [CrossRef]
20. Pavel, M.A.; Lam, C.; Kashyap, P.; Salehi-Najafabadi, Z.; Singh, G.; Yu, Y. Analysis of the Cell Surface Expression of Cytokine Receptors using the Surface Protein Biotinylation Method. *Methods Mol. Biol.* **2014**, *1172*, 185–192.
21. Gadient, R.A.; Patterson, P.H. Leukemia Inhibitory Factor, Interleukin 6, and Other Cytokines using the GP130 Transducing Receptor: Roles in Inflammation and Injury. *Stem Cells* **1999**, *17*, 127–137. [CrossRef] [PubMed]
22. Ruddy, M.J.; Shen, F.; Smith, J.B.; Sharma, A.; Gaffen, S.L. Interleukin-17 Regulates Expression of the CXC Chemokine LIX/CXCL5 in Osteoblasts: Implications for Inflammation and Neutrophil Recruitment. *J. Leukocyte Biol.* **2004**, *76*, 135–144. [CrossRef] [PubMed]
23. Capelli, A.; Di Stefano, A.; Gnemmi, I.; Balbo, P.; Cerutti, C.; Balbi, B.; Lusuardi, M.; Donner, C. Increased MCP-1 and MIP-1β in Bronchoalveolar Lavage Fluid of Chronic Bronchitics. *Eur. Respir. J.* **1999**, *14*, 160–165. [CrossRef] [PubMed]
24. Zhu, J.; Qiu, Y.S.; Majumdar, S.; Gamble, E.; Matin, D.; Turato, G.; Fabbri, L.M.; Barnes, N.; Saetta, M.; Jeffery, P.K. Exacerbations of Bronchitis: Bronchial Eosinophilia and Gene Expression for Interleukin-4, Interleukin-5, and Eosinophil Chemoattractants. *Am. J. Respir. Crit. Care Med.* **2001**, *164*, 109–116. [CrossRef] [PubMed]
25. Coussens, L.M.; Werb, Z. Inflammation and Cancer. *Nature* **2002**, *420*, 860–867. [CrossRef] [PubMed]
26. Kyama, C.; Mihalyi, A.; Simsa, P.; Mwenda, J.; Tomassetti, C.; Meuleman, C.; D'Hooghe, T. Non-Steroidal Targets in the Diagnosis and Treatment of Endometriosis. *Curr. Med. Chem.* **2008**, *15*, 1006–1017. [CrossRef]
27. Appelmann, I.; Liersch, R.; Kessler, T.; Mesters, R.M.; Berdel, W.E. Angiogenesis inhibition in cancer therapy: Platelet-derived growth factor (PDGF) and vascular endothelial growth factor (VEGF) and their receptors: Biological functions and role in malignancy. *Recent Results Cancer Res.* **2010**, *180*, 51–81.
28. Dace, D.S.; Khan, A.A.; Stark, J.L.; Kelly, J.; Cross, A.H.; Apte, R.S. Interleukin-10 Overexpression Promotes Fas-Ligand-Dependent Chronic Macrophage-Mediated Demyelinating Polyneuropathy. *PLoS ONE* **2009**, *4*, e7121. [CrossRef]
29. Stout, B.A.; Melendez, K.; Seagrave, J.; Holtzman, M.J.; Wilson, B.; Xiang, J.; Tesfaigzi, Y. STAT1 Activation Causes Translocation of Bax to the Endoplasmic Reticulum during the Resolution of Airway Mucous Cell Hyperplasia by IFN-Gamma. *J. Immunol.* **2007**, *178*, 8107–8116. [CrossRef]
30. Tabas, I.; Seimon, T.; Timmins, J.; Li, G.; Lim, W. Macrophage Apoptosis in Advanced Atherosclerosis. *Ann. N.Y. Acad. Sci.* **2009**, *1173* (Suppl. 1), E40. [CrossRef]
31. Wang, X.Z.; Ron, D. Stress-Induced Phosphorylation and Activation of the Transcription Factor CHOP (GADD153) by p38 MAP Kinase. *Science* **1996**, *272*, 1347–1349. [CrossRef] [PubMed]
32. Endo, M.; Mori, M.; Akira, S.; Gotoh, T. C/EBP Homologous Protein (CHOP) is Crucial for the Induction of Caspase-11 and the Pathogenesis of Lipopolysaccharide-Induced Inflammation. *J. Immunol.* **2006**, *176*, 6245–6253. [CrossRef] [PubMed]

biomedicines

MDPI

Review

Implications of Breast Cancer Chemotherapy-Induced Inflammation on the Gut, Liver, and Central Nervous System

Taurean Brown [1,2,3], DeLawrence Sykes [4] and Antiño R. Allen [1,2,3,*]

1 Division of Radiation Health, University of Arkansas for Medical Sciences, Little Rock, AR 72205, USA; TBrown8@uams.edu
2 Department of Pharmaceutical Sciences, University of Arkansas for Medical Sciences, Little Rock, AR 72205, USA
3 Department of Neurobiology & Developmental Sciences, University of Arkansas for Medical Sciences, Little Rock, AR 72205, USA
4 Department of Biology, Pomona College, Claremont, CA 91711, USA; delawerence.sykes@pomona.edu
* Correspondence: aallen@uams.edu; Tel.: +1-501-686-7335

Abstract: Breast Cancer is still one of the most common cancers today; however, with advancements in diagnostic and treatment methods, the mortality and survivorship of patients continues to decrease and increase, respectively. Commonly used treatments today consist of drug combinations, such as doxorubicin and cyclophosphamide; docetaxel, doxorubicin, and cyclophosphamide; or doxorubicin, cyclophosphamide, and paclitaxel. Although these combinations are effective at destroying cancer cells, there is still much to be understood about the effects that chemotherapy can have on normal organ systems such as the nervous system, gastrointestinal tract, and the liver. Patients can experience symptoms of cognitive impairments or "chemobrain", such as difficulty in concentrating, memory recollection, and processing speed. They may also experience gastrointestinal (GI) distress symptoms such as diarrhea and vomiting, as well as hepatotoxicity and long term liver damage. Chemotherapy treatment has also been shown to induce peripheral neuropathy resulting in numbing, pain, and tingling sensations in the extremities of patients. Interestingly, researchers have discovered that this array of symptoms that cancer patients experience are interconnected and mediated by the inflammatory response.

Keywords: cyclophosphamide; doxorubicin; docetaxel; paclitaxel

Citation: Brown, T.; Sykes, D.; Allen, A.R. Implications of Breast Cancer Chemotherapy-Induced Inflammation on the Gut, Liver, and Central Nervous System. *Biomedicines* **2021**, *9*, 189. https://doi.org/10.3390/biomedicines9020189

Academic Editor: Juan Gambini

Received: 15 December 2020
Accepted: 10 February 2021
Published: 13 February 2021

1. Introduction

Breast cancer is one of the most common cancers in the world and one of the leading causes of mortality among women worldwide [1]. Although incidences of breast cancer are increasing in countries such as the United States, related mortality continues to decrease, and survivorship continues to increase [1]. In 1975, the breast cancer death rate for women aged 30 to 79 was 48.3 deaths per 100,000 women; however, by the year 2000, the breast cancer death rate dropped to 38.0 deaths per 100,000 women [2]. In the year 2010, the average annual percentage change for breast cancer related deaths decreased by 2.9 percent and this trend is expected to continue well on into the year 2030 [3]. These recent trends are largely due to improved prevention, detection, and treatment methods over the last several decades. However, despite these positive trends in survivorship, we are still trying to understand the implications of current treatment methods on the long-term health and quality of life of breast cancer patients.

One of the oldest and most commonly used treatment methods for breast cancer and cancer, in general, is chemotherapy. Using chemotherapy to treat cancer has a long history that has its underpinnings in the 1940s, based on observations made previously during the First World War. Mustard gas, which had been used as a biological weapon, was observed to reduce white blood cell counts in soldiers, and consequently, scientists theorized that this agent could be used to treat cancer. As a result, experiments began to assess the ability of mustard agents to treat lymphoma bearing mice [4,5]. Upon noticeable regressions of the lymphoma in the mice, a less volatile form of mustard gas (mustine) was used to treat a human patient with non-Hodgkin's lymphoma with some limited success [6]. In the decades following, chemotherapy garnered skepticism as methods such as surgery and radiotherapy were prioritized for treating cancer; however, with the eventual plateau of cure rates by these other methods and the continued development of chemotherapy treatments, chemotherapy soon began to develop into what we know today.

Breast cancer was largely responsible for the resurgence of the use of chemotherapy both in conjunction with and after surgery. In the 1970s, chemotherapy was adapted for breast cancer with the first reports of the efficacy of combining cyclophosphamide, methotrexate, and fluorouracil (CMF) as an adjuvant treatment [4,5]. This discovery was important not only for the management of breast cancer but also for the practice of implementing drug combinations into cancer treatment as a supplement to surgery. Although the use of anthracycline agents (doxorubicin) to treat metastatic breast cancer was described in the 1960s, it was only in the 1990s that the combination of doxorubicin and cyclophosphamide (AC) became a standard treatment regimen in breast cancer treatment [7,8]. The rationale for introducing anthracyclines in breast cancer treatment was to reduce the duration of treatment, the number of hospital visits, nausea, and to improve the efficacy of CMF treatment [9]. Development of taxanes similarly began in the 1970s; however, the inclusion of drugs such as paclitaxel and docetaxel in combination with anthracycline treatments did not occur until the late 1990s and early 2000s [10–14]. The addition of taxanes in conjunction with AC treatment has been shown to significantly improve the efficacy of treatment and the overall survival among women with breast cancer compared to just AC alone [14,15].

Today, the most commonly used breast cancer treatments consist of one of two combination treatments: docetaxel (Taxotere), doxorubicin (Adriamycin), and cyclophosphamide (TAC) or doxorubicin, cyclophosphamide, and paclitaxel (Taxol) (AC-T). Despite the substantial evidence for the effectiveness of these combinations in treating breast cancer, much is still unknown about the long-term implications of these treatment methods on patient health. A prime example of this is the phenomenon of chemotherapy-induced cognitive impairment colloquially known as "chemobrain." Chemobrain is defined by the experience of cognitive deficits such as impaired processing speed, memory retention, and concentration after or during chemotherapy treatment. Currently, the mechanisms behind the neurobiological damage that induces chemobrain are still not fully understood. Recent research has provided evidence to suggest that the inflammation response plays an essential role in chemotherapy-induced behavioral comorbidities as well as a host of other neurological disorders [16]. In this review, we will discuss the relationship between breast cancer chemotherapy-induced inflammation and the central and peripheral nervous systems with a particular focus on the effect of peripheral-organ inflammation on neurological outcomes. Additionally, we will discuss a few current potential anti-inflammatory therapeutic options that may help attenuate neurological deficits inflicted by breast cancer chemotherapy.

2. Chemobrain and Inflammation: What Is the Connection?

Chemobrain is a condition in cancer patients described as cognitive impairment or decline following chemotherapy treatment. Initial concerns over the cognitive deficits associated with chemotherapeutics began as early as the late 1950s and accelerated in the 1980s as more evidence for this condition was identified [17,18]. Over the last 40 years, chemobrain has remained a concern in cancer patients as evidenced by the continued research on the phenomenon [19]. It is estimated that between 13% and 78% of breast cancer patients report experiencing measurable cognitive impairment both during and after chemotherapy treatment [20–22]. Typically, most breast cancer patients report a wide range of cognitive impairment, which includes deficits in memory retention, executive function, reaction time, and processing speed. Longitudinal studies have also shown that chemobrain symptoms can persist as long as 2 to 20 years after chemotherapy treatment [23–27]. Similar behavioral deficits have been observed in animal models. For example, several studies using the Y-maze spontaneous alternation task have observed deficits in short-term memory in rodent models after administration of both cyclophosphamide and doxorubicin [28,29]. Other studies have assessed short-term memory using the novel object recognition test, which tests a rodent's natural curiosity to investigate novel stimuli, and found a lowered preference score for the novel object in rodents administered a cocktail of CMF [30]. Similarly, impairments in long-term spatial memory have been observed using the Morris Water Maze in rodents that were administered either CMF or AC-T [31,32].

Despite this knowledge, there is currently a lack of understanding of the underlying mechanisms that induce the chemobrain phenotype. The secondary damage that chemotherapeutics can enact on the body and its various organ systems has been well established in the literature. Though they are effective at killing cancer, many current treatments lack the specificity to only attack cancer cells and consequently inflict damage on normal healthy tissue. For example, doxorubicin, a commonly used drug in breast cancer treatment, has long been implicated in inducing cumulative and dose-dependent cardiotoxicity resulting in severe cardiomyopathy or congestive heart failure through mechanisms such as apoptosis, oxidative stress, and mitochondrial damage [33–35].

Unfortunately, the central nervous system (CNS) is not entirely exempt from these untargeted side effects of chemotherapeutics. One innate form of defense the brain has against direct non-targeted tissue damage from chemotherapeutic drugs is the blood–brain barrier (BBB), a microvascular semi-permeable filtration system of the CNS that prevents the passage of pathogens and toxins from the bloodstream into the brain [36]. This normally beneficial barrier can also present an obstacle to the delivery of drugs to the central nervous system, such as in the treatment of brain cancers. To bypass this limitation, several different methods have been developed to increase the permeability of drugs through the BBB [37]. However, in cases where we do not want to directly treat or affect the CNS, such as in breast cancer treatment, we still observe damage or impairments in CNS functions such as chemobrain. Generally, most commonly used breast cancer chemotherapeutics such as doxorubicin and taxanes do not readily cross the BBB with the exception of cyclophosphamide and fluorouracil [38–41]. Since most of these drugs cannot damage the CNS directly, the sustaining damage they inflict comes indirectly through various mechanisms, most notably inflammation.

Inflammation is the body's normal immune response to external damage, pathogens, or chemical or radioactive irritants. The inflammatory response is mediated predominantly by cytokines, small protein signaling molecules responsible for regulating inflammation in response to infection, injury, or wound healing. Cytokine dysregulation and subsequent sustained inflammation is an important factor in many disease states, such as cardiovascular disease, pulmonary disease, cancer, and neurological disorders [42]. Chemotherapy has been implicated in inducing inflammation by disrupting normal cytokine regulation in both human and rodent models as well as inducing monocytic migration to areas of inflammation both within the body and the CNS [43,44]. Migrating monocytes can cluster and produce pro-inflammatory cytokines resulting in dysregulation of normal cytokine production. Cytokine dysregulation is a detrimental feature of cancer treatment, as the chemotherapy can result in damage to all tissues, inflicting sustained damage to normal tissue both directly and indirectly. Recently, researchers have begun to investigate this relationship between peripheral inflammation in various organ systems and the brain to explain the mechanisms behind conditions such as chemobrain. In the next few sections, we will discuss how chemotherapy can induce inflammation in peripheral organs such as the gut and liver and cause neurological comorbidities (Figure 1).

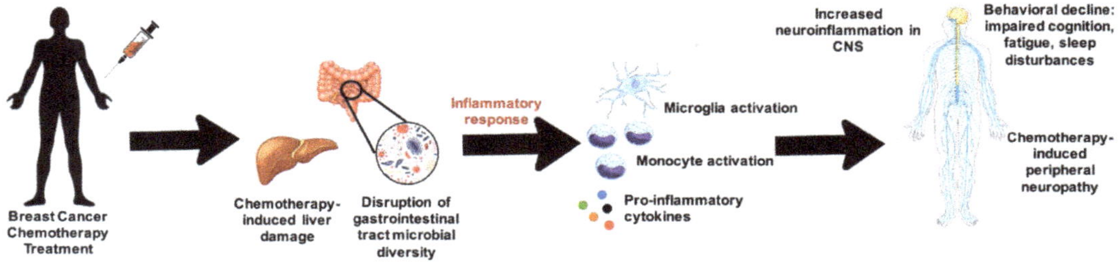

Figure 1. Overview of how breast cancer chemotherapy can damage the liver and disrupt microbial diversity within the gastrointestinal tract and cause inflammatory mediated damage on the nervous system.

3. Gut-Brain Axis and Inflammation

The human gastrointestinal (GI) tract contains a complex ecosystem of microbes estimated to number over 1014 [45]. The microbes that inhabit the GI tract collectively encode 100 times more unique genes than the human genome. These microbes expand on the metabolic capabilities found within the human genome and significantly influence neurology, immunity, endocrinology, disease states, and clinical outcomes [46]. The ability of the CNS to affect the GI tract has long been characterized; however, the ability of the microbiota within the GI tract to impact CNS functioning is a relatively new concept. Links between the microbiota of the GI tract and the brain have been observed in various neurological disorders, such as Parkinson's disease, schizophrenia, autism, depression, anxiety, and Alzheimer's disease [47–50].

The connection between the GI tract and the nervous system are currently explained fundamentally by disruptions in the microbial diversity within the gut. Different microbes existing within the gut produce byproducts that are essential for normal bodily homeostasis as well as regulation of metabolic and immune processes. In cancer patients, chemotherapy often results in the reduction of important microbes within the gut such as the butyrate-producing bacteria Faecalibacterium and Roseburia [51]. Butyrate is a microbial byproduct that has anti-inflammatory properties. The effects of chemotherapy have been examined in numerous animal models. Although rodents have a different microbial composition, a similar pathophysiology can be characterized in mice and humans after chemotherapy, including, crypt ablation, villus blunting, epithelial atrophy of the small and large intestine with accompanied mucosal damage and mucosal degradation [52,53]. One study found that chemotherapeutic drugs increased β-glucuronidase-producing bacteria in a rodent model, causing the reactivation of chemotherapeutics in the GI tract and contributing to intestinal toxicity, mucositis, and diarrhea [54]. Changes in GI microbial composition have also been observed in various neurological conditions. For instance, in a mouse model of Alzheimer's disease, animals had a decrease in Allobaculum and Akkermansia and an increase in Rikenellaceae relative to the wild type control animals [55]. Similar findings were observed in a clinical study that reported notable changes in the microbial diversity in the guts of Alzheimer patients, which was marked by a decrease in Firmicutes and an increase in Bacteroidetes [56]. Chemotherapy has frequently been linked to gastrointestinal complications due to a variety of symptoms in cancer patients such as diarrhea, constipation, and vomiting [57–59]. The severity of these types of symptoms can result in dosage adjustments, delays in treatments, or discontinuation of treatments, causing poor clinical outcomes.

In addition to the disruption of gut microflora, these chemotherapeutic agents can also produce intestinal inflammation. Gastrointestinal inflammation has been implicated extensively as the link between the gut and CNS. One proposed mechanism of action is that decreases in microbial diversity and irritation of the intestinal lining subsequently results in the increased permeability of the intestines. This can result in infiltration of peripheral immune cells into the intestine, causing activation of immune cells and the release of pro-inflammatory cytokines that induce peripheral inflammation as well as neuroinflammation in the brain, resulting in behavioral impairments [60]. Neuroinflammation is one of the primary mechanisms thought to underlie long-term cognitive dysfunction in aging and neurological disorders such as chemobrain [61]. Peripheral cytokines released from the gut and nearby tissue as a result of chemotherapy are thought to travel through the bloodstream, bypassing the BBB, and directly inducing inflammation in brain tissue. Some research even suggests that this prolonged cytokine expression could damage the integrity of the BBB allowing for chemotherapeutic agents to more readily pass and damage brain tissue directly [62]. The gut microbiota have a dual role being both helpful and harmful as a consequence of the dysbiosis caused by chemotherapeutic treatment. Certain clusters can contribute to pathophysiology as a secondary effect of treatment. Chemotherapy induced mucosal inflammation of the gastrointestinal tract, termed mucositis, adversely impacts some intestinal microbes. For example, conventional mice show increased inflammation and higher intestinal epithelial permeability compared to germ free mice post mucositis induction [63]. The increased inflammation and permeability results from an increased number of lesions in the epithelium of conventional mice which ultimately increased susceptibility to the harmful effects of some gut microbes that opt to be facultatively opportunistic. These results provide evidence for the key role that gut microbes play in the development and progression of mucositis.

Gut microbiota complexity is also suspected to either directly or indirectly influence microglia, the immune cells within the CNS. Germ-free mice exhibited impairments in microglial maturation and function that were restored when microbiota or short fatty chain acids were introduced into the mice [64]. In addition to increased cytokine expression, increased microglial activation in brain regions responsible for mood regulation and cognition have been observed in behavioral disorders such as major depression disorder [65,66]. Peripheral cytokine expression induced by chemotherapy is also suspected to induce localized neuroinflammation by stimulating/activating other neuronal cells, such as astrocytes, oligodendrocytes, and neurons resulting in localized cytokine/chemokine release and consequent cognitive impairment [67].

4. Liver-Brain Inflammation Axis

The connection between the liver and the brain is another emerging area of research as is the liver's contribution to chemobrain. The liver is unique in that it services as a barrier between the gut and the body; additionally, peripheral organ centered inflammation changes neural transmission of the CNS thereby altering behavior [68]. Several mechanisms have been elucidated for crosstalk between the liver and the brain, underscoring the role the liver plays in facilitating communication between the brain and the periphery. Such as the GI tract, the connection between the liver and brain is suspected to be mediated by the immune system due to acute liver damage. Chemotherapy-induced hepatotoxicity has long been a concern in cancer treatment. This is because many chemotherapeutic drugs require optimal liver functioning in order to be metabolized, which can consequently induce liver damage. Several common breast cancer drugs, such as methotrexate, doxorubicin, and cyclophosphamide have been cited with various levels of hepatotoxicity [69]. Cyclophosphamide and doxorubicin have also been implicated in causing drug-induced liver injury conditions such as sinusoidal obstruction syndrome [70,71]. Even taxanes such as docetaxel and paclitaxel as well as 5 F-U have been found to induce liver injury through the accumulation of fat globules in hepatocytes [71]. Most chemotherapeutic drugs are lipophilic and are readily taken up by the liver, which can result in irreversible hepatocellular damage through the recruitment of inflammatory cells [69]. Another unique feature of the liver is reflected in the heterogeneous nature of its cellular composition. Roughly 80% of cells in the liver are hepatocytes with the remaining cells consisting of non-parenchymal cells such as intracellular hepatocytes, stellate cells, and Kupffer cells [68]. The liver contains the largest population of Kupffer cells (a type of macrophage) in the body. Liver inflammation is usually characterized by the activation of Kupffer cells and the production of pro-inflammatory cytokines, such as NF-α, IL-1β, and IL-6 [72,73]. The liver's peripheral connection to the brain in the context of inflammation has been described in four different pathways. First, the neural pathway describes the connection between the CNS and the liver via the vagus nerve. The liver is innervated by vagal afferents that can respond to immune mediators such as proinflammatory cytokines [74,75]. Vagal nerve afferents express cytokine receptors in addition to having macrophages within its fibers that can also respond to cytokines, which could directly induce inflammation in the CNS [76]. One study found that induced peripheral inflammation in human subjects resulted in increased activity within an area of the vagus during a high performance word task, which was correlated with increased fatigue [77]. However, recent studies suggest a decreased importance of this pathway in prolonged peripheral inflammation as liver transplants (requires denervation of the liver) in Hepatitis C patients have not been shown to improve long term behavioral outcomes [78]. Second, circulating cytokines released by the liver can also directly interact with receptors on cerebral endothelial cells. TNF-alpha and IL-beta mediated signaling in the liver can induce activation of NF-κB signaling resulting in signal cascade events that can activate immune cells such as microglia within the brain parenchyma inducing inflammation [68,74]. Third, circulating cytokines from the liver can also induce immune responses via circumventricular organs and the choroid plexus, regions of the brain that lack a BBB. Fourth, circulating cytokines from the liver can also trigger monocyte transmigration into the brain in response to the activation of microglia. Once activated microglia can produce the monocyte chemoattractant protein 1(MCP-1), triggering the recruitment of monocytes into the brain resulting in an inflammation cascade event [74]. Whatever the mechanism of action it is evident that chemotherapy induced liver injury is a serious issue that can directly impact other organ systems such as the CNS. Liver induced brain inflammation has also been reported to affect cognitive outcomes and cause many different behavioral comorbidities, such as fatigue, difficulty concentrating, sleep disturbances, or memory impairment [68,79–81].

5. Chemotherapy-Induced Peripheral Neuropathy

In addition to the aforementioned effects on the CNS, chemotherapeutic agents can also affect the sensory, motor, and autonomic functions of the peripheral nervous system (PNS). Chemotherapy-induced peripheral neuropathy (CIPN) is characterized by damage to nerves that control movement and sensory processing for extremities such as the arms, legs, and feet. CIPN usually has a range of symptoms including numbness, tingling, altered touch sensation, spontaneous painful sensations, impaired balance or movement, constipation, and impaired sexual or urinary function [82,83]. CIPN is becoming increasingly more relevant in clinical settings with reported incidences of 68.1% when measured in the first month after chemotherapy, 60.0% at 3 months, and 30.0% at and after 6 months [84,85]. Some risk factors of CIPN in cancer patients can include genetic predisposition, history of smoking, and the overall sum of chemotherapeutics received [84,85]. Several types of chemotherapeutic agents are known to induce CIPN, most notably, taxanes (paclitaxel and docetaxel), which are frequently used within breast cancer treatment [86]. Although docetaxel and paclitaxel are unable to cross the BBB, CIPN is a dose-limiting adverse side effect of treatment [86]. There are several suggested mechanisms believed to contribute to this condition; however, one prime candidate is neuronal damage by way of immune-mediated processes. Chemotherapeutics such as taxanes can induce peripheral inflammation by inducing the release of pro-inflammatory cytokines within tissues affected by the drug. Peripheral cytokine release can then activate immune-associated cells within the CNS (macrophages, monocytes, astrocytes, and microglia) causing neuroinflammation [87,88]. Once activated immune-associated cells of the CNS can cluster and increase levels of pro-inflammatory cytokines, which can result in nociceptor sensitization and hyperexcitability of peripheral neurons [89]. Evidence of this mechanism of action is further supported by a study that showed that CIPN can be prevented in paclitaxel-treated rodents by treatment with an inhibitor of macrophages, monocytes, and microglia [90].

This inflammatory cascade induced by taxanes may also play a role in axon degeneration, which may contribute to the CIPN phenotype [89]. One study found that a decrease in the level of the chemokine MCP and subsequent decreased activation of its receptor C Chemokine Receptor 2 (CCR2) decreases nerve degeneration as well as CIPN-such as behaviors in rodents [91].

6. Therapeutic Strategies for Chemotherapy-Induced Inflammation

The conditions caused by chemotherapy-induced inflammation and damage to the CNS and PNS are all likely multifactorial and involve several of the mechanisms outlined above as well as others not explicitly outlined in this review such as oxidative stress damage. In terms of therapeutic strategies specific to combating chemotherapy-induced inflammation, there are a few options; however, the efficacy of all of these treatments have yet to fully be determined. One strategy that researchers have implemented in order to treat chemotherapy-induced cognitive impairment is to directly target the CNS by manipulating mechanisms involved in neuroinflammation as well as restoring cognitive performance via cognitive strengthening exercises. Ginkgo biloba is one compound that has been used to treat cognitive impairments observed after breast cancer specifically [92]. Ginkgo biloba is a compound isolated from the leaves of the ginkgo tree and has been widely used over the counter for its mental health benefits as well as neuroprotective properties [93]. Ginkgo biloba neuroprotective properties stem from its manipulation of pathways such as Nrf2/HO2 and CRMP2 [94]. Both of these pathways have been implicated in manipulating inflammatory processes such as the recruitment of immune cells to sites of inflammation within the body and CNS [95,96]. Chemotherapy has also been implicated in reducing neurogenesis within the brain via oxidative or inflammatory processes, which has been linked to cognitive impairment due to decreasing in synaptic plasticity. Interestingly, ginkgo biloba has also been shown to induce neurogenesis via the CRMP2 thus this compound may be beneficial if administered simultaneously with chemotherapy treatment [94]. Non-medical approaches such as cognitive therapy for cancer patients have also become increasingly more commonplace to help patients cope with cognitive decline after treatment. This can include behavior training strategies in memory retention, attention span, self-awareness, relaxation, meditation, and computer simulated activities [97–102].

For inflammation induced within the GI tract, one method of treatment is the implementation of prebiotics, probiotics, and postbiotics supplementation. Prebiotics are nondigestible ingredients that support the growth of beneficial bacteria in the GI tract and probiotics are supplements that contain beneficial GI bacteria. Pairing probiotics with cancer treatment has been shown to ease GI issues, intestinal inflammation, and intestinal permeability while increasing the microbial diversity in cancer patients [103]. Probiotics also have been shown to improve behavioral outcomes in clinical trials of patients with depression, anxiety, and Alzheimer's disease [104–107]. There is less research on prebiotic supplementation; however, some studies have shown evidence of improved sleep behaviors and reduction of mood comorbidities in rodents and humans respectively [108,109]. Recently, the potential of metabolite-based therapeutic strategies or "postbiotics" as a method to treat microbial disruptions within the GI tract has been investigated. It is theorized that the intestinal microbiota of the gut impact host physiology through the secretion of small metabolites that modulate intricate cellular functions of the host organism [110–112]. The approach of this therapy is to not specifically target microbial composition in the gut but rather administer or inhibit metabolites in order to counteract the negative side effects of microbiome disruptions [113]. In addition, some studies have implicated the importance of dietary choices and exercise in improving microbiome health and neuronal health [114,115]. For example, alpha linoleic acid (ALA) an omega-3 polyunsaturated acid isolated from plant sources such as walnuts and soybean oil has been well documented in its role in brain development, anti-inflammatory, and antioxidative activities particularly in Alzheimer's models [116,117]. ALA diet supplementation has been noted to improve cognitive performance in Alzheimer's models through the inhibition of pro-inflammatory cytokines as well as decreasing oxidative stress levels [118,119]. Approaching correcting disruptions in microbial communities in the GI tract from these different perspectives could potentially reduce GI tract inflammation induced in chemotherapy treatment and subsequently improve behavioral outcomes of cancer patients.

Anti-inflammatory therapies for liver inflammation are limited; however, there has been some evidence of promise in a few drug treatments. Some studies have investigated the potential of inhibiting the recruitment of monocyte-derived, inflammatory macrophages into the liver with drugs such as cenicriviroc [120–122]. Chrysin has been found in rats to have a protective effect on cyclophosphamide-induced hepatotoxicity, inflammation, and apoptosis [123]. Garlic extract has been shown to have protective effects against hematological alterations, immunosuppression, hepatic oxidative stress, and renal damage in part due to decreasing cytokine levels in serum of rats [124]. Similarly, geraniol has been found to protect against cyclophosphamide-induced hepatotoxicity in rats through mediation of MAPK and PPAR-y signaling pathways by way of reducing inflammation markers [125]. Ganglion is another potential therapeutic option for cyclophosphamide-induced liver hepatotoxicity by activating Nrf2 signaling and consequently attenuating oxidative damage, inflammation, and apoptosis in rats [126]. Ganoderic acid has also been found to attenuate hepatotoxicity by reducing cytokine levels in both serum and livers within mice [127].

As for CIPN there are a few potential therapeutic options. As mentioned earlier, researchers suspect monocytic migration and subsequent inflammation induced by these cells as key contributors of CIPN [44]. As such, researchers have begun to investigate the potential of targeting the receptors of these monocytic cells as well as their chemokine stimulants in order to treat CIPN. However, manipulation of these mechanisms for the purpose of CIPN treatment still remains in the preclinical stage. There is some promise though in other related pathological conditions. Monoclonal antibodies have been used to target colony stimulating factor 1, which is a molecule that regulates the differentiation of macrophages and has been used to treat solid tumors with some success in clinical trials [128]. Another humanized monoclonal antibody against CX3CL1 has been used to clinically treat rheumatoid arthritis and Crohn's disease [129]. Thus, manipulation of monocyte migration processes may be a successful avenue for CIPN treatment. Some other candidate drugs for treatment of CIPN are metformin and minocycline [130–132]. Metformin although widely used as an anti-diabetic drug has been shown to reduce CIPN-such as symptoms (mechanical allodynia) in rodents treated with paclitaxel [133,134]. The anti-inflammatory effect of metformin works by decreasing pro-inflammatory cytokines and suppressing macrophage activity [135]. Minocycline functions similarly by inhibiting the activation of monocytes and decreases the release of pro-inflammatory cytokines [136,137]. One pilot study conducted on breast cancer patients found that administration of the drug did not improve general paclitaxel-induced sensory neuropathy symptoms (numbness, tingling, burning pain), but did decrease the average pain score and fatigue compared to the placebo group [138]. The use of medicinal herbs as a therapeutic approach to CIPN is also a growing area of research. Rosmarinic acid, a compound isolated from the plant rosemary, has also been shown to have anti-inflammatory properties and has been used for centuries to treat inflammatory conditions such as rheumatoid arthritis [139]. Several studies have found rosmarinic acid to be quite effective at attenuating neuropathic pain within rodents via the downregulation of pro-inflammatory markers [140–142]. Cannabinoids are a group of compounds isolated from the Cannabis sativa plant that mediate their effects through cannabinoid receptors and are a novel therapeutic target for inflammation. Δ9-tetrahydrocannabinol (THC) and cannabidiol (CBD) are the two active cannabinoid compounds found within the plant. Cannabinoid receptors such as CB1 and CB2 are predominantly expressed in the brain and on immune cells indicating they may play a useful role in regulating inflammation [143]. There have been a few clinical studies that investigated the effectiveness of THC/CBD sprays as a treatment method for neuropathic pain within cancer patients and have observed measurable reductions in pain of patients [144–146]. Although the clinical efficacy of these treatments is still to be determined they are all certainly great candidates as therapeutic strategies, neuroprotectants, and anti-inflammatory agents for chemotherapy-induced inflammatory organ damage.

7. Conclusions

Breast cancer is still one of the most common cancers and leading cause of mortality due to cancer in women; however, with scientific advancements in treatment and diagnostic methods, the life expectancy of breast cancer patients has improved. Despite improvements in treatment methods, such as chemotherapy, the quality of life of breast cancer patients is still a relevant topic of study as we are still discovering that some common treatments produce long-term side effects on the nervous system such as chemobrain and CIPN. More research is needed to truly understand the complex relationship mediated by the immune system between organ systems such as the GI tract, liver, and the nervous system. Continuing to delineate this complex relationship between these organ systems and the CNS will allow for the discovery of novel therapeutic approaches that will help improve the quality of life of breast cancer patient's post-treatment.

Author Contributions: Writing—original draft preparation, T.B., D.S. and A.R.A.; writing—review and editing, T.B., D.S., A.R.A.; funding acquisition, A.R.A. All authors have read and agreed to the published version of the manuscript.

Funding: This work was supported by Grant under NIH P20 GM109005 (A.R.A.). The funders had no role in study. Approval date: 15 March 2020.

Institutional Review Board Statement: Not applicable.

Informed Consent Statement: Not applicable.

Data Availability Statement: Not applicable.

Conflicts of Interest: The authors declare no conflict of interest.

References

1. Day, S.; Bevers, T.B.; Palos, G.R.; Rodriguez, M.A. American Cancer Society/American Society of Clinical Oncology Breast Cancer Survivorship Care Guideline. *Breast Dis. Year Book Q.* **2016**, *4*, 327–329. [CrossRef]
2. Berry, D.A.; Cronin, K.A.; Plevritis, S.K.; Fryback, D.G.; Clarke, L.; Zelen, M.; Mandelbatt, J.S.; Yakolev, A.Y.; Habbema, D.F.; Feuer, E.J. Effect of screening and adjuvant therapy on mortality from breast cancer. *N. Engl. J. Med.* **2005**, *353*, 1784–1792. [CrossRef]
3. Rahib, L.; Smith, B.D.; Aizenberg, R.; Rosenzweig, A.B.; Fleshman, J.M.; Matrisian, L.M. Projecting cancer incidence and deaths to 2030: The unexpected burden of thyroid, liver, and pancreas cancers in the United States. *Cancer Res.* **2014**, *74*, 2913–2921. [CrossRef]
4. DeVita, V.T., Jr.; Chu, E. A history of cancer chemotherapy. *Cancer Res.* **2008**, *68*, 8643–8653. [CrossRef] [PubMed]
5. Bonadonna, G.; Brusamolino, E.; Valagussa, P.; Rossi, A.; Brugnatelli, L.; Brambilla, C.; De Lena, M.; Tancini, G.; Bajetta, E.; Musumeci, R.; et al. Combination chemotherapy as an adjuvant treatment in operable breast cancer. *N. Engl. J. Med.* **1976**, *294*, 405–410. [CrossRef] [PubMed]
6. Goodman, L.S.; Wintrobe, M.M. Nitrogen mustard therapy; use of methyl-bis (beta-chloroethyl) amine hydrochloride and tris (beta-chloroethyl) amine hydrochloride for Hodgkin's disease, lymphosarcoma, leukemia and certain allied and miscellaneous disorders. *J. Am. Med. Assoc.* **1946**, *132*, 126–132. [CrossRef]
7. Fisher, B.; Brown, A.M.; Dimitrov, N.V.; Poisson, R.; Redmond, C.; Margolese, R.G.; Bowman, D.; Wolmark, N.; Wicerham, D.L.; Kardinal, C.G. Two months of doxorubicin-cyclophosphamide with and without interval reinduction therapy compared with 6 months of cyclophosphamide, methotrexate, and fluorouracil in positive-node breast cancer patients with tamoxifen-nonresponsive tumors: Results from the National Surgical Adjuvant Breast and Bowel Project B-15. *J. Clin. Oncol.* **1990**, *8*, 1483–1496.
8. Bonadonna, G.; Monfardini, S.; De Lena, M.; Fossati-Bellani, F. Clinical evaluation of adriamycin, a new antitumour antibiotic. *Br. Med. J.* **1969**, *3*, 503–506. [CrossRef]
9. Verrill, M. Chemotherapy for early-stage breast cancer: A brief history. *Br. J. Cancer* **2009**, *101*, S2. [CrossRef]

10. Wani, M.C.; Taylor, H.L.; Wall, M.E.; Coggon, P.; McPhail, A.T. Plant antitumor agents. VI. The isolation and structure of taxol, a novel antileukemic and antitumor agent from Taxus brevifolia. *J. Am. Chem. Soc.* **1971**, *93*, 2325–2327. [CrossRef] [PubMed]
11. Mamounas, E.P.; Bryant, J.; Lembersky, B.; Fehrenbacher, L.; Sedlacek, S.M.; Fisher, B.; Wickerham, D.L.; Yothers, G.; Soran, A.; Wolmark, N. Paclitaxel after doxorubicin plus cyclophosphamide as adjuvant chemotherapy for node-positive breast cancer: Results from NSABP B-28. *J. Clin. Oncol.* **2005**, *23*, 3686–3696. [CrossRef]
12. Henderson, I.C.; Berry, D.A.; Demetri, G.D.; Cirrincione, C.T.; Goldstein, L.J.; Martino, S.; Ingle, J.N.; Cooper, M.R.; Hayes, D.F.; Tkaczuk, K.H.; et al. Improved outcomes from adding sequential Paclitaxel but not from escalating Doxorubicin dose in an adjuvant chemotherapy regimen for patients with node-positive primary breast cancer. *J. Clin. Oncol.* **2003**, *21*, 976–983. [CrossRef]
13. Bear, H.D.; Anderson, S.; Smith, R.E.; Geyer, C.E.; Mamounas, E.P.; Fisher, B.; Brown, A.M.; Robidoux, A.; Margolese, R.; Kahlenberg, M.S.; et al. Sequential Preoperative or Postoperative Docetaxel Added to Preoperative Doxorubicin Plus Cyclophosphamide for Operable Breast Cancer: National Surgical Adjuvant Breast and Bowel Project Protocol B-27. *J. Clin. Oncol.* **2006**, *24*, 2019–2027. [CrossRef] [PubMed]
14. Martin, M.; Pienkowski, T.; Mackey, J.; Pawlicki, M.; Guastalla, J.; Weaver, C.; Tomiak, E.; Al-Tweigeri, T.; Chap, L.; Juhos, E.; et al. Adjuvant Docetaxel for Node-Positive Breast Cancer. *N. Engl. J. Med.* **2005**, *352*, 2302–2313. [CrossRef] [PubMed]
15. Watanabe, T.; Kuranami, M.; Inoue, K.; Masuda, N.; Aogi, K.; Ohno, S.; Iwata, H.; Mukai, H.; Uemura, Y.; Ohashi, Y. Comparison of an AC-taxane versus AC-free regimen and paclitaxel versus docetaxel in patients with lymph node-positive breast cancer: Final results of the National Surgical Adjuvant Study of Breast Cancer 02 trial, a randomized comparative phase 3 study. *Cancer* **2017**, *123*, 759–768. [CrossRef] [PubMed]
16. Joshi, G.; Aluise, C.D.; Cole, M.P.; Sultana, R.; Pierce, W.M.; Vore, M.; St, Clair, D.K.; Butterfield, D.A. Alterations in brain antioxidant enzymes and redox proteomic identification of oxidized brain proteins induced by the anti-cancer drug adriamycin: Implications for oxidative stress-mediated chemobrain. *Neuroscience* **2010**, *166*, 796–807. [CrossRef]
17. Silberfarb, P.M.; Philibert, D.; Levine, P.M. Psychosocial aspects of neoplastic disease: II. Affective and cognitive effects of chemotherapy in cancer patients. *Am. J. Psychiatry* **1980**, *137*, 597–601.
18. Silberfarb, P.M. Chemotherapy and cognitive defects in cancer patients. *Annu. Rev. Med.* **1983**, *34*, 35–46. [CrossRef]
19. Moore, H.C.F. An overview of chemotherapy-related cognitive dysfunction, or "chemobrain". *Oncology* **2014**, *28*, 797–804.
20. Ahles, T.A.; Root, J.C.; Ryan, E.L. Cancer- and cancer treatment-associated cognitive change: An update on the state of the science. *J. Clin. Oncol.* **2012**, *30*, 3675–3686. [CrossRef]
21. Ahles, T.A.; Saykin, A.J.; McDonald, B.C.; Li, Y.; Furstenberg, C.T.; Hanscom, B.S.; Mulrooney, T.J.; Schwartz, G.N.; Kaufman, P.A. Longitudinal assessment of cognitive changes associated with adjuvant treatment for breast cancer: Impact of age and cognitive reserve. *J. Clin. Oncol.* **2010**, *28*, 4434–4440. [CrossRef]
22. Wefel, J.S.; Saleeba, A.K.; Buzdar, A.U.; Meyers, C.A. Acute and late onset cognitive dysfunction associated with chemotherapy in women with breast cancer. *Cancer* **2010**, *116*, 3348–3356. [CrossRef]
23. Ahles, T.A.; Saykin, A.J.; Furstenberg, C.T.; Cole, B.; Mott, L.A.; Skalla, K.; Whedon, M.B.; Bivens, S.; Mitchell, T.; Greenberg, E.R.; et al. Neuropsychologic Impact of Standard-Dose Systemic Chemotherapy in Long-Term Survivors of Breast Cancer and Lymphoma. *J. Clin. Oncol.* **2002**, *20*, 485–493. [CrossRef]
24. Saykin, A.J.; Ahles, T.A.; McDonald, B.C. Mechanisms of chemotherapy-induced cognitive disorders: Neuropsychological, pathophysiological, and neuroimaging perspectives. *Semin. Clin. Neuropsychiatry* **2003**, *8*, 201–216.
25. Schagen, S.B.; Muller, M.J.; Boogerd, W.; Rosenbrand, R.M.; van Rhijn, D.; Rodenhuis, S.; Van Dam, F.S. Late effects of adjuvant chemotherapy on cognitive function:a follow-up study in breast cancer patients. *Ann. Oncol.* **2002**, *13*, 1387–1397. [CrossRef] [PubMed]
26. Silverman, D.H.S.; Dy, C.J.; Castellon, S.A.; Lai, J.; Pio, B.S.; Abraham, L.; Waddell, K.; Petersen, L.; Phelps, M.E.; Ganz, P.A. Altered frontocortical, cerebellar, and basal ganglia activity in adjuvant-treated breast cancer survivors 5–10 years after chemotherapy. *Breast Cancer Res. Treat.* **2007**, *103*, 303–311. [CrossRef]
27. Koppelmans, V.; Breteler, M.M.B.; Boogerd, W.; Seynaeve, C.; Gundy, C.; Schagen, S.B. Neuropsychological performance in survivors of breast cancer more than 20 years after adjuvant chemotherapy. *J. Clin. Oncol.* **2012**, *30*, 1080–1086. [CrossRef]
28. Kitamura, Y.; Kanemoto, E.; Sugimoto, M.; Machida, A.; Nakamura, Y.; Naito, N.; Kanzaki, H.; Miyazaki, I.; Asanuma, M.; Sendo, T. Influence of nicotine on doxorubicin and cyclophosphamide combination treatment-induced spatial cognitive impairment and anxiety-like behavior in rats. *Naunyn Schmiedebergs Arch. Pharmacol.* **2017**, *390*, 369–378. [CrossRef] [PubMed]
29. Salas-Ramirez, K.Y.; Bagnall, C.; Frias, L.; Abdali, S.A.; Ahles, T.A.; Hubbard, K. Doxorubicin and cyclophosphamide induce cognitive dysfunction and activate the ERK and AKT signaling pathways. *Behav. Brain Res.* **2015**, *292*, 133–141. [CrossRef] [PubMed]
30. Briones, T.L.; Woods, J. Dysregulation in myelination mediated by persistent neuroinflammation: Possible mechanisms in chemotherapy-related cognitive impairment. *Brain Behav. Immun.* **2014**, *35*, 23–32. [CrossRef] [PubMed]
31. Anderson, J.E.; Trujillo, M.; McElroy, T.; Groves, T.; Alexander, T.; Kiffer, F.; Antiño, A. Early Effects of Cyclophosphamide, Methotrexate, and 5-Fluorouracil on Neuronal Morphology and Hippocampal-Dependent Behavior in a Murine Model. *Toxicol. Sci.* **2020**, *173*, 156–170. [CrossRef]

32. McElroy, T.; Brown, T.; Kiffer, F.; Wang, J.; Byrum, S.D.; Oberley-Deegan, R.E.; Antiño, A. Assessing the Effects of Redox Modifier MnTnBuOE-2-PyP 5+ on Cognition and Hippocampal Physiology Following Doxorubicin, Cyclophosphamide, and Paclitaxel Treatment. *Int. J. Mol. Sci.* **2020**, *21*, 1867. [CrossRef] [PubMed]
33. Zhao, L.; Zhang, B. Doxorubicin induces cardiotoxicity through upregulation of death receptors mediated apoptosis in cardiomyocytes. *Sci. Rep.* **2017**, *7*, 44735. [CrossRef]
34. Koleini, N.; Kardami, E. Autophagy and mitophagy in the context of doxorubicin-induced cardiotoxicity. *Oncotarget* **2017**, *8*, 46663–46680. [CrossRef] [PubMed]
35. Volkova, M.; Russell, R. Anthracycline Cardiotoxicity: Prevalence, Pathogenesis and Treatment. *Curr. Cardiol. Rev.* **2011**, *7*, 214–220. [CrossRef]
36. Daneman, R.; Prat, A. The blood-brain barrier. *Cold Spring Harb. Perspect. Biol.* **2015**, *7*, a020412. [CrossRef] [PubMed]
37. Arvanitis, C.D.; Ferraro, G.B.; Jain, R.K. The blood–brain barrier and blood–tumour barrier in brain tumours and metastases. *Nat. Rev. Cancer* **2020**, *20*, 26–41. [CrossRef] [PubMed]
38. Sardi, I.; la Marca, G.; Cardellicchio, S.; Giunti, L.; Malvagia, S.; Genitori, L.; Massimino, M.; Martino, M.D.; Giovannini, M.G. Pharmacological modulation of blood-brain barrier increases permeability of doxorubicin into the rat brain. *Am. J. Cancer Res.* **2013**, *3*, 424–432. [PubMed]
39. Li, A.-J.; Zheng, Y.-H.; Liu, G.-D.; Liu, W.-S.; Cao, P.-C.; Bu, Z.-F. Efficient delivery of docetaxel for the treatment of brain tumors by cyclic RGD-tagged polymeric micelles. *Mol. Med. Rep.* **2015**, *11*, 3078–3086. [CrossRef]
40. Awad, A.; Stüve, O. Cyclophosphamide in multiple sclerosis: Scientific rationale, history and novel treatment paradigms. *Ther. Adv. Neurol. Disord.* **2009**, *2*, 50–61. [CrossRef]
41. Formica, V.; Leary, A.; Cunningham, D.; Chua, Y.J. 5-Fluorouracil can cross brain-blood barrier and cause encephalopathy: Should we expect the same from capecitabine? A case report on capecitabine-induced central neurotoxicity progressing to coma. *Cancer Chemother. Pharmacol.* **2006**, *58*, 276–278. [CrossRef]
42. Arulselvan, P.; Fard, M.T.; Tan, W.S.; Gothai, S.; Fakurazi, S.; Norhaizan, M.E.; Kumar, S.S. Role of Antioxidants and Natural Products in Inflammation. *Oxid. Med. Cell. Longev.* **2016**, *2016*, 5276130. [CrossRef] [PubMed]
43. Vyas, D.; Laput, G.; Vyas, A.K. Chemotherapy-enhanced inflammation may lead to the failure of therapy and metastasis. *OncoTargets Ther.* **2014**, *7*, 1015–1023. [CrossRef] [PubMed]
44. Montague, K.; Malcangio, M. The Therapeutic Potential of Monocyte/Macrophage Manipulation in the Treatment of Chemotherapy-Induced Painful Neuropathy. *Front. Mol. Neurosci.* **2017**, *10*, 397. [CrossRef] [PubMed]
45. Thursby, E.; Juge, N. Introduction to the human gut microbiota. *Biochem. J.* **2017**, *474*, 1823–1836. [CrossRef]
46. Ervin, S.M.; Ramanan, S.V.; Bhatt, A.P. Relationship Between the Gut Microbiome and Systemic Chemotherapy. *Dig. Dis. Sci.* **2020**, *65*, 874–884. [CrossRef]
47. Foster, J.A.; McVey Neufeld, K.-A. Gut-brain axis: How the microbiome influences anxiety and depression. *Trends Neurosci.* **2013**, *36*, 305–312. [CrossRef]
48. Krajmalnik-Brown, R.; Lozupone, C.; Kang, D.-W.; Adams, J.B. Gut bacteria in children with autism spectrum disorders: Challenges and promise of studying how a complex community influences a complex disease. *Microb. Ecol. Health Dis.* **2015**, *26*, 26914. [CrossRef]
49. Severance, E.G.; Yolken, R.H.; Eaton, W.W. Autoimmune diseases, gastrointestinal disorders and the microbiome in schizophrenia: More than a gut feeling. *Schizophr. Res.* **2016**, *176*, 23–35. [CrossRef]
50. Gerhardt, S.; Mohajeri, M.H. Changes of Colonic Bacterial Composition in Parkinson's Disease and Other Neurodegenerative Diseases. *Nutrients* **2018**, *10*, 708. [CrossRef]
51. Montassier, E.; Batard, E.; Massart, S.; Gastinne, T.; Carton, T.; Caillon, J.; Fresne, S.L.; Caroff, N.; Hardcuin, J.B.; Moreau, P.; et al. 16S rRNA Gene Pyrosequencing Reveals Shift in Patient Faecal Microbiota During High-Dose Chemotherapy as Conditioning Regimen for Bone Marrow Transplantation. *Microb. Ecol.* **2014**, *67*, 690–699. [CrossRef] [PubMed]
52. McQuade, R.M.; Stojanovska, V.; Abalo, R.; Bornstein, J.C.; Nurgali, K. Chemotherapy-Induced Constipation and Diarrhea: Pathophysiology, Current and Emerging Treatments. *Front. Pharmacol.* **2016**, *7*, 414. [CrossRef] [PubMed]
53. Sangild, P.T.; Shen, R.L.; Pontoppidan, P.; Rathe, M. Animal models of chemotherapy-induced mucositis: Translational relevance and challenges. *Am. J. Physiol. Gastrointest. Liver Physiol.* **2018**, *314*, G231–G246. [CrossRef]
54. Stringer, A.M.; Gibson, R.J.; Bowen, J.M.; Logan, R.M.; Ashton, K.; Yeoh, A.S.J.; Al-Dasooqui, N.; Keefe, D.M.K. Irinotecan-induced mucositis manifesting as diarrhoea corresponds with an amended intestinal flora and mucin profile. *Int. J. Exp. Pathol.* **2009**, *90*, 489–499. [CrossRef] [PubMed]
55. Harach, T.; Marungruang, N.; Duthilleul, N.; Cheatham, V.; Mc Coy, K.D.; Frisoni, G.; Neher, J.J.; Fåk, F.; Jucker, M.; Lasser, T.; et al. Reduction of Abeta amyloid pathology in APPPS1 transgenic mice in the absence of gut microbiota. *Sci. Rep.* **2017**. [CrossRef] [PubMed]
56. Vogt, N.M.; Kerby, R.L.; Dill-McFarland, K.A.; Harding, S.J.; Merluzzi, A.P.; Johnson, S.C.; Carlsson, C.M.; Asthana, S.; Zetterberg, H.; Blennow, K.; et al. Gut microbiome alterations in Alzheimer's disease. *Sci. Rep.* **2017**, *7*, 13537. [CrossRef]
57. Stein, A.; Voigt, W.; Jordan, K. Chemotherapy-induced diarrhea: Pathophysiology, frequency and guideline-based management. *Ther. Adv. Med. Oncol.* **2010**, *2*, 51–63. [CrossRef]

58. Farrell, C.; Brearley, S.G.; Pilling, M.; Molassiotis, A. The impact of chemotherapy-related nausea on patients' nutritional status, psychological distress and quality of life. *Support. Care Cancer* **2013**, *21*, 59–66. [CrossRef]
59. Talley, N.J.; Phillips, S.F.; Haddad, A.; Miller, L.J.; Twomey, C.; Zinsmeister, A.R.; MacCarty, R.L.; Ciociola, A. GR 38032F (Ondansetron), a selective 5HT3 receptor antagonist, slows colonic transit in healthy man. *Dig. Dis. Sci.* **1990**, *35*, 477–480. [CrossRef]
60. Jordan, K.R.; Loman, B.R.; Bailey, M.T.; Pyter, L.M. Gut microbiota-immune-brain interactions in chemotherapy-associated behavioral comorbidities. *Cancer* **2018**, *124*, 3990–3999. [CrossRef]
61. Glass, C.K.; Saijo, K.; Winner, B.; Marchetto, M.C.; Gage, F.H. Mechanisms Underlying Inflammation in Neurodegeneration. *Cell* **2010**, *140*, 918–934. [CrossRef]
62. Ren, X.; St Clair, D.K.; Butterfield, D.A. Dysregulation of cytokine mediated chemotherapy induced cognitive impairment. *Pharmacol. Res.* **2017**, *117*, 267–273. [CrossRef] [PubMed]
63. Pedroso, S.H.S.P.; Vieira, A.T.; Bastos, R.W.; Oliveira, J.S.; Cartelle, C.T.; Arantes, R.M.E.; Soares, P.M.G.; Generoso, S.V.; Cardoso, V.N.; Teixeira, M.M.; et al. Evaluation of mucositis induced by irinotecan after microbial colonization in germ-free mice. *Microbiology* **2015**, *161*, 1950–1960. [CrossRef]
64. Erny, D.; Hrabě de Angelis, A.L.; Jaitin, D.; Wieghofer, P.; Staszewski, O.; David, E.; Keren-Shaul, H.; Mahlakoiv, T.; Jakobshagen, K.; Buch, T.; et al. Host microbiota constantly control maturation and function of microglia in the CNS. *Nat. Neurosci.* **2015**, *18*, 965–977. [CrossRef]
65. Torres-Platas, S.G.; Cruceanu, C.; Chen, G.G.; Turecki, G.; Mechawar, N. Evidence for increased microglial priming and macrophage recruitment in the dorsal anterior cingulate white matter of depressed suicides. *Brain Behav. Immun.* **2014**, *42*, 50–59. [CrossRef]
66. Tonelli, L.H.; Stiller, J.; Rujescu, D.; Giegling, I.; Schneider, B.; Maurer, K.; Schnabel, A.; Möller, H.; Chen, H.H.; Postolache, T.T. Elevated cytokine expression in the orbitofrontal cortex of victims of suicide. *Acta Psychiatr. Scand.* **2008**, *117*, 198–206. [CrossRef]
67. Wang, X.-M.; Walitt, B.; Saligan, L.; Tiwari, A.F.Y.; Cheung, C.W.; Zhang, Z.-J. Chemobrain: A critical review and causal hypothesis of link between cytokines and epigenetic reprogramming associated with chemotherapy. *Cytokine* **2015**, *72*, 86–96. [CrossRef] [PubMed]
68. D'Mello, C.; Swain, M.G. Liver–brain interactions in inflammatory liver diseases: Implications for fatigue and mood disorders. *Brain Behav. Immun.* **2014**, *35*, 9–20. [CrossRef]
69. Ramadori, G.; Cameron, S. Effects of systemic chemotherapy on the liver. *Ann. Hepatol.* **2010**, *9*, 133–143. [CrossRef]
70. Seo, A.N.; Kim, H. Sinusoidal obstruction syndrome after oxaliplatin-based chemotherapy. *Clin. Mol. Hepatol.* **2014**, *20*, 81–84. [CrossRef]
71. Sharma, A.; Houshyar, R.; Bhosale, P.; Choi, J.-I.; Gulati, R.; Lall, C. Chemotherapy induced liver abnormalities: An imaging perspective. *Clin. Mol. Hepatol.* **2014**, *20*, 317–326. [CrossRef] [PubMed]
72. Barak, V.; Selmi, C.; Schlesinger, M.; Blank, M.; Agmon-Levin, N.; Kalickman, I.; Gershwin, M.E.; Shoenfeld, Y. Serum inflammatory cytokines, complement components, and soluble interleukin 2 receptor in primary biliary cirrhosis. *J. Autoimmun.* **2009**, *33*, 178–182. [CrossRef] [PubMed]
73. Loppnow, H.; Werdan, K.; Werner, C. The enhanced plasma levels of soluble tumor necrosis factor receptors (sTNF-R1; sTNF-R2) and interleukin-10 (IL-10) in patients suffering from chronic heart failure are reversed in patients treated with beta-adrenoceptor antagonist. *Auton. Autacoid Pharmacol.* **2002**, *22*, 83–92. [CrossRef]
74. D'Mello, C.; Swain, M.G. Liver-brain inflammation axis. *Am. J. Physiol. Gastrointest. Liver Physiol.* **2011**, *301*, G749–G761. [CrossRef] [PubMed]
75. Metz, C.N.; Pavlov, V.A. Vagus nerve cholinergic circuitry to the liver and the gastrointestinal tract in the neuroimmune communicatome. *Am. J. Physiol. Gastrointest. Liver Physiol.* **2018**, *315*, G651–G658. [CrossRef] [PubMed]
76. Ek, M.; Kurosawa, M.; Lundeberg, T.; Ericsson, A. Activation of vagal afferents after intravenous injection of interleukin-1beta: Role of endogenous prostaglandins. *J. Neurosci.* **1998**, *18*, 9471–9479. [CrossRef] [PubMed]
77. Harrison, N.A.; Brydon, L.; Walker, C.; Gray, M.A.; Steptoe, A.; Dolan, R.J.; Critchley, H.D. Neural origins of human sickness in interoceptive responses to inflammation. *Biol. Psychiatry* **2009**, *66*, 415–422. [CrossRef]
78. Van Ginneken, B.T.J.; van den Berg-Emons, R.J.G.; van der Windt, A.; Tilanus, H.W.; Metselaar, H.J.; Stam, H.J.; Kazemier, G. Persistent fatigue in liver transplant recipients: A two-year follow-up study. *Clin. Transplant.* **2010**, *24*, E10–E16. [CrossRef] [PubMed]
79. Forton, D. Hepatitis C and cognitive impairment in a cohort of patients with mild liver disease. *Hepatology* **2002**, *35*, 433–439. [CrossRef] [PubMed]
80. Newton, J.L.; Hollingsworth, K.G.; Taylor, R.; El-Sharkawy, A.M.; Khan, Z.U.; Pearce, R.; Sutcliffe, K.; Okonkwo, O.; Davidson, A.; Burt, J.; et al. Cognitive impairment in primary biliary cirrhosis: Symptom impact and potential etiology. *Hepatology* **2008**, *48*, 541–549. [CrossRef]
81. Newton, J.L.; John Gibson, G.; Tomlinson, M.; Wilton, K.; Jones, D. Fatigue in primary biliary cirrhosis is associated with excessive daytime somnolence. *Hepatology* **2006**, *44*, 91–98. [CrossRef] [PubMed]
82. Bernhardson, B.-M.; Tishelman, C.; Rutqvist, L.E. Chemosensory Changes Experienced by Patients Undergoing Cancer Chemotherapy: A Qualitative Interview Study. *J. Pain Symptom Manag.* **2007**, *34*, 403–412. [CrossRef] [PubMed]

83. Mols, F.; van de Poll-Franse, L.V.; Vreugdenhil, G.; Beijers, A.J.; Kieffer, J.M.; Aaronson, N.K.; Husson, O. Reference data of the European Organisation for Research and Treatment of Cancer (EORTC) QLQ-CIPN20 Questionnaire in the general Dutch population. *Eur. J. Cancer* **2016**, *69*, 28–38. [CrossRef] [PubMed]
84. Seretny, M.; Currie, G.L.; Sena, E.S.; Ramnarine, S.; Grant, R.; MacLeod, M.R.; Colvin, L.A.; Fallon, M. Incidence, prevalence, and predictors of chemotherapy-induced peripheral neuropathy: A systematic review and meta-analysis. *Pain* **2014**, *155*, 2461–2470. [CrossRef] [PubMed]
85. Flatters, S.J.L.; Dougherty, P.M.; Colvin, L.A. Clinical and preclinical perspectives on Chemotherapy-Induced Peripheral Neuropathy (CIPN): A narrative review. *Br. J. Anaesth.* **2017**, *119*, 737–749. [CrossRef]
86. Starobova, H.; Vetter, I. Pathophysiology of Chemotherapy-Induced Peripheral Neuropathy. *Front. Mol. Neurosci.* **2017**. [CrossRef] [PubMed]
87. Ruiz-Medina, J.; Baulies, A.; Bura, S.A.; Valverde, O. Paclitaxel-induced neuropathic pain is age dependent and devolves on glial response. *Eur. J. Pain* **2013**, *17*, 75–85. [CrossRef] [PubMed]
88. Lees, J.G.; Makker, P.G.S.; Tonkin, R.S.; Abdulla, M.; Park, S.B.; Goldstein, D.; Moalem-Taylor, G. Immune-mediated processes implicated in chemotherapy-induced peripheral neuropathy. *Eur. J. Cancer* **2017**, *73*, 22–29. [CrossRef]
89. Zajączkowska, R.; Kocot-Kępska, M.; Leppert, W.; Wrzosek, A.; Mika, J.; Wordliczek, J. Mechanisms of Chemotherapy-Induced Peripheral Neuropathy. *Int. J. Mol. Sci.* **2019**, *20*, 1451. [CrossRef]
90. Liu, C.-C.; Lu, N.; Cui, Y.; Yang, T.; Zhao, Z.-Q.; Xin, W.-J.; Liu, X.-G. Prevention of Paclitaxel-Induced Allodynia by Minocycline: Effect on Loss of Peripheral Nerve Fibers and Infiltration of Macrophages in Rats. *Mol. Pain* **2010**, *6*, 1744–8069. [CrossRef]
91. Zhang, H.; Boyette-Davis, J.A.; Kosturakis, A.K.; Li, Y.; Yoon, S.-Y.; Walters, E.T.; Dougherty, P.M. Induction of monocyte chemoattractant protein-1 (MCP-1) and its receptor CCR2 in primary sensory neurons contributes to paclitaxel-induced peripheral neuropathy. *J. Pain* **2013**, *14*, 1031–1044. [CrossRef]
92. Morean, D.F.; O'Dwyer, L.; Cherney, L.R. Therapies for Cognitive Deficits Associated With Chemotherapy for Breast Cancer: A Systematic Review of Objective Outcomes. *Arch. Phys. Med. Rehabil.* **2015**, *96*, 1880–1897. [CrossRef] [PubMed]
93. Deutsch, J.E.; Anderson, E.Z. *Complementary Therapies for Physical Therapy*; Elsevier Inc.: Amsterdam, The Netherlands, 2008. [CrossRef]
94. Nada, S.E.; Shah, Z.A. Preconditioning with Ginkgo biloba (EGb 761®) provides neuroprotection through HO1 and CRMP2. *Neurobiol. Dis.* **2012**, *46*, 180–189. [CrossRef] [PubMed]
95. Ahmed, S.M.U.; Luo, L.; Namani, A.; Wang, X.J.; Tang, X. Nrf2 signaling pathway: Pivotal roles in inflammation. *Biochim. Biophys. Acta Mol. Basis Dis.* **2017**, *1863*, 585–597. [CrossRef]
96. Giraudon, P.; Nicolle, A.; Cavagna, S.; Benetollo, C.; Marignier, R.; Varrin-Doyer, M. Insight into the role of CRMP2 (collapsin response mediator protein 2) in T lymphocyte migration. *Cell Adhes. Migr.* **2013**, *7*, 38–43. [CrossRef] [PubMed]
97. Ercoli, L.M.; Castellon, S.A.; Hunter, A.M.; Kwan, L.; Kahn-Mills, B.A.; Cernin, P.A.; Leuchter, A.F.; Ganz, P.A. Assessment of the feasibility of a rehabilitation intervention program for breast cancer survivors with cognitive complaints. *Brain Imaging Behav.* **2013**, *7*, 543–553. [CrossRef]
98. Ferguson, R.J.; Ahles, T.A.; Saykin, A.J.; McDonald, B.C.; Furstenberg, C.T.; Cole, B.F.; Mott, L.A. Cognitive-behavioral management of chemotherapy-related cognitive change. *Psychooncology* **2007**, *16*, 772–777. [CrossRef]
99. Milbury, K.; Chaoul, A.; Biegler, K.; Wangyal, T.; Spelman, A.; Meyers, C.A.; Arun, B.; Palmer, J.L.; Taylor, J.; Cohen, L. Tibetan sound meditation for cognitive dysfunction: Results of a randomized controlled pilot trial. *Psychooncology* **2013**, *22*, 2354–2363. [CrossRef]
100. Ferguson, R.J.; McDonald, B.C.; Rocque, M.A.; Furstenberg, C.T.; Horrigan, S.; Ahles, T.A.; Saykin, A.J. Development of CBT for chemotherapy-related cognitive change: Results of a waitlist control trial. *Psychooncology* **2012**, *21*, 176–186. [CrossRef]
101. Poppelreuter, M.; Weis, J.; Bartsch, H.H. Effects of specific neuropsychological training programs for breast cancer patients after adjuvant chemotherapy. *J. Psychosoc. Oncol.* **2009**, *27*, 274–296. [CrossRef]
102. Kesler, S.; Hadi Hosseini, S.M.; Heckler, C.; Janelsins, M.; Palesh, O.; Mustian, K.; Morrow, G. Cognitive training for improving executive function in chemotherapy-treated breast cancer survivors. *Clin. Breast Cancer* **2013**, *13*, 299–306. [CrossRef]
103. Liu, Z.; Qin, H.; Yang, Z.; Xia, Y.; Liu, W.; Yang, J.; Jiang, Y.; Zhang, H.; Yang, Z.; Wang, Y.; et al. Randomised clinical trial: The effects of perioperative probiotic treatment on barrier function and post-operative infectious complications in colorectal cancer surgery—A double-blind study. *Aliment. Pharmacol. Ther.* **2011**, *33*, 50–63. [CrossRef] [PubMed]
104. Huang, R.; Wang, K.; Hu, J. Effect of Probiotics on Depression: A Systematic Review and Meta-Analysis of Randomized Controlled Trials. *Nutrients* **2016**, *8*, 483. [CrossRef] [PubMed]
105. Akkasheh, G.; Kashani-Poor, Z.; Tajabadi-Ebrahimi, M.; Jafari, P.; Akbari, H.; Taghizadeh, M.; Memarzadeh, M.R.; Asemi, Z.; Esmaillzadeh, A. Clinical and metabolic response to probiotic administration in patients with major depressive disorder: A randomized, double-blind, placebo-controlled trial. *Nutrition* **2016**, *32*, 315–320. [CrossRef] [PubMed]
106. McKean, J.; Naug, H.; Nikbakht, E.; Amiet, B.; Colson, N. Probiotics and Subclinical Psychological Symptoms in Healthy Participants: A Systematic Review and Meta-Analysis. *J. Altern. Complement. Med.* **2017**, *23*, 249–258. [CrossRef]
107. Akbari, E.; Asemi, Z.; Kakhaki, R.D.; Bahmani, F.; Kouchaki, E.; Tamtaji, O.R.; Hamidi, G.A.; Salami, M. Effect of Probiotic Supplementation on Cognitive Function and Metabolic Status in Alzheimer's Disease: A Randomized, Double-Blind and Controlled Trial. *Front. Aging Neurosci.* **2016**. [CrossRef]

108. Thompson, R.S.; Roller, R.; Mika, A.; Greenwood, B.N.; Knight, R.; Chichlowski, M.; Berg, B.M.; Fleshner, M. Dietary Prebiotics and Bioactive Milk Fractions Improve NREM Sleep, Enhance REM Sleep Rebound and Attenuate the Stress-Induced Decrease in Diurnal Temperature and Gut Microbial Alpha Diversity. *Front. Behav. Neurosci.* **2017**, *10*, 240. [CrossRef]
109. Schmidt, K.; Cowen, P.J.; Harmer, C.J.; Tzortzis, G.; Errington, S.; Burnet, P.W.J. Prebiotic intake reduces the waking cortisol response and alters emotional bias in healthy volunteers. *Psychopharmacology* **2015**, *232*, 1793–1801. [CrossRef]
110. Franzosa, E.A.; Sirota-Madi, A.; Avila-Pacheco, J.; Fornelos, N.; Haiser, H.J.; Reinker, S.; Vatanen, T.; Hall, A.B.; Mallick, H.; Mclver, L.J.; et al. Author Correction: Gut microbiome structure and metabolic activity in inflammatory bowel disease. *Nat. Microbiol.* **2019**, *4*, 898. [CrossRef] [PubMed]
111. Skelly, A.N.; Sato, Y.; Kearney, S.; Honda, K. Mining the microbiota for microbial and metabolite-based immunotherapies. *Nat. Rev. Immunol.* **2019**, *19*, 305–323. [CrossRef]
112. Blacher, E.; Levy, M.; Tatirovsky, E.; Elinav, E. Microbiome-Modulated Metabolites at the Interface of Host Immunity. *J. Immunol.* **2017**, *198*, 572–580. [CrossRef]
113. Wong, A.C.; Levy, M. New Approaches to Microbiome-Based Therapies. *mSystems* **2019**, *4*. [CrossRef]
114. Monda, V.; Villano, I.; Messina, A.; Valenzano, A.; Esposito, T.; Moscatelli, F.; Viggiano, A.; Cibelli, G.; Chieffi, S.; Monda, M.; et al. Exercise Modifies the Gut Microbiota with Positive Health Effects. *Oxid. Med. Cell. Longev.* **2017**, *2017*, 3831972. [CrossRef]
115. Gentile, F.; Doneddu, P.E.; Riva, N.; Nobile-Orazio, E.; Quattrini, A. Diet, Microbiota and Brain Health: Unraveling the Network Intersecting Metabolism and Neurodegeneration. *Int. J. Mol. Sci.* **2020**, *21*, 7471. [CrossRef]
116. Monaco, A.; Ferrandino, I.; Boscaino, F.; Cocca, E.; Cigliano, L.; Maurano, F.; Luongo, D.; Spagnuolo, M.S.; Rossi, M.; Bergamo, P. Conjugated linoleic acid prevents age-dependent neurodegeneration in a mouse model of neuropsychiatric lupus via the activation of an adaptive response. *J. Lipid Res.* **2018**, *59*, 48–57. [CrossRef]
117. Whelan, J.; Fritsche, K. Linoleic acid. *Adv. Nutr.* **2013**, *4*, 311–312. [CrossRef]
118. Lee, A.Y.; Lee, M.H.; Lee, S.; Cho, E.J. Alpha-Linolenic Acid from Perilla frutescens var. japonica Oil Protects Aβ-Induced Cognitive Impairment through Regulation of APP Processing and Aβ Degradation. *J. Agric. Food Chem.* **2017**, *65*, 10719–10729. [CrossRef]
119. Khan, M.S.; Muhammad, T.; Ikram, M.; Kim, M.O. Dietary Supplementation of the Antioxidant Curcumin Halts Systemic LPS-Induced Neuroinflammation-Associated Neurodegeneration and Memory/Synaptic Impairment via the JNK/NF-κB/Akt Signaling Pathway in Adult Rats. *Oxidative Med. Cell. Longev.* **2019**, 1–23. [CrossRef] [PubMed]
120. Krenkel, O.; Puengel, T.; Govaere, O.; Abdallah, A.T.; Mossanen, J.C.; Kohlhepp, M.; Liepelt, A.; Lefebvre, E.; Luedde, T.; Hellerbrand, C.; et al. Therapeutic inhibition of inflammatory monocyte recruitment reduces steatohepatitis and liver fibrosis. *Hepatology* **2018**, *67*, 1270–1283. [CrossRef] [PubMed]
121. Weiskirchen, R.; Tacke, F. Liver Fibrosis: From Pathogenesis to Novel Therapies. *Dig. Dis.* **2016**, *34*, 410–422. [CrossRef] [PubMed]
122. Anstee, Q.M.; Neuschwander-Tetri, B.A.; Wong, V.W.-S.; Abdelmalek, M.F.; Younossi, Z.M.; Yuan, J.; Pecoraro, M.L.; Seyedkazemi, S.; Fischer, L.; Bedossa, P.; et al. Cenicriviroc for the treatment of liver fibrosis in adults with nonalcoholic steatohepatitis: AURORA Phase 3 study design. *Contemp. Clin. Trials* **2020**, *89*, 105922. [CrossRef] [PubMed]
123. Temel, Y.; Kucukler, S.; Yıldırım, S.; Caglayan, C.; Kandemir, F.M. Protective effect of chrysin on cyclophosphamide-induced hepatotoxicity and nephrotoxicity via the inhibition of oxidative stress, inflammation, and apoptosis. *Naunyn Schmiedebergs Arch. Pharmacol.* **2020**, *393*, 325–337. [CrossRef]
124. El-Sebaey, A.M.; Abdelhamid, F.M.; Abdalla, O.A. Protective effects of garlic extract against hematological alterations, immunosuppression, hepatic oxidative stress, and renal damage induced by cyclophosphamide in rats. *Environ. Sci. Pollut. Res. Int.* **2019**, *26*, 15559–15572. [CrossRef]
125. Mohammed, M.J.; Tadros, M.G.; Michel, H.E. Geraniol protects against cyclophosphamide-induced hepatotoxicity in rats: Possible role of MAPK and PPAR-γ signaling pathways. *Food Chem. Toxicol.* **2020**, *139*, 111251. [CrossRef]
126. Aladaileh, S.H.; Abukhalil, M.H.; Saghir, S.A.; Hanieh, H.; Alfwuaires, M.A.; Almaiman, A.A.; Bin-Jumah, M.; Mahmoud, A.Y. Galangin Activates Nrf2 Signaling and Attenuates Oxidative Damage, Inflammation, and Apoptosis in a Rat Model of Cyclophosphamide-Induced Hepatotoxicity. *Biomolecules* **2019**, *9*, 346. [CrossRef] [PubMed]
127. Lixin, X.; Lijun, Y.; Songping, H. Ganoderic acid A against cyclophosphamide-induced hepatic toxicity in mice. *J. Biochem. Mol. Toxicol.* **2019**, *33*, e22271. [CrossRef] [PubMed]
128. Panni, R.Z.; Linehan, D.C.; DeNardo, D.G. Targeting tumor-infiltrating macrophages to combat cancer. *Immunotherapy* **2013**, *5*, 1075–1087. [CrossRef] [PubMed]
129. Imai, T.; Yasuda, N. Therapeutic intervention of inflammatory/immune diseases by inhibition of the fractalkine (CX3CL1)-CX3CR1 pathway. *Inflamm. Regen.* **2016**, *36*, 9. [CrossRef]
130. Kim, H.-S.; Suh, Y.-H. Minocycline and neurodegenerative diseases. *Behav. Brain Res.* **2009**, *196*, 168–179. [CrossRef]
131. Garrido-Mesa, N.; Zarzuelo, A.; Gálvez, J. Minocycline: Far beyond an antibiotic. *Br. J. Pharmacol.* **2013**, *169*, 337–352. [CrossRef] [PubMed]
132. Hu, L.-Y.; Mi, W.-L.; Wu, G.-C.; Wang, Y.-Q.; Mao-Ying, Q.-L. Prevention and Treatment for Chemotherapy-Induced Peripheral Neuropathy: Therapies Based on CIPN Mechanisms. *Curr. Neuropharmacol.* **2019**, *17*, 184–196. [CrossRef] [PubMed]

133. Mao-Ying, Q.-L.; Kavelaars, A.; Krukowski, K.; Huo, X.-J.; Zhou, W.; Price, T.J.; Cleeland, C.; Heijnen, C.J. The Anti-Diabetic Drug Metformin Protects against Chemotherapy-Induced Peripheral Neuropathy in a Mouse Model. *PLoS ONE* **2014**, e100701. [CrossRef]
134. Melemedjian, O.K.; Yassine, H.N.; Shy, A.; Price, T.J. Proteomic and Functional Annotation Analysis of Injured Peripheral Nerves Reveals ApoE as a Protein Upregulated by Injury that is Modulated by Metformin Treatment. *Mol. Pain* **2013**, *9*, 1744–8069. [CrossRef]
135. Huang, N.-L.; Chiang, S.-H.; Hsueh, C.-H.; Liang, Y.-J.; Chen, Y.-J.; Lai, L.-P. Metformin inhibits TNF-alpha-induced IkappaB kinase phosphorylation, IkappaB-alpha degradation and IL-6 production in endothelial cells through PI3K-dependent AMPK phosphorylation. *Int. J. Cardiol.* **2009**, *134*, 169–175. [CrossRef] [PubMed]
136. Huang, C.-Y.; Chen, Y.-L.; Li, A.H.; Lu, J.-C.; Wang, H.-L. Minocycline, a microglial inhibitor, blocks spinal CCL2-induced heat hyperalgesia and augmentation of glutamatergic transmission in substantia gelatinosa neurons. *J. Neuroinflamm.* **2014**, *11*, 7. [CrossRef]
137. Ledeboer, A.; Sloane, E.M.; Milligan, E.D.; Frank, M.G.; Mahony, J.H.; Maier, S.F.; Watkins, L.R. Minocycline attenuates mechanical allodynia and proinflammatory cytokine expression in rat models of pain facilitation. *Pain* **2005**, *115*, 71–83. [CrossRef] [PubMed]
138. Pachman, D.R.; Dockter, T.; Zekan, P.J.; Fruth, B.; Ruddy, K.J.; Ta, L.E.; Lafky, J.M.; Dentchev, T.; Le-Lindqwister, N.A.; Sikov, W.M.; et al. A pilot study of minocycline for the prevention of paclitaxel-associated neuropathy: ACCRU study RU221408I. *Support Care Cancer* **2017**, *25*, 3407–3416. [CrossRef] [PubMed]
139. Ghasemian, M.; Owlia, S.; Owlia, M.B. Review of Anti-Inflammatory Herbal Medicines. *Adv. Pharmacol. Sci.* **2016**, 1–11. [CrossRef]
140. Rahbardar, M.G.; Amin, B.; Mehri, S.; Mirnajafi-Zadeh, S.J.; Hosseinzadeh, H. Anti-inflammatory effects of ethanolic extract of Rosmarinus officinalis L. and rosmarinic acid in a rat model of neuropathic pain. *Biomed. Pharmacother.* **2017**, *86*, 441–449. [CrossRef]
141. Rahbardar, M.G.; Amin, B.; Mehri, S.; Mirnajafi-Zadeh, S.J.; Hosseinzadeh, H. Rosmarinic acid attenuates development and existing pain in a rat model of neuropathic pain: An evidence of anti-oxidative and anti-inflammatory effects. *Phytomedicine* **2018**, *40*, 59–67. [CrossRef]
142. Ghasemzadeh, M.R.; Amin, B.; Mehri, S.; Mirnajafi-Zadeh, S.J.; Hosseinzadeh, H. Effect of alcoholic extract of aerial parts of Rosmarinus officinalis L. on pain, inflammation and apoptosis induced by chronic constriction injury (CCI) model of neuropathic pain in rats. *J. Ethnopharmacol.* **2016**, *194*, 117–130. [CrossRef] [PubMed]
143. Nagarkatti, P.; Pandey, R.; Rieder, S.A.; Hegde, V.L.; Nagarkatti, M. Cannabinoids as novel anti-inflammatory drugs. *Future Med. Chem.* **2009**, *1*, 1333–1349. [CrossRef]
144. Johnson, J.R.; Lossignol, D.; Burnell-Nugent, M.; Fallon, M.T. An open-label extension study to investigate the long-term safety and tolerability of THC/CBD oromucosal spray and oromucosal THC spray in patients with terminal cancer-related pain refractory to strong opioid analgesics. *J. Pain Symptom. Manag.* **2013**, *46*, 207–218. [CrossRef] [PubMed]
145. Serpell, M.; Ratcliffe, S.; Hovorka, J.; Schofield, M.; Taylor, L.; Lauder, H.; Ehler, E. A double-blind, randomized, placebo-controlled, parallel group study of THC/CBD spray in peripheral neuropathic pain treatment. *Eur. J. Pain* **2014**, *18*, 999–1012. [CrossRef] [PubMed]
146. Hoggart, B.; Ratcliffe, S.; Ehler, E.; Simpson, K.H.; Hovorka, J.; Lejčko, J.; Taylor, L.; Lauder, H.; Serpell, M. A multicentre, open-label, follow-on study to assess the long-term maintenance of effect, tolerance and safety of THC/CBD oromucosal spray in the management of neuropathic pain. *J. Neurol.* **2015**, *262*, 27–40. [CrossRef]

biomedicines

MDPI

Review

Can Exercise-Induced Muscle Damage Be a Good Model for the Investigation of the Anti-Inflammatory Properties of Diet in Humans?

Spyridon Methenitis [1], Ioanna Stergiou [2,3], Smaragdi Antonopoulou [3] and Tzortzis Nomikos [3,*]

1 Sports Performance Laboratory, School of Physical Education & Sports Science, National and Kapodistrian University of Athens, 17237 Athens, Greece; smetheni@phed.uoa.gr
2 Bioiatriki, Ergometric and Nutrition Center, 11526 Athens, Greece; joannste23@gmail.com
3 Department of Nutrition & Dietetics, School of Health Sciences and Education, Harokopio University, 17671 Athens, Greece; antonop@hua.gr
* Correspondence: tnomikos@hua.gr

Abstract: Subclinical, low-grade, inflammation is one of the main pathophysiological mechanisms underlying the majority of chronic and non-communicable diseases. Several methodological approaches have been applied for the assessment of the anti-inflammatory properties of nutrition, however, their impact in human body remains uncertain, because of the fact that the majority of the studies reporting anti-inflammatory effect of dietary patterns, have been performed under laboratory settings and/or in animal models. Thus, the extrapolation of these results to humans is risky. It is therefore obvious that the development of an inflammatory model in humans, by which we could induce inflammatory responses to humans in a regulated, specific, and non-harmful way, could greatly facilitate the estimation of the anti-inflammatory properties of diet in a more physiological way and mechanistically relevant way. We believe that exercise-induced muscle damage (EIMD) could serve as such a model, either in studies investigating the homeostatic responses of individuals under inflammatory stimuli or for the estimation of the anti-inflammatory or pro-inflammatory potential of dietary patterns, foods, supplements, nutrients, or phytochemicals. Thus, in this review we discuss the possibility of exercise-induced muscle damage being an inflammation model suitable for the assessment of the anti-inflammatory properties of diet in humans.

Keywords: oxidative stress; experimental model; anti-inflammatory diets; inflammatory response; chronic inflammation; low grade chronic inflammation; inflammatory models

Citation: Methenitis, S.; Stergiou, I.; Antonopoulou, S.; Nomikos, T. Can Exercise-Induced Muscle Damage Be a Good Model for the Investigation of the Anti-Inflammatory Properties of Diet in Humans?. *Biomedicines* **2021**, *9*, 36. https://doi.org/10.3390/biomedicines9010036

Received: 9 November 2020
Accepted: 29 December 2020
Published: 5 January 2021

Publisher's Note: MDPI stays neutral with regard to jurisdictional claims in published maps and institutional affiliations.

1. Introduction

Subclinical, low-grade, inflammation is one of the main pathophysiological mechanisms underlying the majority of chronic and non-communicable diseases [1–5]. It is therefore obvious that non-pharmacological interventions, such as dietary ones, aiming to modulate immune system, without compromising it, could serve as efficient ways of prevention while at the same time they could act complementarily to standard medication. In the last two decades, several dietary patterns different food items, phytochemicals, nutraceuticals, and supplements are promoted with the claim of possessing anti-inflammatory properties [6–11]. However, the impact of the above interventions in the immune system of humans remains uncertain since the majority of the studies have been performed under laboratory settings (e.g., cell culture and/or animal testing). Thus, the extrapolation of these results to humans is risky [12,13]. In addition, the majority of the clinical trials, exploring the "anti-inflammatory" effect of dietary/supplementation patterns on human subjects, assess their effectiveness based on their impact on a limited panel of inflammatory biochemical markers, mainly under controlled, fasted, non-stressed conditions. According to this, it will be of interest if we could assess the pro-inflammatory and/or anti-inflammatory profile of different dietary interventions, by developing inflammatory models, in humans, which could induce a transient inflammatory response to volunteers in a regulated and predicted fashion. The development of inflammatory conditions in humans, could be achieved, either by pharmaceutical or medical interventions, or by intentional injuries such as mechanical trauma, toxins, unhealthy lifestyles, and burns. Of course, the majority of these approaches have several ethical restraints that impair the development of such models. In contrast, ethical, controlled, and well-established models, to induce transient inflammation in humans, are certain exercise/training modalities, which are known to induce elevations of inflammatory-, oxidative stress-, and muscle-damage-related blood markers [14,15], impair clinical phenotypes, and alter metabolic procedures [16–19]. In this review article we discuss the possibility of exercise-induced muscle damage (EIMD) being a model of acute inflammation suitable for the assessment of the anti-inflammatory properties of diet in humans.

2. The Protective Anti-Inflammatory Role of Nutrition in Chronic Diseases

The inflammatory responses are integral parts of the normal innate immune response conferring protection to infection and initiating mechanisms of repair and regeneration of damaged tissues [20,21]. Under acute inflammatory conditions, recognition receptors activate several signaling cascades, leading to the release of pro- and anti-inflammatory mediators, which orchestrate the recruitment of neutrophils and monocytes/macrophages to the damaged tissues while at the same time initiate the lysis of inflammation and the repair of tissue [20–23]. However, even a low to moderate chronic activation of inflammatory mechanisms induced either from long-term, persistent infections, autoimmune diseases, and/or increased daily inflammatory insults due to lifestyle (obesity, sedentary lifestyle, smoking, stress) and dietary habits (dense meals rich in simple sugars, trans fatty acids, advanced glycation end-products) overwhelms the anti-inflammatory processes of the immune system resulting in a chronic, sub-clinical inflammation [2,6,24–30]. The biochemical phenotype of this condition is mildly elevated levels of inflammatory mediators in the circulation. For example, C-reactive protein (CRP) levels are raised 2–3 fold under low-grade inflammation while those levels can be increased up to 10–1000 times in acute inflammation [31].

It is well documented that a subclinical activation of the inflammatory mechanisms may be a predisposing risk factor for non-communicable diseases such as cardiovascular disease, cancer, metabolic syndrome, diabetes, depression, dementia, and biological aging in general [1–4,25,32–36]. Actually, subclinical inflammation seems to underlie the link between unhealthy lifestyle with the pathogenesis of chronic diseases [2,23,29]. Taking into account the linear relationship between the levels of subclinical inflammation markers (e.g., CRP) and the risk for chronic diseases it is obvious that even a small attenuation of subclinical inflammation by lifestyle changes may confer protection against those diseases [7,36–39]. Therefore, dietary interventions targeting to reduce inflammation seem to be an efficient way of prevention for diseases with a chronic inflammatory background [7,9,10,30,40–43].

It is now known that prudent dietary patterns, such as the Mediterranean Diet [7,8,39,44,45] and macro/micro-nutrients, have a strong protective effect against non-communicable diseases, with a strong inflammatory profile [10,30,40–43]. For the majority of these studies, the assessment of the anti-inflammatory properties of diet was based on the measurement of few classical circulating markers (CRP, IL-6, TNFα). On the other hand, a plethora of microNutrients, phytochemicals, and supplements failed to attenuate inflammation in humans, despite their strong anti-inflammatory actions in cellular and animal studies [12,13,40,46]. The main reason for this discrepancy is the complexity of the pathophysiology of inflammation in humans which can be poorly replicated by animals or cell culture models. Taking into consideration the controversy between animal and human experimentation it seems that the development of more realistic, novel methodological tools for the study of inflammation directly to humans is highly important.

3. The Development of Inflammation Models in Humans Would Greatly Facilitate the Assessment of the Anti-Inflammatory Properties of Nutrition

Several methodological approaches have been applied for the assessment of the anti-inflammatory properties of nutrition. The majority of them is based on cellular and animal models of inflammation. Cellular models of inflammation include LPS-induced secretion of cytokines, expression of adhesion molecules in the surface of cells, phagocytosis activity, natural killer cells lysing capability against cancer cells etc. Cell-based assays were mainly utilized for the identification of the anti-inflammatory properties of isolated nutrients, extracts, and phytochemicals. Despite their usefulness for screening purposes and mechanistic studies the results of those studies cannot be extrapolated directly to humans [12,13,40,46]. The active dietary ingredients, in vivo, are found in much lower concentrations and in a more complex environment than those used in the cellular studies and in structural forms which may differ from the initial structures in foods due to in vivo metabolism [47].

The rapid growth of genetic engineering enabled the development of a plethora of animal models of inflammation by which the anti-inflammatory properties of diet could be assessed, in a more physiological way. Moreover, animal experiments provide wider access to the immune system (thymus, lymph nodes, bone marrow, peritoneal cavity). However, after many years of studying and working with animals in biomedical research, ethical issues have emerged concerning the reproducibility of animal models and their relevance with human inflammatory diseases [12,13,40,46,48]. The results from animal experiments cannot be easily extrapolated to humans because of the biological differences between species [12,13,40,46,48]. Over and above that, many studies in animal models are of poor methodological design exposing patients to unnecessary risk and wasting research funds. This is justified by the discrepancy between the outcomes of animal experiments and clinical trials [12,46,48].

The majority of human studies, investigating the association between diet and inflammation, are cross-sectional and prospective epidemiological studies [3,49–54]. The outcomes are based on the measurement of a small panel of soluble inflammatory mediators and hematological indices which by no way give a holistic view of the inflammatory system while at the same time is questionable whether the tools of the nutritional assessment are reliable to estimate dietary intakes accurately [3,49–54]. Randomized dietary interventions are the gold standard of human experimentation and several dietary interventions have been so far tried to assess the ability of dietary patterns, supplements, food items, and nutrients to modulate subclinical inflammation [3,49–54]. Although this is the best experimental approach so far, randomized dietary interventions lack mechanistic information since the interpretation of the results is based on the comparison of a limited panel of inflammatory indices, measured under static conditions in biological fluids, before and after the intervention. Even if a dietary intervention is able to favorably modulate inflammatory indices this could be the indirect result of diet on other risk factors of subclinical inflammation (e.g., weight loss) rather than a direct involvement to inflammatory mechanisms. In addition, most dietary intervention studies do not assess clinical phenotypes of inflammation either because they do not exist or they are difficult to be estimated in humans. Finally, most dietary intervention studies measure inflammatory mediators, at one-time point, under fasting and resting conditions which does not allow the assessment of intervention's ability to modulate the response (plasticity) of the immune system under real inflammatory insults. It is therefore obvious that the development of an inflammatory model in humans, by which we could induce inflammatory responses to humans in a regulated, specific, and non-harmful way, could greatly facilitate the estimation of the anti-inflammatory properties of diet in a more physiological and mechanistically relevant way. We believe that exercise-induced muscle damage could serve as such a model, at least for acute/transient, self-limited inflammatory pathophysiological conditions. Considering this, several excellent studies, mainly coming from the field of sports nutrition, have already proven the ability of dietary interventions (protein supplements, phytochemicals, omega-3 fatty acids,

BCAA) to diminish EIMD-induced inflammation, and thus to provide positive effects on muscle morphology/function, athletic performance and recovery, establishing the utility of EIMD as a suitable inflammatory model (for example: [5,14,15,55–70]).

4. Exercise-Induced Muscle Damage's Prototypic Inflammatory Responses in Muscle Tissue

EIMD is a phenomenon that occurs either after a prolonged unaccustomed exercise, or after a very intense, high-demanding exercise (high intensity, long duration, high volume, high frequent, or combination of these), as a consequence of the very high mechanical and metabolic demands during the exercise [14,15,55,65,70–75]. EIMD is classified as a grade 1 muscular injury, characterized by minor ultrastructural muscle disruptions without a permanent defect, such as structural disruption of sarcomeres, disturbed excitation-contraction coupling and calcium signaling, and extended muscle protein degradation [14,15,55,71–82]. Although the pathology of EIMD is usually subclinical, the perceived sensation may vary from mild muscle stiffness to exhausting pain and a temporary reduction in both maximum strength and range of motion until several days after the stimuli [15,83,84]. It is also usually accompanied by sensitivity, swelling, or stiffness during palpation or motion of the damaged muscle, a process which is associated with delayed onset muscle soreness (DOMS) [73,85]. However, this inflammatory environment as a cellular response of muscle tissue damage is of high importance for the proper muscle tissue's repair and regeneration [15,71,76,78,82,85].

The type of exercise and the type of muscle contractions applied are crucial determinants of the damaging and inflammatory responses. It is well established that the eccentric exercise, which involves only lengthening muscle actions, could lead to extensive EIMD and inflammation [15,55,72,74,84,86–88]. During eccentric exercises (isokinetic, downhill running, descending the stairs or a box) muscles are forced to lengthen, when the external forces (external weights, gravity, body weight) acting on them are greater than the forces that muscles can produce. This leads to an overstretching of sarcomeres, beyond their normal lengths [63,72,74,84,88–99]. During extensive sarcomere lengthening, there is a decreased overlapping of actin-myosin filaments, leading to a decreased number of active cross-bridge attachments, and thus to a decreased capability for active force generation [55,72–74,84,90,93,97–103]. In addition, although during eccentric contractions, muscles are capable to produce or absorb greater forces, as it reveals from the force–velocity curve [104], the motor units recruitment order is different between eccentric contractions and concentric, with type II muscle fibers to be recruited from the onset of muscle contraction even if the activation of muscle fibers is reduced compared to when the muscle performs maximal concentric contractions [105–107]. Thus, due to the fewer motor units that are recruited during eccentric contractions, as well as to the stretched and overstretched sarcomeres, where there is a reduced overlap of myosin and actin filaments, muscles are forced to overcome the external loads in a very adverse mechanical environment, in the same time that passive forces are dramatically increased leading to sarcomeres' overstraining and thus a disruption of the sarcomere, probably due to titin-stretch-induced damage [74,84,90,97–99,102,108–110]. In addition, during repeated eccentric contractions, the weaker sarcomeres are the first ones that are affected by the above situations, by remaining over-stretched (probably due to the breakdown of titin) and becoming incapable to continue subsequent contractions [74,84,93,95,97–99,102,108–110]. Hence, the remaining, "stronger" sarcomeres receive even higher loads leading to over-exertion of them, too. This gradually leads to an extensive damage of sarcomeres, breakdown of sarcoplasmic reticulum membranes, and loss of calcium homeostasis in the myocyte [74,84,98,108–110]. At this point, the dramatic increase in cytoplasmic calcium causes activation of several calcium-dependent proteolytic and phospholipolytic processes along with disruption of myofibrillar proteins and sarcolemma of the damaged fibers [74,76,78,84,98,111–118]. In addition, eccentric exercise damages mitochondria, sarcoplasmic, and connective tissue network [55,84,87,98,116,117]. The damage appears to worsen within the days following eccentric exercise, reaching a peak at 24–72 h post exercise depending on the type, intensity and loads of exercise and then gradually disappears within 2 or 3 weeks after exercise [14,15,21,55,66,67,71,72,76,79–90,93,97,116,117].

The inflammatory response, after EIMD, has been characterized quite well and several excellent original and review articles describe it in detail [15,21,71,74,76–79,90,93,119]. However, it should be mentioned that the majority of the mechanistic details presented in Figure 1 are based on cellular and animal studies while the inflammatory response in humans is not fully investigated and well addressed. Briefly, it begins immediately after the main mechanical damage when increased Ca^{2+} concentrations in the cytoplasm lead to degradation of muscle proteins and membrane phospholipids by activation of calpains and phospholipases A2 [114]. Meanwhile, three different types of inflammatory cells enter the injured area after muscle damage, namely, neutrophils and macrophages of type M1 and M2 [the analogs of rats' CD68 (ED1+) and CD163 (ED2+) in humans].

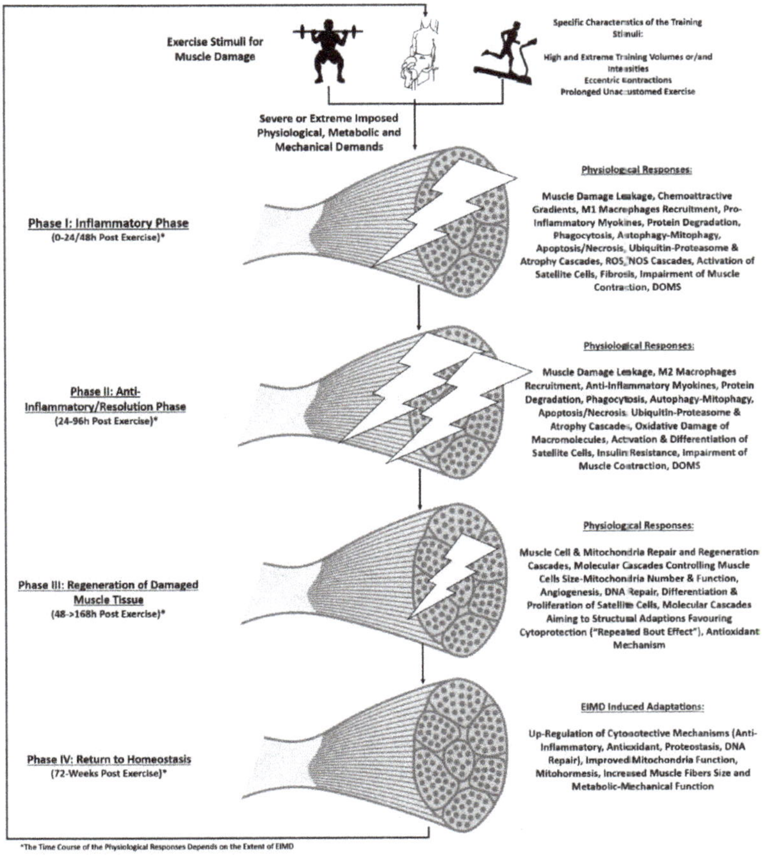

Figure 1. Time course of the physiological responses during exercise-induced muscle damage.

Their main purpose is to degrade the damaged tissue by releasing active oxygen /nitrogen forms, and induce oxidative stress which is crucial for muscle regeneration after EIMD [14,71,76,87,93,117,120–124]. Neutrophils infiltrate the muscle tissue within a few hours and they phagocytose necrotic muscle fibers and cellular "remnant" while they constitute a source of pro-inflammatory myokines such as IL-1 and TNF-α [71,74,76,78,87,115,123–

126]. Twenty-four hours post-EIMD macrophages appear in the damaged muscle tissue remaining for up to 14 days at the injured sites. The first subpopulation of macrophages are the macrophages expressing the ED1+ antigen and can enter into injured muscle fibers to phagocyte remnant cells and eroded myofibrils. The second subpopulation is ED2+ macrophages whose primary function is the secretion of growth factors and cytokines such as IGF-1, IL-6, and PDGF that can regulate proliferation and differentiation of myoblasts. Although, white blood cells are the main mediators of inflammation, fibroblasts and satellite cells are also "recruited" in the damaged area [71,115,127,128]. Fibroblasts have been shown to produce IL-6 and IL-1α, maintaining by this way the inflammatory response, and activating the proliferation of satellite cells to initiate the regeneration of damaged muscle fibers [71,125,128–135]. In addition, EIMD, elicits reactive oxygen and nitrogen species (RONS) which accompany the inflammatory response. According to the extent of muscle damage, RONS can further damage the muscle tissue but they also play a significant role for muscle regeneration and the adaptation of muscle tissues to eccentric exercise by mediating the up-regulation of antioxidant enzymes and the mitohormetic effects of exercise [14,16,18,70,79,120,136–151]. As a consequence of the activation of all the previous mentioned mechanisms in response to EIMD muscle cells' autophagy, apoptosis, and regeneration-adaptation molecular mechanisms are upregulated, to reinforce the regeneration of muscle cells [103,136,141,144,146,148,152–182]. Thus, EIMD is also a successful model to investigate the effect of dietary compounds on the stress-induced mechanisms of autophagy, apoptosis, and regeneration-adaptation molecular cascades. Table 1 summarizes the most common clinical and biochemical indices that are affected by EIMD.

Table 1. Clinical and biochemical indices affected by the inflammatory response after exercise-induced muscle damage.

Physiological Response	Marker
Pain/Delayed Muscle Soreness	Perceived Muscle Soreness by Visual Analog Scale or Algometers
Muscle Function	Rate of Force/Torque Development, Maximum Strength Power, Range of Motion, Muscular Work
Oedema	Limb Circumferences
Oxidative Stress	Protein Carbonyls, MDA, Isoprostanes, GSH/GSSG, Antioxidant Enzymes (Glutathione Peroxidases, Superoxide Dismutase, Catalase), Total Antioxidant Capacity, Antioxidant Vitamins
Muscle Damage	CK, LDH, Myoglobin, T-Troponin, Hydroxyproline, Hydroxylysine
Systemic Inflammation	WBC Count, IL-6, TNF-a, CRP, IL-10, IL-8, IL-1Ra, Lipid Mediators, INF-γ, MCP1, MIP-1

5. Exercise-Induced Muscle Damage and Its Methodological Advantages as an inflammatory Model in Humans

In our opinion, EIMD is a convenient, dynamic, and informative model of inflammation. It can be applied either in studies investigating the homeostatic responses of individuals under inflammatory stimuli or for the estimation of the anti-inflammatory or pro-inflammatory potential of dietary patterns, foods, supplements, nutrients or phytochemicals. The main advantages of EIMD are the following (Figure 2):

i. EIMD can be easily accepted by the volunteers and the bioethics committees. It can be easily induced by different types of exercise/training either in the lower or the upper limbs (see below). The inflammatory response can be applied to all kinds of populations irrespective of their health and training status, age, gender, race, body composition etc. Most importantly, volunteers easily consent to this kind of intervention which is actually just about exercise for them. In addition, most bioethics committees would have no objections to this kind of experimentation in humans.

ii. EIMD can be easily applied to humans in a regulated manner. Exercise scientists can induce muscle damage by forcing muscles to lengthen while generating active tension, with various stimuli. As it has been discussed in the previous section, EIMD can be easily induced through eccentric training after 85 to 300 maximal eccentric contractions, while the magnitude and the extent of EIMD from eccentric exercise, seems to be higher and prolonged (lasting for 72 h until 1–2weeks) compared to other type of exercises [14,15,55,62–64,66,67,70,72,74,79,84,86,88,90,93,94,97,112,113,117,122,132,183–200]. It should be mentioned that eccentric EIMD can be used and recommended for the prevention and/or rehabilitation of many chronic health conditions [94,188,199,201–221] since eccentric exercise has about 2–4 times lower metabolic and cardiovascular demands compared to other types of exercises [96,222]. Therefore, it seems that the use of eccentric exercise is a safe, effective, and regulated way to induce EIMD in all population groups. However, other training stimuli could also be applied. For example, high volume drop jump sessions ($\geq$100 jumps) [223–228], or in general exercises with an increased volume of stretch-lengthening cycle movements [229], prolonged moderate to high intensity running [196,230,231], cycling [232–235], and downhill running [236–240], have been repeatedly reported to induce significant EIMD, lasting for more than 72–96 h post-training. Although traditional resistance training (e.g., 60–80% of 1RM, 4–8 sets per exercise) can induce also EIMD [241–243] and trigger immune [244–249] and inflammation-related molecules (e.g., cytokines and chemokines) responses [245–252], the extent of EIMD is limited or significantly lower and with shorter duration than the above type of exercises, especially compared to eccentric training [74,117,202,253,254]. For most of these exercises, no special instrumentation is required. Independent of the exercise type, EIMD will be stronger and longer if the exercise used is characterized by very high mechanical and metabolic demands, e.g., with high volumes and intensities, fast contraction velocities, high contraction frequencies, short rest periods, and at long muscle lengths [14,15,55,62–67,70–75,79,84,86,88,90,93,97,112,113,117,122,132,183–228]. However, it seems that EIMD is even greater and with longer duration in untrained participants [255] and when a new/different training stimuli (unaccustomed exercise) that voluntaries are not familiar with it is applied [256].

iii. The inflammatory mechanisms underlying EIMD are well defined. The muscle microtrauma, induced by the different types of exercise, but mostly from eccentric exercise, can trigger a typical cascade of inflammatory events that resemble aseptic inflammation after tissue damage (see above). It is therefore easier for researchers to identify the crucial mechanistic points that each intervention could affect.

iv. One of the biggest advantages of EIMD, is that researchers could have the whole picture of the inflammatory response and its lysis in a strict and regulated time course. In contrast, when individuals with already established low-grade, chronic inflammation are recruited, the variability of the clinical and biochemical phenotypes, pharmacology, and medical history is usually large even in well-controlled studies. Thus, even in the best controlled cross sectional studies, the diversity between the participants would have a strong conflicting impact on research outcomes.

v. Biological sampling. Apart from the classical blood or saliva samples, that are usually collected before and several time points after the exercise trial this type of experiments allow you to take samples of the inflamed tissue, namely muscle biopsies. This technique has been used in many studies, investigating either the training-induced adaptations on muscle fibers (for example [89,122,257–263]), or muscle damage-inflammation (for example [63,122,128,231,248,264–271]. Muscle samples for such type of studies are usually obtained with Bergstrom needles from vastus lateralis of lower extremities, under local anesthesia, easy and quite safe for the volunteers, while in the majority of the countries, this is well accepted from the bioethics committees. The main advantage of taking muscle samples is that researchers, can investigate inflammation straight on the inflamed tissue and its cells in contrast to the majority of the studies where the inflammatory mechanisms are inferred by the alteration of biochemical markers in the circulation. Muscle biopsies can provide important information on the extent of sarcomere damage, of intra-cell biochemical-molecular procedures and/or genetic background of EIMD.

vi. The kinetics of clinical phenotypes linked to the inflammatory response can be easily determined. Such phenotypes are delayed-onset muscle soreness, maximum isometric torque, range of motion, limb circumference, and several other types of ergometric tests according to the inflamed limb.

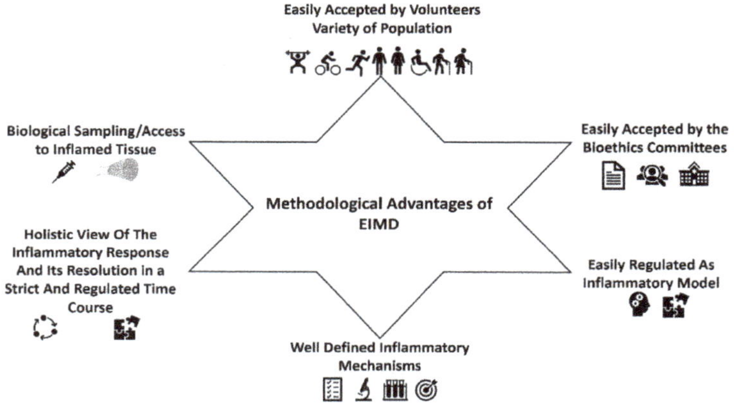

Figure 2. Methodological advantages of exercise-induced muscle damage.

6. Applications of Exercise Induced Muscle Damage as a Model of Inflammation

The EIMD model can serve as a precise model, in studies investigating the effects of nutritional and training interventions, on acute and chronic inflammation conditions, mainly in metabolic-related inflammatory conditions. As for example, EIMD could serve as a useful model in human studies investigating:

i. Acute and chronic inflammations. EIMD inflammatory response share similar pathophysiological and biochemical responses with acute and chronic inflammation. Thus, EIMD could find application in studies investigating the effect of nutrition and/or exercise, in acute and chronic inflammatory conditions such as those observed before and/or during the majority of chronic and non-communicable diseases [1,2,4,5,8,9,20,24,29,32–34,128,272]. For example, the inflammatory status of certain population groups (e.g., obese vs. normal weight) can be better assessed and compared under the dynamic conditions of EIMD. Taking into account that muscle biopsies can also be obtained and then the molecular mechanisms of autophagy, apoptosis and regeneration-adaptation could also be studied [75,103,136,141,144,146,148,152–182].

ii. Considering the pathophysiology behind conditions such as muscle/neurogenic inflammation, atrophy, cachexia, sarcopenia, and chronic muscle protein degradation EIMD can serve as a very reliable and regulated model to investigate how nutrition and or exercise may affect the physiological and biochemical background of those conditions.

iii. Ischemic preconditioning (IPC). After an EIMD stimuli, the following exercise bouts induce lower muscle damage and inflammation, due to the specific muscle adaptations, that minimize the extent of muscle damage, a phenomenon that it is known as "repeated bout effect" (RBE [79,84,273–276]). IPC protective mechanisms are comparable to those of RBE. IPC attained after one to five cycles of intermittent bouts of Ischemia/reperfusion, provide protection against the possibility of subsequent ischemia with longer duration. It has been documented that ROS are the main cardioprotective factor of IPC. Just a single bout of IPC produces a significant amount of ROS from mitochondria which trigger the protective signaling cascade [139]. Almost the same mechanisms seem to induce the RBE after repeated bouts of training sessions [79,84,273–276], providing further support that EIMD is a very good model to investigate the IPC and the hormetic effects of diet on those mechanisms.

iv. Rhabdomyolysis. Rhabdomyolysis is a pathophysiological condition of extensive skeletal muscle cell damage which could be induced from many physical (trauma, strenuous muscle exercise, electrical current) and non-physical causes (metabolic syndrome, drugs, electrolyte imbalance) [277]. This is a frequent phenomenon in patients taking statins, which may lead to unfavorable effects ranging from myalgia or myopathy to rhabdomyolysis and sometimes to acute renal failure [277]. The initial metabolic hypothesis of statin myopathy is that mitochondrial function is reduced while neutral lipids are increased, and ubiquitin proteasome is activated. In this case the activation of ubiquitin induces acceleration of proteolysis leading to muscle break down, atrophy, and necrosis [278]. Again, drug- and non-drug-induced rhabdomyolysis, have the same mechanisms and responses as those founded during an EIMD situation, specifically of those that are observed during the first 24–48 h post-exercise [14,15,18,21,55,63,65,66,71,72,74–80,87,90,93,103,116.117,120–123,136–138,140–144,146,148,152–182,196–198,200,279–285]. Therefore, EIMD can be applied in studies investigating the phenotypes that are more prone to rhabdomyolysis or in studies investigating the protective effects of dietary compounds to it.

v. Fibromyalgia (FM). FM is a complex syndrome characterized by widespread pain that affects many tissues and the presence of allodynia and hyperalgesia [286,287]. Fatigue and functional disorders usually appear during the syndrome [286,287]. Pain is a common feature of EIMD and the physiological-metabolic mechanisms-responses observed in FM are similar to those found during EIMD [288].

7. Conclusions

According to the above, it seems that EIMD is a controlled, highly regulated tool in the hands of researchers, to investigate the ability of different types of nutritional and training interventions to interfere with the progression and lysis of acute inflammatory conditions. It is worth testing if the ability of those interventions to attenuate acute inflammatory responses after EIMD can predict their ability to also act protectively against chronic inflammation although such as link has not been established yet Nevertheless, EIMD allows the assessment of the putative anti-inflammatory, hermetic, or immunomodulatory properties of dietary intervention directly to human beings under real, dynamic conditions.

Author Contributions: Writing—review and editing, S.M., I.S., S.A., and T.N., visualization-supervision: T.N. All authors have read and agreed to the published version of the manuscript.

Funding: The study was funded by the Postgraduate Programme of "Applied Nutrition and Dietetics" of Harokopio University.

Acknowledgments: We would like to thank Cleo Maria Kiourelly for helping with the English Editing.

Conflicts of Interest: The authors declare no conflict of interest.

References

1. Donath, M.; Meier, D.; Böni-Schnetzler, M. Inflammation in the pathophysiology and therapy of cardiometabolic disease. *Endocr. Rev.* **2019**, *40*, 1080–1091. [CrossRef] [PubMed]
2. Saltiel, A.; Olefsky, J. Inflammatory mechanisms linking obesity and metabolic disease. *J. Clin. Investig.* **2017**, *127*, 1–4. [CrossRef]
3. Deng, F.; Shivappa, N.; Tang, Y.; Mann, J.; Hebert, J. Association between diet-related inflammation, all-cause, all-cancer, and cardiovascular disease mortality, with special focus on prediabetics: Findings from NHANES III. *Eur. J. Nutr.* **2017**, *56*, 1085–1093. [CrossRef] [PubMed]
4. Fougère, B.; Boulanger, E.; Nourhashémi, F.; Guyonnet, S.; Cesari, M. Chronic inflammation: Accelerator of biological aging. *J. Gerontol. A Biol. Sci. Med. Sci.* **2016**, *72*, 1218–1225. [CrossRef]
5. Draganidis, D.; Karagounis, L.; Athanailidis, I.; Chatzinikolaou, A.; Jamurtas, A.; Fatouros, I. Inflammaging and Skeletal Muscle: Can Protein Intake Make a Difference? *J. Nutr.* **2016**, *146*, 1940–1952. [CrossRef] [PubMed]
6. Torres, S.; Fabersani, E.; Marquez, A.; Gauffin-Cano, P. Adipose tissue inflammation and metabolic syndrome. The proactive role of probiotics. *Eur. J. Nutr.* **2019**, *58*, 27–43. [CrossRef]
7. Razquin, C.; Martinez-Gonzalez, M. A Traditional Mediterranean Diet Effectively Reduces Inflammation and Improves Cardiovascular Health. *Nutrients* **2019**, *11*, 1842. [CrossRef]
8. Koloverou, E.; Panagiotakos, D. Inflammation: A new player in the link between Mediterranean diet and diabetes mellitus: A review. *Curr. Nutr. Rep.* **2017**, *6*, 247–256. [CrossRef]
9. Calder, P.; Bosco, N.; Bourdet-Sicard, R.; Capuron, L.; Delzenne, N.; Doré, J.; Franceschi, C.; Lehtinen, M.; Recker, T.; Salvioli, S. Health relevance of the modification of low grade inflammation in ageing (inflammageing) and the role of nutrition. *Ageing Res. Rev.* **2017**, *40*, 95–119. [CrossRef]
10. Calder, P.; Albers, R.; Antoine, J.; Blum, S.; Bourdet-Sicard, R.; Ferns, G.; Folkerts, G.; Friedmann, P.; Frost, G.; Guarner, F. Inflammatory disease processes and interactions with nutrition. *Br. J. Nutr.* **2009**, *101*, 1–45. [CrossRef]
11. Lankinen, M.; Uusitupa, M.; Schwab, U. Nordic Diet and Inflammation-A Review of Observational and Intervention Studies. *Nutrients* **2019**, *11*, 1396. [CrossRef] [PubMed]
12. Perel, P.; Roberts, I.; Sena, E.; Wheble, P.; Briscoe, C.; Sandercock, P.; Macleod, M.; Mignini, L.; Jayaram, P.; Khan, K. Comparison of treatment effects between animal experiments and clinical trials: Systematic review. *BMJ* **2007**, *334*, 197. [CrossRef] [PubMed]
13. Laman, J.; Kooistra, S.; Clausen, B. Reproducibility issues: Avoiding pitfalls in animal inflammation models. In *Inflammation. Methods in Molecular Biology*; Clausen, B., Laman, J., Eds.; Humana Press: New York, NY, USA, 2017; Volume 1559, pp. 1–17.
14. Margaritelis, N.V.; Paschalis, V.; Theodorou, A.A.; Kyparos, A.; Nikolaidis, M.G. Redox basis of exercise physiology. *Redox Biol.* **2020**, *35*, 101499. [CrossRef]
15. Peake, J.; Neubauer, O.; Della Gatta, P.; Nosaka, K. Muscle damage and inflammation during recovery from exercise. *J. Appl. Physiol.* **2017**, *122*, 559–570. [CrossRef]
16. Parker, L.; Shaw, C.; Stepto, N.; Levinger, I. Exercise and Glycemic Control: Focus on Redox Homeostasis and Redox-Sensitive Protein Signaling. *Front. Endocrinol.* **2017**, *8*. [CrossRef] [PubMed]
17. González, N.; Santivañez, J.; Fuster, B.; Boira, E.; Martinez-Navarro, I.; Bartoll, Ó.; Domingo, C. Quick Recovery of Renal Alterations and Inflammatory Activation after a Marathon. *Kidney Dis.* **2019**, *5*, 259–265. [CrossRef]
18. Koyama, K. Exercise-induced oxidative stress: A tool for "hormesis" and "adaptive response". *J. Sports Med. Phys. Fitness.* **2014**, *3*, 115–120. [CrossRef]
19. Hikida, R.; Staron, R.; Hagerman, F.; Sherman, W.; Costill, D. Muscle fiber necrosis associated with human marathon runners. *J. Neurol. Sci.* **1983**, *59*, 185–203. [CrossRef]
20. Soehnlein, O.; Steffens, S.; Hidalgo, A.; Weber, C. Neutrophils as protagonists and targets in chronic inflammation. *Nat. Rev. Immunol.* **2017**, *17*, 248. [CrossRef]
21. Kajal, H.; Stephen, C.; Elizabeth, D.; Prabha, C.; David, M. Macrophages and the Recovery from Acute and Chronic Inflammation. *Annu. Rev. Physiol.* **2017**, *79*, 567–592. [CrossRef]
22. Salminen, A.; Huuskonen, J.; Ojala, J.; Kauppinen, A.; Kaarniranta, K.; Suuronen, T. Activation of innate immunity system during aging: NF-kB signaling is the molecular culprit of inflamm-aging. *Ageing Res. Rev.* **2008**, *7*, 83–105. [CrossRef] [PubMed]
23. Libby, P. Inflammatory mechanisms: The molecular basis of inflammation and disease. *Nutr. Rev.* **2007**, *65*, S140–S146. [CrossRef] [PubMed]
24. Pietzner, M.; Kaul, A.; Henning, A.; Kastenmüller, G.; Artati, A.; Lerch, M.; Adamski, J.; Nauck, M.; Friedrich, N. Comprehensive metabolic profiling of chronic low-grade inflammation among generally healthy individuals. *BMC Med.* **2017**, *15*, 210. [CrossRef] [PubMed]
25. Soysal, P.; Stubbs, B.; Lucato, P.; Luchini, C.; Solmi, M.; Peluso, R.; Sergi, G.; Isik, A.; Manzato, E.; Maggi, S. Inflammation and frailty in the elderly: A systematic review and meta-analysis. *Ageing Res. Rev.* **2016**, *31*, 1–8. [CrossRef] [PubMed]
26. Lasselin, J.; Capuron, L. Chronic low-grade inflammation in metabolic disorders: Relevance for behavioral symptoms. *Neuroimmunomodulation* **2014**, *21*, 95–101. [CrossRef] [PubMed]
27. Chovatiya, R.; Medzhitov, R. Stress, inflammation, and defense of homeostasis. *Mol. Cell.* **2014**, *54*, 281–288. [CrossRef] [PubMed]
28. Beyer, I.; Mets, T.; Bautmans, I. Chronic low-grade inflammation and age-related sarcopenia. *Curr. Opin. Clin. Nutr. Metab. Care* **2012**, *15*, 12–22. [CrossRef]

29. Monteiro, R.; Azevedo, I. Chronic inflammation in obesity and the metabolic syndrome. *Mediat. Inflamm.* **2010**, *2010*, 289645. [CrossRef]
30. Minihane, A.; Vinoy, S.; Russell, W.; Baka, A.; Roche, H.; Tuohy, K.; Teeling, J.; Blaak, E.; Fenech, M.; Vauzour, D.; et al. Low-grade inflammation, diet composition and health: Current research evidence and its translation. *Br. J. Nutr.* **2015**, *114*, 999–1012. [CrossRef]
31. Chen, Y.; Liu, S.; Leng, S. Chronic Low-grade Inflammatory Phenotype (CLIP) and Senescent Immune Dysregulation. *Clin. Ther.* **2019**, *41*, 400–409. [CrossRef]
32. Nishida, K.; Otsu, K. Inflammation and metabolic cardiomyopathy. *Cardiovasc. Res.* **2017**, *113*, 389–398. [CrossRef] [PubMed]
33. Hotamisligil, G. Inflammation, metaflammation and immunometabolic disorders. *Nature* **2017**, *542*, 177–185. [CrossRef] [PubMed]
34. Kotas, M.; Medzhitov, R. Homeostasis, inflammation, and disease susceptibility. *Cell* **2015**, *160*, 816–827. [CrossRef] [PubMed]
35. Durham, W.J.; Dillon, E.L.; Sheffield-Moore, M. Inflammatory burden and amino acid metabolism in cancer cachexia. *Curr. Opin. Clin. Nutr. Metab. Care* **2009**, *12*, 72–77. [CrossRef]
36. Danesh, J.; Wheeler, J.; Hirschfield, G.; Eda, S.; Eiriksdottir, G.; Rumley, A.; Lowe, G.; Pepys, M.; Gudnason, V. C-reactive protein and other circulating markers of inflammation in the prediction of coronary heart disease. *N. Engl. J. Med.* **2004**, *350*, 1387–1397. [CrossRef]
37. Mills, P.; Hong, S.; Redwine, L.; Carter, S.; Chiu, A.; Ziegler, M.; Dimsdale, J.; Maisel, A. Physical fitness attenuates leukocyte-endothelial adhesion in response to acute exercise. *J. Appl. Physiol.* **2006**, *101*, 785–788. [CrossRef]
38. Petersen, A.M.; Pedersen, B.K. The anti-inflammatory effect of exercise. *J. Appl. Physiol.* **2005**, *98*, 1154–1162. [CrossRef]
39. Schwingshackl, L.; Hoffmann, G. Mediterranean dietary pattern, inflammation and endothelial function: A systematic review and meta-analysis of intervention trials. *Nutr. Metab. Cardiovasc. Dis.* **2014**, *24*, 929–939. [CrossRef]
40. Ricker, M.; Haas, W. Anti-inflammatory diet in clinical practice: A review. *Nutr. Clin. Pract.* **2017**, *32*, 318–325. [CrossRef]
41. Sears, B. Anti-inflammatory diets. *J. Am. Coll. Nutr.* **2015**, *34*, 14–21. [CrossRef]
42. Halliwell, B. *Antioxidant and Anti-Inflammatory Components of Foods*; ILSI Europe: Brussels, Belgium, 2015; p. 34.
43. Galland, L. Diet and inflammation. *Nutr. Clin. Pract.* **2010**, *25*, 634–640. [CrossRef]
44. Arouca, A.; Meirhaeghe, A.; Dallongeville, J.; Moreno, L.; Lourenço, G.; Marcos, A.; Huybrechts, I.; Manios, Y.; Lambrinou, C.; Gottrand, F. Interplay between the Mediterranean diet and C-reactive protein genetic polymorphisms towards inflammation in adolescents. *Clin. Nutr.* **2020**, *39*, 1919–1926. [CrossRef] [PubMed]
45. Nomikos, T.; Fragopoulou, E.; Antonopoulou, S.; Panagiotakos, D. Mediterranean diet and platelet-activating factor; a systematic review. *Clin. Biochem.* **2018**, *60*, 1–10. [CrossRef]
46. Seok, J.; Warren, S.; Cuenca, A.; Mindrinos, M.; Baker, H.; Xu, W.; Richards, D.; McDonald-Smith, G.; Gao, H.; Hennessy, L. Genomic responses in mouse models poorly mimic human inflammatory diseases. *Proc. Natl. Acad. Sci. USA* **2013**, *110*, 3507–3512. [CrossRef] [PubMed]
47. Gambini, J.; Inglés, M.; Olaso, G.; Lopez-Grueso, R.; Bonet-Costa, V.; Gimeno-Mallench, L.; Mas-Bargues, C.; Abdelaziz, K.; Gomez-Cabrera, M.; Vina, J. Properties of resveratrol: In vitro and in vivo studies about metabolism, bioavailability, and biological effects in animal models and humans. *Oxidative Med. Cell. Longev.* **2015**, *2015*. [CrossRef] [PubMed]
48. Webb, D. Animal models of human disease: Inflammation. *Biochem. Pharmacol.* **2014**, *87*, 121–130. [CrossRef] [PubMed]
49. Ahluwalia, N.; Andreeva, V.; Kesse-Guyot, E.; Hercberg, S. Dietary patterns, inflammation and the metabolic syndrome. *Diabetes Metab.* **2013**, *39*, 99–110. [CrossRef]
50. Wang, X.; Ouyang, Y.; Liu, J.; Zhao, G. Flavonoid intake and risk of CVD: A systematic review and meta-analysis of prospective cohort studies. *Br. J. Nutr.* **2014**, *111*, 1–11. [CrossRef]
51. Rangel-Huerta, O.; Aguilera, C.; Mesa, M.; Gil, A. Omega-3 long-chain polyunsaturated fatty acids supplementation on inflammatory biomakers: A systematic review of randomised clinical trials. *Br. J. Nutr.* **2012**, *107*, S159–S170. [CrossRef]
52. Schwingshackl, L.; Christoph, M.; Hoffmann, G. Effects of olive oil on markers of inflammation and endothelial function—a systematic review and meta-analysis. *Nutrients* **2015**, *7*, 7651–7675. [CrossRef]
53. Buyken, A.; Goletzke, J.; Joslowski, G.; Felbick, A.; Cheng, G.; Herder, C.; Brand-Miller, J. Association between carbohydrate quality and inflammatory markers: Systematic review of observational and interventional studies. *Am. J. Clin. Nutr.* **2014**, *99*, 813–833. [CrossRef] [PubMed]
54. Moradi, S.; Issah, A.; Mohammadi, H.; Mirzaei, K. Associations between dietary inflammatory index and incidence of breast and prostate cancer: A systematic review and meta-analysis. *Nutrition* **2018**, *55*, 168–178. [CrossRef] [PubMed]
55. Owens, D.; Twist, C.; Cobley, J.; Howatson, G.; Close, G. Exercise-induced muscle damage: What is it, what causes it and what are the nutritional solutions? *Eur. J. Sport Sci.* **2018**, *19*, 71–85. [CrossRef] [PubMed]
56. Fouré, A.; Bendahan, D. Is branched-chain amino acids supplementation an efficient nutritional strategy to alleviate skeletal muscle damage? A systematic review. *Nutrients* **2017**, *9*, 1047. [CrossRef]
57. Pasiakos, S.; Lieberman, H.; McLellan, T. Effects of protein supplements on muscle damage, soreness and recovery of muscle function and physical performance: A systematic review. *Sports Med.* **2014**, *44*, 655–670. [CrossRef]
58. Cockburn, E.; Bell, P.; Stevenson, E. Effect of milk on team sport performance after exercise-induced muscle damage. *Med. Sci. Sports Exerc.* **2013**, *45*, 1585–1592. [CrossRef]

59. Cockburn, E.; Hayes, P.; French, D.; Stevenson, E.; St Clair Gibson, A. Acute milk-based protein–CHO supplementation attenuates exercise-induced muscle damage. *Appl. Physiol. Nutr. Metab.* **2008**, *33*, 775–783. [CrossRef]
60. Harty, P.; Cottet, M.; Malloy, J.; Kerksick, C. Nutritional and Supplementation Strategies to Prevent and Attenuate Exercise-Induced Muscle Damage: A Brief Review. *Sports Med. Open* **2019**, *5*, 1. [CrossRef]
61. Sousa, M.; Teixeira, V.; Soares, J. Dietary strategies to recover from exercise-induced muscle damage. *Int. J. Food Sci. Nutr.* **2014**, *65*, 151–163. [CrossRef]
62. Margaritelis, N.; Paschalis, V.; Theodorou, A.; Kyparos, A.; Nikolaidis, M. Antioxidants in Personalized Nutrition and Exercise. *Adv. Nutr.* **2018**, *9*, 813–823. [CrossRef]
63. Michailidis, Y.; Karagounis, L.; Terzis, G.; Jamurtas, A.; Spengos, K.; Tsoukas, D.; Chatzinikolaou, A.; Mandalidis, D.; Stefanetti, R.; Papassotiriou, I. Thiol-based antioxidant supplementation alters human skeletal muscle signaling and attenuates its inflammatory response and recovery after intense eccentric exercise. *Am. J. Clin. Nutr.* **2013**, *98*, 233–245. [CrossRef]
64. Paschalis, V.; Theodorou, A.; Margaritelis, N.; Kyparos, A.; Nikolaidis, M. N-acetylcysteine supplementation increases exercise performance and reduces oxidative stress only in individuals with low levels of glutathione. *Free Radic. Biol. Med.* **2017**, *115*, 288–297. [CrossRef] [PubMed]
65. Margaritelis, N.; Theodorou, A.; Paschalis, V.; Veskoukis, A.; Dipla, K.; Zafeiridis, A.; Panayiotou, G.; Vrabas, I.S.; Kyparos, A.; Nikolaidis, M. Adaptations to endurance training depend on exercise-induced oxidative stress: Exploiting redox inter-individual variability. *Acta Physiol.* **2017**, *222*, e12972. [CrossRef] [PubMed]
66. Kotsis, Y.; Mikellidi, A.; Aresti, C.; Persia, E.; Sotiropoulos, A.; Panagiotakos, D.; Antonopoulou, S.; Nomikos, T. A low-dose, 6-week bovine colostrum supplementation maintains performance and attenuates inflammatory indices following a Loughborough Intermittent Shuttle Test in soccer players. *Eur. J. Nutr.* **2018**, *57*, 1181–1195. [CrossRef] [PubMed]
67. Kotsis, Y.; Methenitis, S.; Mikellidi, A.; Aresti, C.; Persia, E.; Antonopoulou, S.; Nomikos, T. Changes of rate of torque development in soccer players after a Loughborough Intermittent Shuttle Test: Effect of bovine colostrum supplementation. *Isokinet. Exerc. Sci.* **2020**, *28*, 59–72. [CrossRef]
68. Bongiovanni, T.; Genovesi, F.; Nemmer, M.; Carling, C.; Alberti, G.; Howatson, G. Nutritional interventions for reducing the signs and symptoms of exercise-induced muscle damage and accelerate recovery in athletes: Current knowledge, practical application and future perspectives. *Eur. J. Appl. Physiol.* **2020**, *120*, 1965–1996. [CrossRef]
69. Panza, V.P.; Diefenthaeler, F.; Da Silva, E. Benefits of dietary phytochemical supplementation on eccentric exercise-induced muscle damage: Is including antioxidants enough? *Nutrition* **2015**, *31*, 1072–1082. [CrossRef]
70. Margaritelis, N.; Paschalis, V.; Theodorou, A.; Kyparos, A.; Nikolaidis, M. Antioxidant supplementation, redox deficiencies and exercise performance: A falsification design. *Free Radic. Biol. Med.* **2020**, *158*, 44–52. [CrossRef]
71. Paulsen, G.; Mikkelsen, U.R.; Raastad, T.; Peake, J. Leucocytes, cytokines and satellite cells: What role do they play in muscle damage and regeneration following eccentric exercise? *Exerc. Immunol. Rev.* **2012**, *18*, 42–97.
72. Jamurtas, A.; Fatouros, I. Eccentric Exercise, Muscle Damage and Oxidative Stress. In *An International Perspective on Topics in Sports Med. and Sports Injury*; Zaslav, K., Ed.; IntechOpen: London, UK, 2012; pp. 113–130. [CrossRef]
73. Clarkson, P.M.; Hubal, M.J. Exercise-induced muscle damage in humans. *Am. J. Phys. Med. Rehabil.* **2002**, *81*, S52–S69. [CrossRef]
74. Proske, U.; Morgan, D. Muscle damage from eccentric exercise: Mechanism, mechanical signs, adaptation and clinical applications. *J. Physiol.* **2001**, *537*, 333–345. [CrossRef] [PubMed]
75. Methenitis, S. A Brief Review on Concurrent Training: From Laboratory to the Field. *Sports* **2018**, *6*, 127. [CrossRef] [PubMed]
76. Chazaud, B. Inflammation during skeletal muscle regeneration and tissue remodeling: Application to exercise-induced muscle damage management. *Immunol. Cell Biol.* **2016**, *94*, 140–145. [CrossRef] [PubMed]
77. Malm, C. Exercise-induced muscle damage and inflammation: Fact or fiction? *Acta Physiol. Scand.* **2001**, *171*, 233–239. [CrossRef] [PubMed]
78. Tidball, J.; Villalta, A. Regulatory interactions between muscle and the immune system during muscle regeneration. *Am. J. Physiol. Regul. Integr. Comp. Physiol.* **2010**, *298*, R1173–R1187. [CrossRef]
79. Margaritelis, N.; Theodorou, A.; Baltzopoulos, V.; Maganaris, C.; Paschalis, V.; Kyparos, A.; Nikolaidis, M. Muscle damage and inflammation after eccentric exercise: Can the repeated bout effect be removed? *Physiol. Rep.* **2015**, *3*, e12648. [CrossRef]
80. Tokinoya, K.; Ishikura, K.; Ra, S.; Ebina, K.; Miyakawa, S.; Ohmori, H. Relationship between early-onset muscle soreness and indirect muscle damage markers and their dynamics after a full marathon. *J. Exerc. Sci. Fit.* **2020**, *18*, 115–121. [CrossRef]
81. Carmona, G.; Roca, E.; Guerrero, M.; Cussó, R.; Bàrcena, C.; Mateu, M.; Cadefau, J. Fibre-type-specific and Mitochondrial Biomarkers of Muscle Damage after Mountain Races. *Int. J. Sports Med.* **2019**, *40*, 253–262. [CrossRef]
82. Flann, K.L.; LaStayo, P.C.; McClain, D.A.; Hazel, M.; Lindstedt, S.L. Muscle damage and muscle remodeling: No pain, no gain? *J. Exp. Biol.* **2011**, *214*, 674–679. [CrossRef]
83. Baumert, P.; Lake, M.J.; Stewart, C.E.; Drust, B.; Erskine, R.M. Genetic variation and exercise-induced muscle damage: Implications for athletic performance, injury and ageing. *Eur. J. Appl. Physiol.* **2016**, *116*, 1595–1625. [CrossRef]
84. Hyldahl, R.; Hubal, M. Lengthening our perspective: Morphological, cellular, and molecular responses to eccentric exercise. *Muscle Nerve.* **2014**, *49*, 155–170. [CrossRef]
85. Cheung, K.; Hume, P.; Maxwell, L. Delayed onset muscle soreness. *Sports Med.* **2003**, *33*, 145–164. [CrossRef] [PubMed]

86. Paschalis, V.; Koutedakis, Y.; Jamurtas, A.; Mougios, V.; Baltzopoulos, V. Equal volumes of high and low intensity of eccentric exercise in relation to muscle damage and performance. *J. Strength Cond. Res.* **2005**, *19*, 184–188. [CrossRef] [PubMed]
87. Kerksick, C.M.; Willoughby, D.; Kouretas, D.; Tsatsakis, A. Intramuscular responses with muscle damaging exercise and the interplay between multiple intracellular networks: A human perspective. *Food Chem. Toxicol.* **2013**, *61*, 136–143. [CrossRef] [PubMed]
88. Peake, J.; Nosaka, K.; Suzuki, K. Characterization of inflammatory responses to eccentric exercise in humans. *Exerc. Immunol. Rev.* **2005**, *11*, 64–85. [PubMed]
89. Methenitis, S.; Mpampoulis, T.; Spiliopoulou, P.; Papadimas, G.; Papadopoulos, C.; Chalari, E.; Evangelidou, E.; Stasinaki, A.N.; Nomikos, T.; Terzis, G. Muscle fiber composition, jumping performance and rate of force development adaptations induced by different power training volumes in females. *Appl. Physiol. Nutr. Metab.* **2020**, *45*, 996–1006. [CrossRef] [PubMed]
90. Hody, S.; Croisier, J.; Bury, T.; Rogister, B.; Leprince, P. Eccentric muscle contractions: Risks and benefits. *Front. Physiol.* **2019**, *10*. [CrossRef]
91. Bogdanis, G.; Tsoukos, A.; Brown, L.; Selima, E.; Veligekas, P.; Spengos, K.; Terzis, G. Muscle fiber and performance changes after fast eccentric complex training. *Med. Sci. Sports Exerc.* **2018**, *50*, 729–738. [CrossRef]
92. Tinwala, F.; Cronin, J.; Haemmerle, E.; Ross, A. Eccentric Strength Training: A Review of the Available Technology. *Strength Cond. J.* **2017**, *39*, 32–47. [CrossRef]
93. Douglas, J.; Pearson, S.; Ross, A.; McGuigan, M. Eccentric exercise: Physiological characteristics and acute responses. *Sports Med.* **2017**, *47*, 663–675. [CrossRef]
94. Douglas, J.; Pearson, S.; Ross, A.; McGuigan, M. Chronic Adaptations to Eccentric Training: A Systematic Review. *Sports Med.* **2016**, *47*, 917–941. [CrossRef] [PubMed]
95. Vogt, M.; Hoppeler, H. Eccentric exercise: Mechanisms and effects when used as training regime or training adjunct. *J. Appl. Physiol.* **2014**, *116*, 1446–1454. [CrossRef] [PubMed]
96. Isner-Horobeti, M.E.; Dufour, S.P.; Vautravers, P.; Geny, B.; Coudeyre, E.; Richard, R. Eccentric exercise training: Modalities, applications and perspectives. *Sports Med.* **2013**, *43*, 483–512. [CrossRef] [PubMed]
97. Proske, U.; Allen, T. Damage to skeletal muscle from eccentric exercise. *Exerc. Sport Sci. Rev.* **2005**, *33*, 98–104. [CrossRef]
98. Nishikawa, K. Eccentric contraction: Unraveling mechanisms of force enhancement and energy conservation. *J. Exp. Biol.* **2016**, *219*, 189–196. [CrossRef] [PubMed]
99. Lieber, R. Biomechanical response of skeletal muscle to eccentric contractions. *J. Sport Health Sci.* **2018**, *7*, 294–309. [CrossRef]
100. Gordon, A.; Huxley, A.; Julian, F. The variation in isometric tension with sarcomere length in vertebrate muscle fibres. *J. Physiol.* **1966**, *184*, 170–192. [CrossRef]
101. Maganaris, C. Force–length characteristics of in vivo human skeletal muscle. *Acta Physiol. Scand.* **2001**, *172*, 279–285. [CrossRef]
102. Leonard, T.; Herzog, W. Regulation of muscle force in the absence of actin-myosin-based cross-bridge interaction. *Am. J. Physiol. Cell Physiol.* **2010**, *299*, C14–C20. [CrossRef]
103. Krüger, M.; Kötter, S. Titin, a Central Mediator for Hypertrophic Signaling, Exercise-Induced Mechanosignaling and Skeletal Muscle Remodeling. *Front. Physiol.* **2016**, *7*. [CrossRef]
104. Bottinelli, R.; Canepari, M.; Pellegrino, M.A.; Reggiani, C. Force-velocity properties of human skeletal muscle fibres: Myosin heavy chain isoform and temperature dependence. *J. Physiol.* **1996**, *495 Pt 2*, 573–586. [CrossRef]
105. Babault, N.; Pousson, M.; Ballay, Y.; Van Hoecke, J. Activation of human quadriceps femoris during isometric, concentric, and eccentric contractions. *J. Appl. Physiol.* **2001**, *91*, 2628–2634. [CrossRef] [PubMed]
106. Enoka, R.M. Eccentric contractions require unique activation strategies by the nervous system. *J. Appl. Physiol.* **1996**, *81*, 2339–2346. [CrossRef] [PubMed]
107. Aagaard, P. Spinal and supraspinal control of motor function during maximaleccentric muscle contraction: Effects of resistance training. *J. Sport Health Sci.* **2018**, *7*, 282–293. [CrossRef]
108. Morgan, D.; Allen, D. Early events in stretch-induced muscle damage. *J. Appl. Physiol.* **1999**, *87*, 2007–2015. [CrossRef] [PubMed]
109. Lieber, R.; Friden, J. Muscle damage is not a function of muscle force but active muscle strain. *J. Appl. Physiol.* **1993**, *74*, 520–526. [CrossRef] [PubMed]
110. Friden, J.; Lieber, R. Structural and mechanical basis of exercise-induced muscle injury. *Med. Sci. Sports Exerc.* **1992**, *24*, 521–530. [CrossRef]
111. Lee, K.; Ochi, E.; Song, H.; Nakazato, K. Activation of AMP-activated protein kinase induce expression of FoxO1, FoxO3a, and myostatin after exercise-induced muscle damage. *Biochem. Biophys. Res. Commun.* **2015**, *466*, 289–294. [CrossRef]
112. Jiménez-Jiménez, R.; Cuevas, M.; Almar, M.; Lima, E.; García-López, D.; De Paz, J.; González-Gallego, J. Eccentric training impairs NF-κB activation and over-expression of inflammation-related genes induced by acute eccentric exercise in the elderly. *Mech. Ageing Dev.* **2008**, *129*, 313–321. [CrossRef]
113. Murphy, R.; Goodman, C.; McKenna, M.; Bennie, J.; Leikis, M.; Lamb, G. Calpain-3 is autolyzed and hence activated in human skeletal muscle 24 h following a single bout of eccentric exercise. *J. Appl. Physiol.* **2007**, *103*, 926–931. [CrossRef]
114. Belcastro, A.; Shewchuk, L.; Raj, D. Exercise-induced muscle injury: A calpain hypothesis. *Mol. Cell. Biochem.* **1998**, *179*, 135–145. [CrossRef] [PubMed]

115. Charge, S.; Rudnicki, M. Cellular and molecular regulation of muscle regeneration. *Physiol. Rev.* **2004**, *84*, 209–238. [CrossRef] [PubMed]
116. Kim, J.; Lee, J.; Kim, S.; Ryu, H.Y.; Cha, K.; Sung, D.J. Exercise-induced rhabdomyolysis mechanisms and prevention: A literature review. *J. Sport Health Sci.* **2016**, *5*, 324–333. [CrossRef] [PubMed]
117. Franchi, M.; Reeves, N.; Narici, M. Skeletal Muscle Remodeling in Response to Eccentric vs. Concentric Loading: Morphological, Molecular, and Metabolic Adaptations. *Front. Physiol.* **2017**, *8*. [CrossRef] [PubMed]
118. Ulbricht, A.; Gehlert, S.; Leciejewski, B.; Schiffer, T.; Bloch, W.; Höhfeld, J. Induction and adaptation of chaperone-assisted selective autophagy CASA in response to resistance exercise in human skeletal muscle. *Autophagy* **2015**, *11*, 538–546. [CrossRef]
119. Philippou, A.; Bogdanis, G.; Maridaki, M.; Halapas, A.; Sourla, A.; Koutsilieris, M. Systemic cytokine response following exercise-induced muscle damage in humans. *Clin. Chem. Lab. Med.* **2009**, *47*, 777–782. [CrossRef]
120. Cheng, A.; Yamada, T.; Rassier, D.; Andersson, D.; Westerblad, H.; Lanner, J. Reactive oxygen/nitrogen species and contractile function in skeletal muscle during fatigue and recovery. *J. Physiol.* **2016**, *594*, 5149–5160. [CrossRef]
121. Zuo, L.; Pannell, B. Redox Characterization of Functioning Skeletal Muscle. *Front. Physiol.* **2015**, *6*. [CrossRef]
122. Wright, C.R.; Brown, E.L.; Della Gatta, P.A.; Fatouros, I.G.; Karagounis, L.G.; Terzis, G.; Mastorakos, G.; Michailidis, Y.; Mandalidis, D.; Spengos, K.; et al. Regulation of Granulocyte Colony-Stimulating Factor and Its Receptor in Skeletal Muscle Is Dependent Upon the Type of Inflammatory Stimulus. *J. Interferon Cytokine Res.* **2015**, *35*, 710–719. [CrossRef]
123. Tidball, J. Inflammatory processes in muscle injury and repair. *Am. J. Physiol. Regul. Integr. Comp. Physiol.* **2005**, *288*, R345–R353. [CrossRef]
124. Brunelli, S.; Rovere-Querini, P. The immune system and the repair of skeletal muscle. *Pharmacol. Res.* **2008**, *58*, 117–121. [CrossRef] [PubMed]
125. Toth, K.; McKay, B.; De Lisio, M.; Little, J.; Tarnopolsky, M.; Parise, G. IL-6 induced STAT3 signalling is associated with the proliferation of human muscle satellite cells following acute muscle damage. *PLoS ONE* **2011**, *6*, e17392. [CrossRef] [PubMed]
126. Costamagna, D.; Costelli, P.; Sampaolesi, M.; Penna, F. Role of Inflammation in Muscle Homeostasis and Myogenesis. *Mediat. Inflamm.* **2015**, *501*, 805172. [CrossRef] [PubMed]
127. Pedersen, K.; Steensberg, A.; Keller, P.; Keller, C.; Fischer, C.; Hiscock, N.; Van Hall, G.; Plomgaard, P.; Febbraio, M. Muscle-derived interleukin-6: Lipolytic, anti-inflammatory and immune regulatory effects. *Pflug. Arch.* **2003**, *446*, 9–16. [CrossRef]
128. Perandini, L.; Chimin, P.; Lutkemeyer, D.S.; Câmara, N. Chronic inflammation in skeletal muscle impairs satellite cells function during regeneration: Can physical exercise restore the satellite cell niche? *FEBS J.* **2018**, *285*, 1973–1984. [CrossRef]
129. Hawke, T.; Garry, D. Myogenic satellite cells: Physiology to molecular biology. *J. Appl. Physiol.* **2001**, *91*, 534–551. [CrossRef] [PubMed]
130. Serrano, A.; Baeza-Raja, B.; Perdiguero, E.; Jardí, M.; Muñoz-Cánoves, P. Interleukin-6 is an essential regulator of satellite cell-mediated skeletal muscle hypertrophy. *Cell Metab.* **2008**, *7*, 33–44. [CrossRef]
131. Muñoz-Cánoves, P.; Scheele, C.; Pedersen, B.; Serrano, A. Interleukin-6 myokine signaling in skeletal muscle: A double-edged sword? *FEBS J.* **2013**, *280*, 4131–4148. [CrossRef] [PubMed]
132. Cermak, N.; Snijders, T.; McKay, B.; Parise, G.; Verdijk, L.; Tarnopolsky, M.; Gibala, M.; Van Loon, L.J. Eccentric exercise increases satellite cell content in type II muscle fibers. *Med. Sci. Sports Exerc.* **2013**, *45*, 230–237. [CrossRef]
133. Dumont, N.; Bentzinger, F.; Sincennes, M.C.; Rudnicki, M. Satellite cells and skeletal muscle regeneration. *Compr. Physiol.* **2015**. [CrossRef]
134. Furuichi, Y.; Fujii, N. Mechanism of satellite cell regulation by myokines. *J. Sports Med. Phys. Fitness.* **2017**, *6*, 311–316. [CrossRef]
135. Snijders, T.; Verdijk, L.; Beelen, M.; McKay, B.; Parise, G.; Kadi, F.; Van Loon, L. A single bout of exercise activates skeletal muscle satellite cells during subsequent overnight recovery. *Exp. Physiol.* **2012**, *97*, 762–773. [CrossRef] [PubMed]
136. Morales-Alamo, D.; Calbet, J.A. AMPK signaling in skeletal muscle during exercise: Role of reactive oxygen and nitrogen species. *Free Radic. Biol. Med.* **2016**, *98*, 68–77. [CrossRef] [PubMed]
137. Thirupathi, A.; Pinho, R. Effects of reactive oxygen species and interplay of antioxidants during physical exercise in skeletal muscles. *J. Physiol. Biochem.* **2018**, *74*, 359–367. [CrossRef] [PubMed]
138. Aguiló, A.; Tauler, P.; Fuentespina, E.; Tur, J.; Córdova, A.; Pons, A. Antioxidant response to oxidative stress induced by exhaustive exercise. *Physiol. Behav.* **2005**, *84*, 1–7. [CrossRef] [PubMed]
139. Alleman, R.; Katunga, L.; Nelson, M.; Brown, D.; Anderson, E. The "Goldilocks Zone" from a redox perspective—Adaptive vs. deleterious responses to oxidative stress in striated muscle. *Front. Physiol.* **2014**, *5*. [CrossRef]
140. Cooper, C.; Vollaard, N.B.; Choueiri, T.; Wilson, M. Exercise, free radicals and oxidative stress. *Biochem. Soc. Trans.* **2002**, *30*, 280–284. [CrossRef]
141. Filomeni, G.; De Zio, D.; Cecconi, F. Oxidative stress and autophagy: The clash between damage and metabolic needs. *Cell Death Differ.* **2015**, *22*, 377–388. [CrossRef]
142. Pittaluga, M.; Parisi, P.; Sabatini, S.; Ceci, R.; Caporossi, D.; Catani, M.V.; Savini, I.; Avigliano, L. Cellular and biochemical parameters of exercise-induced oxidative stress: Relationship with training levels. *Free Radic. Res.* **2006**, *40*, 607–614. [CrossRef]
143. Steinbacher, P.; Eckl, P. Impact of oxidative stress on exercising skeletal muscle. *Biomolecules* **2015**, *5*, 356–377. [CrossRef]
144. Ferraro, E.; Giammarioli, A.; Chiandotto, S.; Spoletini, I.; Rosano, G. Exercise-induced skeletal muscle remodeling and metabolic adaptation: Redox signaling and role of autophagy. *Antioxid. Redox Signal.* **2014**, *21*, 154–176. [CrossRef] [PubMed]

145. Fyfe, J.J.; Bishop, D.; Stepto, N. Interference between Concurrent Resistance and Endurance Exercise: Molecular Bases and the Role of Individual Training Variables. *Sports Med.* **2014**, *44*, 743–762. [CrossRef] [PubMed]
146. Fyfe, J.J.; Bishop, D.; Zacharewicz, E.; Russell, A.; Stepto, N. Concurrent exercise incorporating high-intensity interval or continuous training modulates mTORC1 signaling and microRNA expression in human skeletal muscle. *Am. J. Physiol. Regul. Integr. Comp. Physiol.* **2016**, *310*, R1297–R1311. [CrossRef] [PubMed]
147. Olesen, J.; Kiilerich, K.; Pilegaard, H. PGC-1α-mediated adaptations in skeletal muscle. *Pflug. Arch.* **2010**, *460*, 153–162. [CrossRef] [PubMed]
148. Joshua, D.; Rebecca, W.; Zhen, Y. Molecular mechanisms for mitochondrial adaptation to exercise training in skeletal muscle. *FASEB J.* **2016**, *30*, 13–22. [CrossRef]
149. Lundby, C.; Jacobs, R. Adaptations of skeletal muscle mitochondria to exercise training. *Exp. Physiol.* **2016**, *101*, 17–22. [CrossRef]
150. Seene, T.; Kaasik, P.; Seppet, E. Changes in Myofibrillar and Mitochondrial Compartments during Increased Activity: Dependance from Oxidative Capacity of Muscle. *Health* **2017**, *9*, 779. [CrossRef]
151. Yan, Z.; Okutsu, M.; Akhtar, Y.; Lira, V. Regulation of exercise-induced fiber type transformation, mitochondrial biogenesis, and angiogenesis in skeletal muscle. *J. Appl. Physiol.* **2011**, *110*, 264–274. [CrossRef]
152. Rodney, G.; Pal, R.; Abo-Zahrah, R. Redox regulation of autophagy in skeletal muscle. *Free Radic. Biol. Med.* **2016**, *98*, 103–112. [CrossRef]
153. Vainshtein, A.; Grumati, P.; Sandri, M.; Bonaldo, P. Skeletal muscle, autophagy, and physical activity: The ménage à trois of metabolic regulation in health and disease. *J. Mol. Med.* **2014**, *92*, 127–137. [CrossRef]
154. Tam, B.; Siu, P. Autophagic Cellular Responses to Physical Exercise in Skeletal Muscle. *Sports Med.* **2014**, *44*, 625–640. [CrossRef] [PubMed]
155. Martin-Rincon, M.; Morales-Alamo, D.; Calbet, J. Exercise-mediated modulation of autophagy in skeletal muscle. *Scand. J. Med. Sci. Sports* **2018**, *28*, 772–781. [CrossRef]
156. Fritzen, A.; Madsen, A.; Kleinert, M.; Treebak, J.; Lundsgaard, A.; Jensen, T.; Richter, E.; Wojtaszewski, J.; Kiens, B.; Frøsig, C. Regulation of autophagy in human skeletal muscle: Effects of exercise, exercise training and insulin stimulation. *J. Physiol.* **2016**, *594*, 745–761. [CrossRef] [PubMed]
157. Gao, H.; Li, Y. Distinct signal transductions in fast- and slow- twitch muscles upon denervation. *Physiol. Rep.* **2018**, *6*, e13606. [CrossRef]
158. Schwalm, C.; Jamart, C.; Benoit, N.; Naslain, D.; Prémont, C.; Prévet, J.; Van Thienen, R.; Deldicque, L.; Francaux, M. Activation of autophagy in human skeletal muscle is dependent on exercise intensity and AMPK activation. *FASEB J.* **2015**, *29*, 3515–3526. [CrossRef] [PubMed]
159. Rocchi, A.; He, C. Regulation of Exercise-Induced Autophagy in Skeletal Muscle. *Curr. Pathobiol. Rep.* **2017**, *5*, 177–186. [CrossRef]
160. Halling, J.; Pilegaard, H. Autophagy-Dependent Beneficial Effects of Exercise. *Cold Spring Harb. Perspect. Med.* **2017**, *7*. [CrossRef]
161. Vainshtein, A.; Hood, D. The regulation of autophagy during exercise in skeletal muscle. *J. Appl. Physiol.* **2016**, *120*, 664–673. [CrossRef]
162. Codina-Martínez, H.; Fernández-García, B.; Díez-Planelles, C.; Fernández, Á.; Higarza, S.; Fernández-Sanjurjo, M.; Díez-Robles, S.; Iglesias-Gutiérrez, E.; Tomás-Zapico, C. Autophagy is required for performance adaptive response to resistance training and exercise-induced adult neurogenesis. *Scand. J. Med. Sci. Sports* **2020**, *30*, 238–253. [CrossRef]
163. Martin-Rincon, M.; Pérez-López, A.; Morales-Alamo, D.; Perez-Suarez, I.; De Pablos-Velasco, P.; Perez-Valera, M.; Perez-Regalado, S.; Martinez-Canton, M.; Gelabert-Rebato, M.; Juan-Habib, J. Exercise Mitigates the Loss of Muscle Mass by Attenuating the Activation of Autophagy during Severe Energy Deficit. *Nutrients* **2019**, *11*, 2824. [CrossRef]
164. Brandt, N.; Gunnarsson, T.; Bangsbo, J.; Pilegaard, H. Exercise and exercise training-induced increase in autophagy markers in human skeletal muscle. *Physiol. Rep.* **2018**, *6*, e13651. [CrossRef] [PubMed]
165. Moberg, M.; Hendo, G.; Jakobsson, M.; Mattsson, M.; Ekblom-Bak, E.; Flockhart, M.; Pontén, M.; Söderlund, K.; Ekblom, B. Increased autophagy signaling but not proteasome activity in human skeletal muscle after prolonged low-intensity exercise with negative energy balance. *Physiol. Rep.* **2017**, *5*, e13518. [CrossRef] [PubMed]
166. Hentilä, J.; Ahtiainen, J.P.; Paulsen, G.; Raastad, T.; Häkkinen, K.; Mero, A.A.; Hulmi, J.J. Autophagy is induced by resistance exercise in young men, but unfolded protein response is induced regardless of age. *Acta Physiol.* **2018**, *224*, e13069. [CrossRef] [PubMed]
167. Ahtiainen, J. Physiological and Molecular Adaptations to Strength Training. In *Concurrent Aerobic and Strength Training: Scientific Basics and Practical Applications*; Schumann, M., Rønnestad, B.R., Eds.; Springer International Publishing: Cham, Switzerland, 2019; pp. 51–73. [CrossRef]
168. Anthony, S.; Henri, B.; Guillaume, P.; Robin, C. Autophagy is essential to support skeletal muscle plasticity in response to endurance exercise. *Am. J. Physiol. Regul. Integr. Comp. Physiol.* **2014**, *307*, R956–R969. [CrossRef]
169. Saxton, R.; Sabatini, D. mTOR signaling in growth, metabolism, and disease. *Cell* **2017**, *168*, 960–976. [CrossRef]
170. Haun, C.; Mumford, P.; Roberson, P.; Romero, M.; Mobley, C.; Kephart, W.; Anderson, R.; Colquhoun, R.; Muddle, T.; Luera, M. Molecular, neuromuscular, and recovery responses to light versus heavy resistance exercise in young men. *Physiol. Rep.* **2017**, *5*, e13457. [CrossRef]

171. Smiles, W.; Areta, J.; Coffey, V.; Phillips, S.; Moore, D.; Stellingwerff, T.; Burke, L.; Hawley, J.; Camera, D. Modulation of autophagy signaling with resistance exercise and protein ingestion following short-term energy deficit. *Am. J. Physiol. Regul. Integr. Comp. Physiol.* **2015**, *309*, R603–R612. [CrossRef]
172. Sakuma, K.; Yamaguchi, A. Molecular Mechanisms Controlling Skeletal Muscle Mass. In *Muscle Cell and Tissue*; IntechOpen: London, UK, 2015.
173. Schiaffino, S.; Dyar, K.; Ciciliot, S.; Blaauw, B.; Sandri, M. Mechanisms regulating skeletal muscle growth and atrophy. *FEBS J.* **2013**, *280*, 4294–4314. [CrossRef]
174. Fernandez-Gonzalo, R.; Lundberg, T.R.; Tesch, P.A. Acute molecular responses in untrained and trained muscle subjected to aerobic and resistance exercise training versus resistance training alone. *Acta Physiol.* **2013**, *209*, 283–294. [CrossRef]
175. De Souza, E.O.; Tricoli, V.; Roschel, H.; Brum, P.C.; Bacurau, A.V.; Ferreira, J.C.; Aoki, M.S.; Neves-Jr, M.; Aihara, A.Y.; Da Rocha Correa Fernandes, A. Molecular adaptations to concurrent training. *Int. J. Sports Med.* **2013**, *34*, 207–213. [CrossRef]
176. Powell, J.; Pollizzi, K.; Heikamp, E.; Horton, M. Regulation of immune responses by mTOR. *Annu. Rev. Immunol.* **2012**, *30*, 39–68. [CrossRef]
177. Hulmi, J.; Walker, S.; Ahtiainen, J.P.; Nyman, K.; Kraemer, W.J.; Häkkinen, K. Molecular signaling in muscle is affected by the specificity of resistance exercise protocol. *Scand. J. Med. Sci. Sports* **2010**, *22*, 240–248. [CrossRef] [PubMed]
178. Laplante, M.; Sabatini, D.M. mTOR signaling at a glance. *J. Cell Sci.* **2009**, *122*, 3589–3594. [CrossRef] [PubMed]
179. Weihrauch, M.; Handschin, C. Pharmacological targeting of exercise adaptations in skeletal muscle: Benefits and pitfalls. *Biochem. Pharmacol.* **2017**, *147*, 211–220. [CrossRef] [PubMed]
180. Herzig, S.; Shaw, R. AMPK: Guardian of metabolism and mitochondrial homeostasis. *Nat. Rev. Mol. Cell Biol.* **2018**, *19*, 121–135. [CrossRef] [PubMed]
181. Hardie, G.; Schaffer, B.; Brunet, A. AMPK: An energy-sensing pathway with multiple inputs and outputs. *Trends Cell Biol.* **2016**, *26*, 190–201. [CrossRef]
182. Combes, A.; Dekerle, J.; Webborn, N.; Watt, P.; Bougault, V.; Daussin, F. Exercise-induced metabolic fluctuations influence AMPK, p38-MAPK and CaMKII phosphorylation in human skeletal muscle. *Physiol. Rep.* **2015**, *3*, e12462. [CrossRef]
183. Chalari, E.; Methenitis, S.; Arnaoutis, G.; Stergiou, I.; Kampouropoulou, C.; Karampelas, E.; Prousinoudi, N.; Argyropoulou, V.; Nomikos, T. Different Kinetics of Oxidative Stress and Inflammatory Markers after Eccentric Exercise in Upper and Lower Limbs. *Proceedings* **2019**, *25*, 17. [CrossRef]
184. Franz, A.; Behringer, M.; Nosaka, K.; Buhren, B.; Schrumpf, H.; Mayer, C.; Zilkens, C.; Schumann, M. Mechanisms underpinning protection against eccentric exercise-induced muscle damage by ischemic preconditioning. *Med. Hypotheses* **2017**, *98*, 21–27. [CrossRef]
185. Chen, T.; Tseng, W.; Huang, G.; Chen, H.; Tseng, K.; Nosaka, K. Superior Effects of Eccentric to Concentric Knee Extensor Resistance Training on Physical Fitness, Insulin Sensitivity and Lipid Profiles of Elderly Men. *Front. Physiol.* **2017**, *8*. [CrossRef]
186. Tajra, V.; Tibana, R.; Vieira, D.; De Farias, D.; Teixeira, T.; Funghetto, S.; Silva, A.; De Sousa, N.; Willardson, J.; Karnikowski, M. Identification of high responders for interleukin-6 and creatine kinase following acute eccentric resistance exercise in elderly obese women. *J. Sci. Med. Sport* **2014**, *17*, 662–666. [CrossRef] [PubMed]
187. Franchi, M.; Atherton, P.; Reeves, N.; Flück, M.; Williams, J.; Mitchell, W.; Selby, A.; Valls, R.B.; Narici, M. Architectural, functional and molecular responses to concentric and eccentric loading in human skeletal muscle. *Acta Physiol.* **2014**, *210*, 642–654. [CrossRef] [PubMed]
188. Paschalis, V.; Nikolaidis, M.; Theodorou, A.; Panayiotou, G.; Fatouros, I.; Koutedakis, Y.; Jamurtas, A. A weekly bout of eccentric exercise is sufficient to induce health-promoting effects. *Med. Sci. Sports Exerc.* **2011**, *43*, 64–73. [CrossRef] [PubMed]
189. Chen, T.; Lin, K.; Chen, H.; Lin, M.; Nosaka, K. Comparison in eccentric exercise-induced muscle damage among four limb muscles. *Eur. J. Appl. Physiol.* **2011**, *111*, 211–223. [CrossRef] [PubMed]
190. Paschalis, V.; Nikolaidis, M.; Theodorou, A.; Giakas, G.; Jamurtas, A.; Koutedakis, Y. Eccentric exercise affects the upper limbs more than the lower limbs in position sense and reaction angle. *J. Sports Sci.* **2010**, *28*, 33–43. [CrossRef]
191. Paschalis, V.; Nikolaidis, M.; Giakas, G.; Theodorou, A.; Sakellariou, G.; Fatouros, I.; Koutedakis, Y.; Jamurtas, A. Beneficial changes in energy expenditure and lipid profile after eccentric exercise in overweight and lean women. *Scand. J. Med. Sci. Sports* **2010**, *20*, e103–e111. [CrossRef]
192. Saka, T.; Akova, B.; Yazici, Z.; Sekir, U.; Gür, H.; Ozarda, Y. Difference in the magnitude of muscle damage between elbow flexors and knee extensors eccentric exercises. *J. Sports Sci. Med.* **2009**, *8*, 107–115.
193. Mahoney, D.J.; Safdar, A.; Parise, G.; Melov, S.; Fu, M.; MacNeil, L.; Kaczor, J.; Payne, E.; Tarnopolsky, M. Gene expression profiling in human skeletal muscle during recovery from eccentric exercise. *Am. J. Physiol. Regul. Integr. Comp. Physiol.* **2008**, *294*, R1901–R1910. [CrossRef]
194. Jamurtas, A.; Theocharis, V.; Tofas, T.; Tsiokanos, A.; Yfanti, C.; Paschalis, V.; Koutedakis, Y.; Nosaka, K. Comparison between leg and arm eccentric exercises of the same relative intensity on indices of muscle damage. *Eur. J. Appl. Physiol.* **2005**, *95*, 179–185. [CrossRef]
195. Feasson, L.; Stockholm, D.; Freyssenet, D.; Richard, I.; Duguez, S.; Beckmann, J.; Denis, C. Molecular adaptations of neuromuscular disease-associated proteins in response to eccentric exercise in human skeletal muscle. *J. Physiol.* **2002**, *543*, 297–306. [CrossRef]

196. Fatouros, I.; Jamurtas, A.; Nikolaidis, M.G.; Destouni, A.; Michailidis, Y.; Vrettou, C.; Douroudos, I.; Avloniti, A.; Chatzinikolaou, A.; Taxildaris, K. Time of sampling is crucial for measurement of cell-free plasma DNA following acute aseptic inflammation induced by exercise. *Clin. Biochem.* **2010**, *43*, 1368–1370. [CrossRef] [PubMed]
197. Margaritelis, N.; Theodorou, A.; Paschalis, V.; Veskoukis, A.; Dipla, K.; Zafeiridis, A.; Panayiotou, G.; Vrabas, I.; Kyparos, A.; Nikolaidis, M. Experimental verification of regression to the mean in Redox Biol.: Differential responses to exercise. *Free Radic. Res.* **2016**, *50*, 1237–1244. [CrossRef] [PubMed]
198. Nikolaidis, M.; Jamurtas, A.Z. Blood as a reactive species generator and redox status regulator during exercise. *Arch. Biochem. Biophys.* **2009**, *490*, 77–84. [CrossRef] [PubMed]
199. Nikolaidis, M.; Paschalis, V.; Giakas, G.; Fatouros, I.; Sakellariou, G.; Theodorou, A.; Koutedakis, Y.; Jamurtas, A. Favorable and prolonged changes in blood lipid profile after muscle-damaging exercise. *Med. Sci. Sports Exerc.* **2008**, *40*, 1483–1489. [CrossRef] [PubMed]
200. Sakelliou, A.; Fatouros, I.; Athanailidis, I.; Tsoukas, D.; Chatzinikolaou, A.; Draganidis, D.; Jamurtas, A.; Liacos, C.; Papassotiriou, I.; Mandalidis, D. Evidence of a redox-dependent regulation of immune responses to exercise-induced inflammation. *Oxidative Med. Cell. Longev.* **2016**, *2016*. [CrossRef] [PubMed]
201. Higbie, E.J.; Cureton, K.J.; Warren, G.L.; Prior, B.M. Effects of concentric and eccentric training on muscle strength, cross-sectional area, and neural activation. *J. Appl. Physiol.* **1996**, *81*, 2173–2181. [CrossRef]
202. Vikne, H.; Refsnes, P.E.; Ekmark, M.; Medbø, J.I.; Gundersen, V.; Gundersen, K. Muscular performance after concentric and eccentric exercise in trained men. *Med. Sci. Sports Exerc.* **2006**, *38*, 1770–1781. [CrossRef]
203. Roig, M.; O'Brien, K.; Kirk, G.; Murray, R.; McKinnon, P.; Shadgan, B.; Reid, D.W. The effects of eccentric versus concentric resistance training on muscle strength and mass in healthy adults: A systematic review with meta-analyses. *Br. J. Sports Med.* **2009**, *43*, 556–568. [CrossRef]
204. Nickols-Richardson, S.M.; Miller, L.E.; Wootten, D.F.; Ramp, W.K.; Herbert, W.G. Concentric and eccentric isokinetic resistance training similarly increases muscular strength, fat-free soft tissue mass, and specific bone mineral measurements in young women. *Osteoporos. Int.* **2007**, *18*, 789–796. [CrossRef]
205. Walker, S.; Blazevich, A.J.; Haff, G.G.; Tufano, J.J.; Newton, R.U.; Häkkinen, K. Greater Strength Gains after Training with Accentuated Eccentric than Traditional Isoinertial Loads in Already Strength-Trained Men. *Front. Physiol.* **2016**, *7*. [CrossRef]
206. Mike, J.; Cole, N.; Herrera, C.; VanD'usseldorp, T.; Kravitz, L.; Kerksick, C. The Effects of Eccentric Contraction Duration on Muscle Strength, Power Production, Vertical Jump, and Soreness. *J. Strength Cond. Res.* **2017**, *31*, 773–736. [CrossRef] [PubMed]
207. LaStayo, P.; Marcus, R.; Dibble, L.; Frajacomo, F.; Lindstedt, S. Eccentric exercise in rehabilitation: Safety, feasibility, and application. *J. Appl. Physiol.* **2014**, *116*, 1426–1434. [CrossRef] [PubMed]
208. Andersen, L.L.; Zeeman, P.; Jørgensen, J.R.; Bech-Pedersen, D.T.; Sørensen, J.; Kjær, M.; Andersen, J.L. Effects of intensive physical rehabilitation on neuromuscular adaptations in adults with poststroke hemiparesis. *J. Strength Cond. Res.* **2011**, *25*, 2808–2817. [CrossRef] [PubMed]
209. Mitchell, K.; Taivassalo, T.; Narici, M.; Franchi, M. Eccentric Exercise and the Critically ILL Patient. *Front. Physiol.* **2017**, *8*, 120. [CrossRef] [PubMed]
210. Okamoto, T.; Masuhara, M.; Ikuta, K. Effects of eccentric and concentric resistance training on arterial stiffness. *J. Hum. Hypertens.* **2006**, *20*, 348–354. [CrossRef]
211. Melo, R.C.; Quitério, R.J.; Takahashi, A.C.; Silva, E.; Martins, L.; Catai, A.M. High eccentric strength training reduces heart rate variability in healthy older men. *Br. J. Sports Med.* **2008**, *42*, 59–63. [CrossRef]
212. Dos Santos, E.S.; Asano, R.Y.; Filho, G.I.; Lopes, N.L.; Panelli, P.; Nascimento, D.; Collier, S.R.; Prestes, J. Acute and chronic cardiovascular response to 16 weeks of combined eccentric or traditional resistance and aerobic training in elderly hypertensive women: A randomized controlled trial. *J. Strength Cond. Res.* **2014**, *28*, 3073–3084. [CrossRef]
213. Takahashi, A.C.; Melo, R.C.; Quitério, R.J.; Silva, E.; Catai, A.M. The effect of eccentric strength training on heart rate and on its variability during isometric exercise in healthy older men. *Eur. J. Appl. Physiol.* **2009**, *105*, 315–323. [CrossRef]
214. Hawkins, S.; Schroeder, T.; Wiswell, R.; Jaque, V.; Marcell, T.; Costa, K. Eccentric muscle action increases site-specific osteogenic response. *Med. Sci. Sports Exerc.* **1999**, *31*, 1287–1292. [CrossRef]
215. Mueller, M.; Breil, F.A.; Vogt, M.; Steiner, R.; Lippuner, K.; Popp, A.; Klossner, S.; Hoppeler, H.; Däpp, C. Different response to eccentric and concentric training in older men and women. *Eur. J. Appl. Physiol.* **2009**, *107*, 145–153. [CrossRef]
216. Leszczak, T.J.; Olson, J.M.; Stafford, J.; Di Brezzo, R. Early adaptations to eccentric and high-velocity training on strength and functional performance in community-dwelling older adults. *J. Strength Cond. Res.* **2013**, *27*, 442–448. [CrossRef]
217. Selva Raj, I.; Bird, S.; Westfold, B.; Shield, A. Effects of eccentrically biased versus conventional weight training in older adults. *Med. Sci. Sports Exerc.* **2012**, *44*, 1167–1176. [CrossRef]
218. Marcus, R.L.; Smith, S.; Morrell, G.; Addison, O.; Dibble, L.E.; Wahoff-Stice, D.; LaStayo, P.C. Comparison of combined aerobic and high-force eccentric resistance exercise with aerobic exercise only for people with type 2 diabetes mellitus. *J. Phys. Ther.* **2008**, *88*, 1345. [CrossRef] [PubMed]
219. Casillas, J.M.; Besson, D.; Hannequin, A.; Gremeaux, V.; Morisset, C.; Tordi, N.; Laurent, Y.; Laroche, D. Effects of an eccentric training personalized by a low rate of perceived exertion on the maximal capacities in chronic heart failure. *Eur. J. Phys. Rehabil. Med.* **2015**, *52*, 159–168. [PubMed]

220. Besson, D.; Joussain, C.; Gremeaux, V.; Morisset, C.; Laurent, Y.; Casillas, J.M.; Laroche, D. Eccentric training in chronic heart failure: Feasibility and functional effects. Results of a comparative study. *Ann. Phys. Rehabil. Med.* **2013**, *56*, 30–40. [CrossRef]
221. Karagiannis, C.; Savva, C.; Mamais, I.; Efstathiou, M.; Monticone, M.; Xanthos, T. Eccentric exercise in ischemic cardiac patients and functional capacity: A systematic review and meta-analysis of randomized controlled trials. *Ann. Phys. Rehabil. Med.* **2016**, *60*, 58–64. [CrossRef]
222. Lastayo, P.C.; Reich, T.E.; Urquhart, M.; Hoppeler, H.; Lindstedt, S.L. Chronic eccentric exercise: Improvements in muscle strength can occur with little demand for oxygen. *Am. J. Physiol. Regul. Integr. Comp. Physiol.* **1999**, *276*, R611–R615. [CrossRef]
223. Bridgeman, L.; Gill, N.; Dulson, D.; McGuigan, M. The Effect of Exercise-Induced Muscle Damage After a Bout of Accentuated Eccentric Load Drop Jumps and the Repeated Bout Effect. *J. Strength Cond. Res.* **2017**, *31*, 386–394. [CrossRef]
224. Skurvydas, A.; Brazaitis, M.; Venckūnas, T.; Kamandulis, S. Predictive value of strength loss as an indicator of muscle damage across multiple drop jumps. *Appl. Physiol. Nutr. Metab.* **2011**, *36*, 353–360. [CrossRef]
225. Howatson, G.; Hoad, M.; Goodall, S.; Tallent, J.; Bell, P.; French, D. Exercise-induced muscle damage is reduced in resistance-trained males by branched chain amino acids: A randomized, double-blind, placebo controlled study. *J. Int. Soc. Sports Nutr.* **2012**, *9*, 20. [CrossRef]
226. Tee, J.; Bosch, A.; Lambert, M. Metabolic Consequences of Exercise-Induced Muscle Damage. *Sports Med.* **2007**, *37*, 827–836. [CrossRef] [PubMed]
227. Tofas, T.; Jamurtas, A.; Fatouros, I.; Nikolaidis, M.; Koutedakis, Y.; Sinouris, E.; Papageorgakopoulou, N.; Theocharis, D. Plyometric Exercise Increases Serum Indices of Muscle Damage and Collagen Breakdown. *J. Strength Cond. Res.* **2008**, *22*, 490–496. [CrossRef] [PubMed]
228. Chatzinikolaou, A.; Fatouros, I.; Gourgoulis, V.; Avloniti, A.; Jamurtas, A.; Nikolaidis, M.; Douroudos, I.; Michailidis, Y.; Beneka, A.; Malliou, P. Time course of changes in performance and inflammatory responses after acute plyometric exercise. *J. Strength Cond. Res.* **2010**, *24*, 1389–1398. [CrossRef] [PubMed]
229. Komi, P.V. Stretch-shortening cycle: A powerful model to study normal and fatigued muscle. *J. Biomech.* **2000**, *33*, 1197–1206. [CrossRef]
230. Peake, J.; Suzuki, K.; Hordern, M.; Wilson, G.; Nosaka, K.; Coombes, J. Plasma cytokine changes in relation to exercise intensity and muscle damage. *Eur. J. Appl. Physiol.* **2005**, *95*, 514–521. [CrossRef] [PubMed]
231. Marklund, P.; Mattsson, M.; Wåhlin-Larsson, B.; Ponsot, E.; Lindvall, B.; Lindvall, L.; Ekblom, B.; Kadi, F. Extensive inflammatory cell infiltration in human skeletal muscle in response to an ultraendurance exercise bout in experienced athletes. *J. Appl. Physiol.* **2013**, *114*, 66–72. [CrossRef]
232. Peñailillo, L.; Blazevich, A.; Numazawa, H.; Nosaka, K. Metabolic and Muscle Damage Profiles of Concentric versus Repeated Eccentric Cycling. *Med. Sci. Sports Exerc.* **2013**, *45*, 1773–1781. [CrossRef]
233. Nieman, D.; Davis, M.; Henson, D.; Gross, S.; Dumke, C.; Utter, A.; Vinci, D.; Carson, J.; Brown, A.; Mcanulty, S.; et al. Muscle Cytokine mRNA Changes after 2.5 h of Cycling: Influence of Carbohydrate. *Med. Sci. Sports Exerc.* **2005**, *37*, 1283–1290. [CrossRef]
234. González-Bartholin, R.; Mackay, K.; Valladares, D.; Zbinden-Foncea, H.; Nosaka, K.; Peñailillo, L. Changes in oxidative stress, inflammation and muscle damage markers following eccentric versus concentric cycling in older adults. *Eur. J. Appl. Physiol.* **2019**, *119*, 2301–2312. [CrossRef]
235. Li, T.L.; Cheng, P.Y. Alterations of immunoendocrine responses during the recovery period after acute prolonged cycling. *Eur. J. Appl. Physiol.* **2007**, *101*, 539. [CrossRef]
236. Kawanishi, N.; Kato, K.; Takahashi, M.; Mizokami, T.; Otsuka, Y.; Imaizumi, A.; Shiva, D.; Yano, H.; Suzuki, K. Curcumin attenuates oxidative stress following downhill running-induced muscle damage. *Biochem. Biophys. Res. Commun.* **2013**, *441*, 573–578. [CrossRef]
237. Peake, J.; Suzuki, K.; Wilson, G.; Hordern, M.; Nosaka, K.; Mackinnon, L.; Coombes, J. Exercise-Induced Muscle Damage, Plasma Cytokines, and Markers of Neutrophil Activation. *Med. Sci. Sports Exerc.* **2005**, *37*, 737–745. [CrossRef] [PubMed]
238. Park, K.; Lee, M. Effects of unaccustomed downhill running on muscle damage, oxidative stress, and leukocyte apoptosis. *J. Exerc. Nutr. Biochem.* **2015**, *19*, 55–63. [CrossRef] [PubMed]
239. Maeo, S.; Ando, Y.; Kanehisa, H.; Kawakami, Y. Localization of damage in the human leg muscles induced by downhill running. *Sci. Rep.* **2017**, *7*, 5769. [CrossRef]
240. Malm, C.; Sjödin, B.; Sjöberg, B.; Lenkei, R.; Renström, P.; Lundberg, I.; Ekblom, B. Leukocytes, cytokines, growth factors and hormones in human skeletal muscle and blood after uphill or downhill running. *J. Physiol.* **2004**, *556*, 983–1000. [CrossRef]
241. Damas, F.; Libardi, C.; Ugrinowitsch, C. The development of skeletal muscle hypertrophy through resistance training: The role of muscle damage and muscle protein synthesis. *Eur. J. Appl. Physiol.* **2018**, *118*, 485–500. [CrossRef]
242. Damas, F.; Phillips, S.; Libardi, C.; Vechin, F.; Lixandrão, M.; Jannig, P.; Costa, L.; Bacurau, A.; Snijders, T.; Parise, G. Resistance training-induced changes in integrated myofibrillar protein synthesis are related to hypertrophy only after attenuation of muscle damage. *J. Physiol.* **2016**, *594*, 5209–5222. [CrossRef]
243. Damas, F.; Ugrinowitsch, C.; Libardi, C.; Jannig, P.; Hector, A.; McGlory, C.; Lixandrão, M.; Vechin, F.; Montenegro, H.; Tricoli, V. Resistance training in young men induces muscle transcriptome-wide changes associated with muscle structure and metabolism refining the response to exercise-induced stress. *Eur. J. Appl. Physiol.* **2018**, *118*, 2607–2616. [CrossRef]

244. Prestes, J.; Pereira, G.; Tibana, R.; Navalta, J. The acute response of apoptosis and migration to resistance exercise is protocol-dependent. *Int. J. Sports Med.* **2014**, *35*, 1051–1056. [CrossRef]
245. Brown, W.; Davison, G.; McClean, C.; Murphy, M. A Systematic Review of the Acute Effects of Exercise on Immune and Inflammatory Indices in Untrained Adults. *Sports Med. Open* **2015**, *1*, 35. [CrossRef]
246. Calle, M.; Fernandez, M. Effects of resistance training on the inflammatory response. *Nutr. Res. Pract.* **2010**, *4*, 259–269. [CrossRef]
247. Cerqueira, É.; Marinho, D.; Neiva, H.; Lourenço, O. Inflammatory Effects of High and Moderate Intensity Exercise—A Systematic Review. *Front. Physiol.* **2020**, *10*. [CrossRef] [PubMed]
248. Della Gatta, P.; Cameron-Smith, D.; Peake, J. Acute resistance exercise increases the expression of chemotactic factors within skeletal muscle. *Eur. J. Appl. Physiol.* **2014**, *114*, 2157–2167. [CrossRef] [PubMed]
249. Koh, T.; Pizza, F.X. Do inflammatory cells influence skeletal muscle hypertrophy? *Front. Biosci.* **2009**, *E1*, 60–71.
250. Ihalainen, J.; Walker, S.; Paulsen, G.; Häkkinen, K.; Kraemer, W.; Hämäläinen, M.; Vuolteenaho, K.; Moilanen, E.; Mero, A. Acute leukocyte, cytokine and adipocytokine responses to maximal and hypertrophic resistance exercise bouts. *Eur. J. Appl. Physiol.* **2014**, *114*, 2607–2616. [CrossRef] [PubMed]
251. Miles, M.; Kraemer, W.; Nindl, B.; Grove, D.; Leach, S.; Dohi, K.; Marx, J.; Volek, J.; Mastro, A. Strength, workload, anaerobic intensity and the immune response to resistance exercise in women. *Acta Physiol.* **2003**, *178*, 155–163. [CrossRef] [PubMed]
252. Mitchell, C.J.; Churchward-Venne, T.A.; Bellamy, L.; Parise, G.; Baker, S.K.; Phillips, S. Muscular and systemic correlates of resistance training-induced muscle hypertrophy. *PLoS ONE* **2013**, *8*, e78636. [CrossRef]
253. Vissing, K.; Overgaard, K.; Nedergaard, A.; Fredsted, A.; Schjerling, P. Effects of concentric and repeated eccentric exercise on muscle damage and calpain–calpastatin gene expression in human skeletal muscle. *Eur. J. Appl. Physiol.* **2008**, *103*, 323–332. [CrossRef]
254. Hyldahl, R.; Olson, T.; Welling, T.; Groscost, L.; Parcell, A. Satellite cell activity is differentially affected by contraction mode in human muscle following a work-matched bout of exercise. *Front. Physiol.* **2014**, *5*. [CrossRef]
255. Newton, M.; Morgan, G.; Sacco, P.; Chapman, D.; Nosaka, K. Comparison of Responses to Strenuous Eccentric Exercise of the Elbow Flexors Between Resistance-Trained and Untrained Men. *J. Strength Cond. Res.* **2008**, *22*, 597–607. [CrossRef]
256. Margaritelis, N.; Theodorou, A.; Chatzinikolaou, P.; Kyparos, A.; Nikolaidis, M.; Paschalis, V. Eccentric exercise per se does not affect muscle damage biomarkers: Early and late phase adaptations. *Eur. J. Appl. Physiol.* **2020**. [CrossRef] [PubMed]
257. Methenitis, S.; Karandreas, N.; Spengos, K.; Zaras, N.; Stasinaki, A.N.; Terzis, G. Muscle Fiber Conduction Velocity, Muscle Fiber Composition, and Power Performance. *Med. Sci. Sports Exerc.* **2016**, *48*, 1761–1771. [CrossRef] [PubMed]
258. Methenitis, S.; Spengos, K.; Zaras, N.; Stasinaki, A.N.; Papadimas, G.; Karampatsos, G.; Arnaoutis, G.; Terzis, G. Fiber Type Composition And Rate Of Force Development In Endurance And Resistance Trained Individuals. *J. Strength Cond. Res.* **2019**, *33*, 2388–2397. [CrossRef] [PubMed]
259. Methenitis, S.; Zaras, N.; Spengos, K.; Stasinaki, A.N.; Karampatsos, G.; Georgiadis, G.; Terzis, G. Role of Muscle Morphology in Jumping, Sprinting, and Throwing Performance in Participants With Different Power Training Duration Experience. *J. Strength Cond. Res.* **2016**, *30*, 807–817. [CrossRef]
260. Spiliopoulou, P.; Zaras, N.; Methenitis, S.; Papadimas, G.; Papadopoulos, C.; Bogdanis, G.; Terzis, G The effect of concurrent power training and high intensity interval cycling on muscle morphology and performance. *J. Strength Cond. Res.* **2019**. [CrossRef]
261. Terzis, G.; Spengos, K.; Methenitis, S.; Aagaard, P.; Karandreas, N.; Bogdanis, G. Early phase interference between low-intensity running and power training in moderately trained females. *Eur. J. Appl. Physiol.* **2016**, *116*, 1063–1073. [CrossRef]
262. Zacharia, E.; Spiliopoulou, P.; Methenitis, S.; Stasinaki, A.N.; Zaras, N.; Papadopoulos, C.; Papadimas, G.; Karampatsos, G.; Bogdanis, G.; Terzis, G. Changes in muscle power and muscle morphology with different volumes of fast eccentric half-squats. *Sports* **2019**, *7*, 164. [CrossRef]
263. Zaras, N.; Spengos, K.; Methenitis, S.; Papadopoulos, C.; Karampatsos, G.; Georgiadis, G.; Stasinaki, A.N.; Manta, P.; Terzis, G. Effects of Strength vs. Ballistic-Power Training on Throwing Performance. *J. Sports Sci. Med.* **2013**, *12*, 130–137.
264. Abramowitz, M.W.P.; Zhang, K.; Brightwell, K.; Newsom, J.; Kwon, K.; Custodio, M.; Buttar, R.; Farooq, H.; Zaidi, B. Skeletal muscle fibrosis is associated with decreased muscle inflammation and weakness in patients with chronic kidney disease. *Am. J. Physiol. Ren. Physiol.* **2018**, *315*, F1658–F1669. [CrossRef]
265. Levinger, I.; Levinger, P.; Trenerry, M.; Feller, J.; Bartlett, J.; Bergman, N.; McKenna, M.; Cameron-Smith, D. Increased inflammatory cytokine expression in the vastus lateralis of patients with knee osteoarthritis. *Arthritis Rheum.* **2011**, *63*, 1343–1348. [CrossRef]
266. Caldow, M.; Cameron-Smith, D.; Levinger, P.; McKenna, M.; Levinger, I. Inflammatory markers in skeletal muscle of older adults. *Eur. J. Appl. Physiol.* **2013**, *113*, 509–517. [CrossRef] [PubMed]
267. Deyhle, M.; Gier, A.; Evens, K.; Eggett, D.; Nelson, W.; Parcell, A.; Hyldahl, R. Skeletal muscle inflammation following repeated bouts of lengthening contractions in humans. *Front. Physiol.* **2016**, *6*. [CrossRef] [PubMed]
268. Vella, L.; Markworth, J.; Paulsen, G.; Raastad, T.; Peake, J.; Snow, R.; Cameron-Smith, D.; Russell, A. Ibuprofen Ingestion Does Not Affect Markers of Post-exercise Muscle Inflammation. *Front. Physiol.* **2016**, *7*. [CrossRef] [PubMed]
269. Stupka, N.; Tarnopolsky, M.; Yardley, N.; Phillips, S. Cellular adaptation to repeated eccentric exercise-induced muscle damage. *J. Appl. Physiol.* **2001**, *91*, 1669–1678. [CrossRef]
270. Vella, L.; Markworth, J.; Farnfield, M.; Maddipati, K.; Russell, A.; Cameron-Smith, D. Intramuscular inflammatory and resolving lipid profile responses to an acute bout of resistance exercise in men. *Physiol. Rep.* **2019**, *7*, e14108. [CrossRef] [PubMed]

271. Sag, E.; Kale, G.; Haliloglu, G.; Bilginer, Y.; Akcoren, Z.; Orhan, D.; Gucer, S.; Topaloglu, H.; Ozen, S.; Talim, B. Inflammatory milieu of muscle biopsies in juvenile dermatomyositis. *Rheumatol. Int.* **2020**. [CrossRef] [PubMed]
272. Singer, K.; Lumeng, C. The initiation of metabolic inflammation in childhood obesity. *J. Clin. Investig.* **2017**, *127*, 65–73. [CrossRef]
273. Hyldahl, R.; Chen, T.; Nosaka, K. Mechanisms and Mediators of the Skeletal Muscle Repeated Bout Effect. *Exerc. Sport Sci. Rev.* **2017**, *45*, 24–33. [CrossRef] [PubMed]
274. Sieljacks, P.; Matzon, A.; Wernbom, M.; Ringgaard, S.; Vissing, K.; Overgaard, K. Muscle damage and repeated bout effect following blood flow restricted exercise. *Eur. J. Appl. Physiol.* **2016**, *116*, 513–525. [CrossRef]
275. Falvo, M.; Schilling, B.; Bloomer, R.; Smith, W. Repeated bout effect is absent in resistance trained men: An electromyographic analysis. *J. Electromyogr. Kinesiol.* **2009**, *19*, e529–e535. [CrossRef] [PubMed]
276. Mascher, H.; Tannerstedt, J.; Brink-Elfegoun, T.; Ekblom, B.; Gustafsson, T.; Blomstrand, E. Repeated resistance exercise training induces different changes in mRNA expression of MAFbx and MuRF-1 in human skeletal muscle. *Am. J. Physiol. Endocrinol. Metab.* **2008**, *294*, E43–E51. [CrossRef] [PubMed]
277. O'Carroll, C.; Fenwick, R. Rhabdomyolysis: A case-based critical reflection on its causes and diagnosis. *J. Emerg. Nurse* **2020**, *28*. [CrossRef]
278. Phillips, P.; Haas, R. Statin myopathy as a metabolic muscle disease. *Expert Rev. Cardiovasc. Ther.* **2008**, *6*, 971–978. [CrossRef] [PubMed]
279. Camera, D.; Smiles, W.; Hawley, J. Exercise-induced skeletal muscle signaling pathways and human athletic performance. *Free Radic. Biol. Med.* **2016**, *98*, 131–143. [CrossRef] [PubMed]
280. Radak, Z.; Bori, Z.; Koltai, E.; Fatouros, I.; Jamurtas, A.; Douroudos, I.; Terzis, G.; Nikolaidis, M.; Chatzinikolaou, A.; Sovatzidis, A. Age-dependent changes in 8-oxoguanine-DNA glycosylase activity are modulated by adaptive responses to physical exercise in human skeletal muscle. *Free Radic. Biol. Med.* **2011**, *51*, 417–423. [CrossRef]
281. Powers, S.; Nelson, B.; Hudson, M. Exercise-induced oxidative stress in humans: Cause and consequences. *Free Radic. Biol. Med.* **2011**, *51*, 942–950. [CrossRef]
282. Finaud, J.; Lac, G.; Filaire, E. Oxidative stress. *Sports Med.* **2006**, *36*, 327–358. [CrossRef]
283. Radak, Z. *Free Radicals in exeRcise and Aging*; Human Kinetics Europe: Leeds, UK, 2000.
284. Fehrenbach, E.; Northoff, H. Free radicals, exercise, apoptosis, and heat shock proteins. *Exerc. Immunol. Rev.* **2000**, *7*, 66–89.
285. Brancaccio, P.; Lippi, G.; Maffulli, N. Biochemical markers of muscular damage. *Clin. Chem. Lab. Med.* **2010**, *48*, 757–767. [CrossRef]
286. Wolfe, F.; Clauw, D.; Fitzcharles, M.; Goldenberg, D.; Häuser, W.; Katz, R.; Mease, P.; Russell, A.; Russell, I.; Walitt, B. 2016 Revisions to the 2010/2011 fibromyalgia diagnostic criteria. *Semin. Arthritis Rheum.* **2016**, *46*, 319–329. [CrossRef]
287. Atzeni, F.; Talotta, R.; Masala, I.; Giacomelli, C.; Conversano, C.; Nucera, V.; Lucchino, B.; Iannuccelli, C.; Di Franco, M.; Bazzichi, L. One year in review 2019: Fibromyalgia. *Clin. Exp. Rheumatol.* **2019**, *37* (Suppl. 116), 3–10. [PubMed]
288. Littlejohn, G.; Guymer, E. Neurogenic inflammation in fibromyalgia. *Semin. Immunopathol.* **2018**, *40*, 291–300. [CrossRef] [PubMed]

biomedicines

MDPI

Review

Therapeutic Potential of Porcine Liver Decomposition Product: New Insights and Perspectives for Microglia-Mediated Neuroinflammation in Neurodegenerative Diseases

Tamotsu Tsukahara [1,*], Hisao Haniu [2], Takeshi Uemura [2,3] and Yoshikazu Matsuda [4]

1 Department of Pharmacology and Therapeutic Innovation, Nagasaki University Graduate School of Biomedical Sciences, Nagasaki 852-8521, Japan
2 Institute for Biomedical Sciences, Interdisciplinary Cluster for Cutting Edge Research, Shinshu University, Matsumoto 390-8621, Japan; hhaniu@shinshu-u.ac.jp (H.H.); tuemura@shinshu-u.ac.jp (T.U.)
3 Division of Gene Research, Research Center for Supports to Advanced Science, Shinshu University, Nagano 390-8621, Japan
4 Division of Clinical Pharmacology and Pharmaceutics, Nihon Pharmaceutical University, Saitama 362-0806, Japan; yomatsuda@nichiyaku.ac.jp
* Correspondence: ttamotsu@nagasaki-u.ac.jp

Received: 8 October 2020; Accepted: 21 October 2020; Published: 22 October 2020

Abstract: It is widely accepted that microglia-mediated inflammation contributes to the progression of neurodegenerative diseases; however, the precise mechanisms through which these cells contribute remain to be elucidated. Microglia, as the primary immune effector cells of the brain, play key roles in maintaining central nervous system (CNS) homeostasis. Microglia are located throughout the brain and spinal cord and may account for up to 15% of all cells in the brain. Activated microglia express pro-inflammatory cytokines that act on the surrounding brain and spinal cord. Microglia may also play a detrimental effect on nerve cells when they gain a chronic inflammatory function and promote neuropathologies. A key feature of microglia is its rapid morphological change upon activation, characterized by the retraction of numerous fine processes and the gradual acquisition of amoeba-like shapes. These morphological changes are also accompanied by the expression and secretion of inflammatory molecules, including cytokines, chemokines, and lipid mediators that promote systemic inflammation during neurodegeneration. This may be considered a protective response intended to limit further injury and initiate repair processes. We previously reported that porcine liver decomposition product (PLDP) induces a significant increase in the Hasegawa's Dementia Scale-Revised (HDS-R) score and the Wechsler Memory Scale (WMS) in a randomized, double-blind, placebo-controlled study in healthy humans. In addition, the oral administration of porcine liver decomposition product enhanced visual memory and delayed recall in healthy adults. We believe that PLDP is a functional food that aids cognitive function. In this review, we provide a critical assessment of recent reports of lysophospholipids derived from PLDP, a rich source of phospholipids. We also highlight some recent findings regarding bidirectional interactions between lysophospholipids and microglia and age-related neurodegenerative diseases such as dementia and Alzheimer's disease.

Keywords: microglia; porcine liver decomposition product; lysophospholipids; mild cognitive impairment; dementia; neuroinflammation; cytokines; oxygen reactive species

1. Introduction

Amnesic patients with mild cognitive impairment (MCI) are at risk of developing dementia. Approximately 15–20% of people aged 65 or older have MCI [1]. Alzheimer's disease, Lewy body dementia, and vascular dementia are the most common forms of dementia; both are preceded by a stage of cognitive impairment [2,3]. However, some individuals with amnesia and MCI revert to normal cognition or do not deteriorate further. While clinical studies are currently being conducted to identify novel therapeutics to improve symptoms and prevent or delay the progression of MCI to dementia, no therapeutic drugs have been approved for MCI thus far. Therefore, further studies are needed to determine the causes of MCI and risk factors of progression from MCI to dementia. It has been reported that lipids are increasingly recognized for their roles in neuronal function in the brain [4]. Indeed, the healthy human brain is composed of nearly 60% lipids, which is higher than in any other tissue [5]. Their work also showed that the relative abundance of phosphatidylcholine (PC), phosphatidylserine (PS), and phosphatidylethanolamine (PE) varies between the white and gray matter in the brain [5]. Phospholipids are important components of all mammalian cells; they have a variety of biological functions in the brain and serve as precursors for various secondary messengers such as arachidonic acid (AA), eicosapentaenoic acid (EPA), docosahexaenoic acid (DHA), ceramide, phosphatidic acid (PA), and lysophosphatidic acid (LPA). Lysophospholipid mediators have long been recognized as membrane phospholipid metabolites [6]. They belong primarily to one of six classes based on the structure of the lipid headgroup: LPA, lysophosphatidylcholine (LPC), lysophosphatidylethanolamine (LPE), lysophosphatidylglycerol (LPG), lysophosphatidylinositol (LPI), and lysophosphatidylserine (LPS). Each class has distinct biological functions dependent on physiological adaptation and availability of their respective cell surface receptors [7]. Lysophospholipids have been shown to induce a wide variety of biological effects, including cell proliferation, calcium signaling, metabolic activity, inflammatory and anti-inflammatory processes, and neurite formation [8–13]. These effects are generally evoked through receptor–ligand interactions, but this is not always the case. In addition to signaling via receptors, high physiological concentrations of LPC (approximately 150–200 μM in body fluids) suggest that they can alter membrane properties or interact directly with proteins in ways other than saturable binding to a ligand-specific site [13]. Furthermore, lipid head-group specificity in these instances may be due to the net charge of the lipid head groups. This net charge may affect the viscosity of the lipid bilayer or allow interactions with lipolytic enzymes, such as phospholipase A_2 (PLA_2) and phospholipase D (PLD), which convert these structural phospholipids into regulatory messengers and subsequently influence neurotransmission [14]. Previous evidence has indicated that cyclic phosphatidic acid (cPA) is generated in mammalian cells by phospholipase D_2 (PLD_2) from LPC in vitro and in vivo and mimics the effects of activating signaling pathways similar to those of neurotrophin NGF [15]. In addition, cPA effectively attenuates demyelination, glial activation, and motor dysfunction in an animal model of multiple sclerosis [16]. These studies suggested that phospholipids could be promising therapeutic agents for neurodegenerative diseases. Thus, it is critically important to focus our research efforts on PLDP in older individuals.

2. Microglia in Neurodegeneration

Neurodegeneration is an age-dependent progressive deterioration of neuronal components and functions, ultimately leading to cognitive impairment and dementia [17]. These changes occur due to genetic mutations or protein-misfolding diseases such as Alzheimer's disease that can accumulate with age [18]. Many groups have clearly demonstrated the close spatial–temporal relationship network between amyloid fibrils and activated microglia in both Alzheimer's disease patients and animal models [19–21]. Several studies have also indicated that Alzheimer's risk genes determine the microglial response to amyloid-β precursor protein but not to Tau pathology using single microglia sequencing [22,23]. These results suggest that microglia are associated with the progression of Alzheimer's disease. Activation of microglia has been extensively documented as an early event in the pathogenesis of protein-misfolding diseases [24]. These reports suggest that microglia are important aspects of CNS homeostasis and injury repair in aging. Under pathological conditions, such as altered neuronal function, injury, ischemia, and inflammation, microglia become activated, proliferate, and change from a ramified to an amoeboid cell type [25]. Microglial activation has been shown to lead to two opposing cell states, namely classical (M1) and alternative (M2) activation. The M1 phenotype is considered to be a pro-inflammatory state, in which microglial cells produce and release reactive oxygen species (ROS) and cytokines [26]. This is particularly evident in neurodegenerative disorders that involve protein aggregation events such as Alzheimer's disease. Activated microglia play a potentially detrimental role by eliciting the expression of pro-inflammatory cytokines, such as interleukin 1 beta (IL-1β), IL-6, and tumor necrosis factor-alpha (TNF-α), affecting the surrounding brain tissue [27]. Under ischemic stress, microglia are activated and produce high levels of ROS, which are known to induce oxidative injury in neurovascular cells [28]. In contrast, the M2 microglial phenotype is considered an anti-inflammatory effect and is involved in the production and release of pleiotropic cytokines and neurotrophins, such as IL-10, IL-4, and TGF-β, and low levels of pro-inflammatory cytokines. Anti-inflammatory cytokines such as IL-10 and IL-4 induce the M2 phenotype, which possesses neuroprotective properties. Microglia have become more important than ever in demonstrating strong genetic implications for microglia molecules and the immune system (Figure 1). These studies indicate that understanding human microglial function in neurodegenerative diseases may elucidate new targeted therapies.

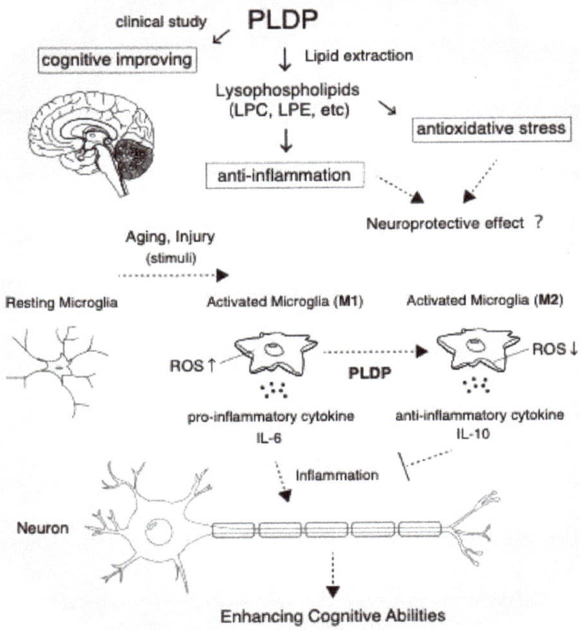

Figure 1. A potential role in the mechanism of action of PLDP in microglial cells. Our previous study suggested that PLDP improve cognitive function at older ages [29], by acting as a rich source of lysophospholipids (LPLs). Total phospholipids were extracted from PLDP using the Bligh and Dyer method,

an analysis of the composition of total phospholipids from PLDP revealed that the most abundant LPLs was LPC and LPE. We measured LPS-mediated anti-inflammatoly cytokines expression and ROS production with or without PLDP-derived LPLs treatment, IL-6 expression and ROS production was decreased.Conversion to the activated microglial phenotype (M1 and M2) is often accompanied by the release of NO and reactive oxygen species (ROS), along with the production of inflammatory cytokines such as IL-1, IL-6, and tumor necrosis factors (TNFs). This inflammatory milieu creates a toxic environment that leads to neuronal dysfunction and death. PLDP is a rich source of lysophospholipids including lysophosphatidylcholine (LPC) and lysophosphatidylethanolamine (LPE). In contrast, anti-inflammatory cytokines such as IL-10 and IL-4 induce the M2 phenotype, which possesses neuroprotective properties. We identified novel cooperative actions of lysophospholipids resulting in inhibition of IL-6 secretion and intracellular ROS accumulation in microglia after LPS-induced neuroinflammation. PLDP represents a promising nutraceutical that could improve cognitive function.

3. Mitochondrial Dysfunction and Neurodegenerative Disease

The inflammatory response is crucial in controlling and counteracting the harmful effects triggered by a variety of insults to the central nervous system. However, severe or chronic neuroinflammation can damage the central nervous system (CNS) because of excessive microglial production of cytokines and other inflammatory mediators, such as ROS. More recently, evidence has emerged for impaired mitochondrial dynamics in neurodegenerative diseases such as Alzheimer's disease. Mitochondria are responsible for ATP generation, ROS formation, intracellular Ca^{2+} homeostasis, and cell death [30]. The mitochondrial cascade hypothesis includes oxidative stress and overproduction of oxidative free radicals such as ROS and reactive nitrogen species [31]. ROS are toxic by-products generated in the mitochondria, and excess ROS may contribute to age-related disease. Impaired mitochondrial function and associated bioenergetic changes alter Alzheimer's disease homeostasis and lead to an accumulation of amyloid β-protein. Damage to mitochondria leads to a deficiency in energy production, oxidative stress, inflammation, and neuronal damage [32]. Microglia are resident macrophages and play a central role in Alzheimer's disease-related inflammation. It has been reported that microglial cells internalize aggregates of the Alzheimer's disease amyloid β-protein via the scavenger receptor CD36 [30]. Microglia have been reported to play a central role as moderators of amyloid β-protein degradation or clearance [33]. Recent evidence indicates that decreased clearance of amyloid β-protein is the driving force leading to its toxic accumulation in Alzheimer's disease. Amyloid β-protein interacts with microglia via CD36 and a heterodimer of toll-like receptor (TLR) 4 and 6. This interaction seems to activate the NLR family pyrin domain containing 3 (NLRP3) inflammasome, which results in the secretion of IL-1β [34]. The resulting overexpression of IL-1β can aggravate the chronic inflammatory response in the CNS [35]. These findings suggest that NLRP3 and IL-1β play important roles in the pathophysiology of Alzheimer's disease.

4. PLDP and Cognitive Improvement

To take advantage of the by-products of the porcine industry, porcine livers are used to obtain protein hydrolyzates. Porcine liver decomposition product (PLDP) is produced by hydrolysis, carried out using commercially available proteases and performed under optimal conditions [29]. After hydrolysis, proteases are heat-inactivated. Following the filtration and washing steps, a filter cake is formed. It has been reported that peptides from porcine liver hydrolyzates have antioxidant and angiotensin-converting enzyme (ACE) inhibitory properties [36]. Reductions in serum cholesterol have been observed following liver phospholipid treatment [37]. These data suggest that the liver has a high nutritional content and offers a good source of protein, lipids, and carbohydrates [38]. Our recent study demonstrated that PLDP can improve cognitive function in older adults by providing a rich source of phospholipids and lysophospholipids [29]. These findings suggest that PLDP is a promising nutraceutical for healthy adults over 40 years of age. We have previously demonstrated that PLDP primarily consists of phospholipids [29]. The components and amount of PLDP administered daily are shown in Table 1. An analysis of the composition of PLDP revealed that the most abundant phospholipids belonged to the PC class. Within this class, PC was the most abundant phospholipid, followed by PE. Other identified phospholipids included PS, PI, and PA. Likewise, extracted ion chromatogram (EIC) analysis of LPCs in the PLDP showed that the most abundant LPC was LPC (18:0). The most abundant LPE was LPE (18:0), while the most abundant LPI detected was LPI (18:0). The most abundant LPS detected was LPS (18:0), and the most abundant LPA detected was LPA (18:0) [39]. PLDP primarily includes phospholipids [29]. Phospholipids are structurally and functionally important cell membrane constituents. Numerous studies have been conducted to examine their role in aging [40], as phospholipids are the primary functional components of neuronal membranes [41]. These results suggest that PLDP represents a promising nutraceutical that could improve cognitive function in healthy adults over 40 years of age. Phospholipids, including PC, PE, PI, PS, and PA, are composed of a diacylglycerol moiety attached to a phosphate group, which in turn is connected to various head groups. Two acyl chains derived from fatty acids are attached to the first and second carbons of the glycerol moiety, denoted as sn-1 and sn-2, respectively [42]. Multiple isoforms of PLA_2 have been reported to hydrolyze PC, PS, and PE at the sn-2 position to form lysophospholipids, including LPA, LPC, LPS, and LPE [43]. Phospholipids are major constituents in the intestinal lumen after meal consumption and products of phospholipid metabolism in the intestine through PLA2- and ATX-mediated pathways [44]. Oral medication administration is one of the preferred routes for patients. Many drugs can be administered orally as capsules, tablets, or liquids. Since oral administration is the most convenient, safest, and least expensive route, it is most often used. Phospholipids derived from food sources (e.g., PLDP), especially complex lipids, are also capable of affecting gastrointestinal function and the enteric nervous system [45]. In addition, the digestive tract releases multiple types of bioactive lipids into the intestinal lumen [46]. Therefore, gastrointestinal inflammation is affected by both dietary lipids and lipid metabolism in the digestive tract [47]. Modulation of gastrointestinal wound repair and acute inflammation by mucus phospholipids in tissue is well understood [48]. In addition, systemic inflammation can increase the levels of pro-inflammatory cytokines in the CNS associated with glial activation in neurodegeneration [49]. LPC and LPA, which are also produced via PC hydrolysis, increase alpha-7 nicotinic acetylcholine receptor signaling and improve cognitive function by increasing long-term potentiation, increasing synaptic excitability [50]. Lysophospholipids mediate signaling, proliferation, neural activity, and inflammation, thus contributing to the regulation of a variety of important pathophysiological processes, including cerebral ischemia, vascular dementia, and Alzheimer's disease [51]. Under normal circumstances, inflammation is a protective response that facilitates the healing process [52]. However, leukocytes and macrophages are found throughout the blood and cytokines are secreted by cells of the nervous system as part of an immune-modulating response that helps to resolve inflammation [53]. Neuroinflammation is a hallmark of all major CNS diseases. The main mediators of neuroinflammation are microglial cells, which are activated during CNS injuries (e.g., stroke and spinal cord injury). Microglial cells initiate a rapid response that involves cell migration, proliferation, and release of cytokines, chemokines, and neurotrophic factors [54]. In addition, microglia can release potent neurotoxins that cause neuronal damage [55]. Since mitochondrial dysfunction is involved in neuroinflammation, repair and support of this organelle is critical in biological systems. Mitochondria have a lipid membrane, similar in composition to the plasma membrane, which can be damaged by the production of reactive oxygen species (ROS). Excess free-radical species adversely modify cell components, exacerbating lipid, protein, and DNA damage that underlie multiple pathogenic conditions. Induced lipid peroxidation also plays a critical role in cell death pathways, including apoptosis [56]. Therefore, exogenous phospholipids can provide an important source of bioactive components for the repair of these membranes [57]. We anticipate that a detailed study of the biological activities of phospholipids identified in PLDP will clarify the currently unknown pathophysiological mechanisms underlying dementia.

Table 1. The components and the amount of PLDP administered daily are shown. PC: phosphatidylcholine, PE: phosphatidylethanolamine, PI: phosphatidylinositol, PS: phosphatidylserine, PA: phosphatidic acid, SM: sphingomyelin, LPC: lysophosphatidylcholine.

Composition		Amount/Day
Phospholipids	PC	16.8 mg
	PE	4.0 mg
	PI	4.0 mg
	PS	1.7 mg
	PA	3.2 mg
	SM	2.2 mg
	LPC	6.7 mg
Cholesterol		4.5 mg
Purine (guanine)		1.4 mg

5. Lysophospholipids and Neuroinflammation

Based on the results of research over the last two decades, lysophospholipids have served not only as structural components of biological membranes, but also as biologically active molecules. They are known to influence a broad variety of processes, including neurogenesis, immunity, vascular development, and regulation of metabolic diseases [15,44,58–60]. With growing interest in the involvement of extracellular lysophospholipids in both normal physiology and pathology, it has become increasingly evident that these small mediators may have therapeutic potential for anti-neurodegenerative indications. It has been demonstrated that the lipopolysaccharide (LPS)-mediated inflammatory response, including increased microglial cytokine production, is significantly suppressed by LPC or LPE exposure [39,61]. Microglial activation leads to the production of pro-inflammatory cytokines, including IL-1, IL-6, and TNF-α [25]. A recent study suggested that LPC treatment attenuated the increased expression of the pro-inflammatory cytokines IL-1β, IL-6, and TNF-α, which suggests that it may be neuroprotective and/or protect against neuroinflammation. Previous studies have suggested that the pro-inflammatory cytokine TNF-α is a primary mediator of the inflammatory response that stimulates the synthesis and release of other cytokines [62]. Our results showed that the LPS-mediated inflammatory response, including the observed increase in microglial cytokine production, was suppressed by LPC exposure. This finding is important given that microglia-mediated neuroinflammation is regarded as a pathological mechanism in many neurodegenerative diseases and a key event accelerating cognitive or functional decline. While the release of these factors is typically intended to prevent further damage to CNS tissues, they may be toxic to certain neurons and other glial cells [25]. These studies suggest that understanding the role of proinflammatory cytokines in neurodegenerative diseases is complicated by cytokines possessing dual roles in neuroprotection and neurodegeneration. For example, IL-6 plays roles in aging, brain injury, dementia, and autoimmune disease [63]. IL-6 is a pleiotropic cytokine that is often undetectable in the normal brain. Its acute release in response to injury is well studied and documented [64]. LPS usually stimulates IL-6 production in both astrocytes and microglia, while TNF-α induces IL-6 in astrocytes, but not microglia [64]. There may be species-specific effects in which LPS mostly affects TNFα, IL-1β, and IL-6 production in microglia rather than in astrocytes, although IL-1β stimulates IL-6 synthesis in astrocytes [65]. Previous studies have also indicated that the anti-inflammatory cytokine IL-10 was induced by LPC or LPE exposure in ventral mesencephalic neurons and microglia in response to LPS stimulation [66,67]. IL-10 is known to inhibit the LPS-induced production of several inflammatory mediators [68]. Furthermore, it is an important modulator of neuronal homeostasis, with anti-inflammatory and neuroprotective functions, which can be released by activated microglia [69]. Neuroinflammation is a major pathogenic condition that affects the onset and progression of neurodegenerative diseases [70]. Inhibition of inflammatory cytokine production may play a role in the anti-inflammatory activity of lysophospholipids, suggesting novel therapeutic applications.

6. Oxidative Stress and Lysophospholipids

Oxidative stress is an important phenomenon caused by an imbalance between the production and degradation of free radicals and ROS in cells, leading to accumulation [71]. ROS are known to damage all cellular macromolecules (lipids, nucleic acids, and proteins). This damage leads to secondary metabolic activities that can be just as damaging as the initial ROS [72]. Oxidative stress seems to be involved in the pathogenesis of both major types of dementia: Alzheimer's disease and vascular dementia [73]. In Alzheimer's disease, oxidative modifications are closely associated with subtle inflammatory processes in the brain [74]. The brain becomes extremely enriched in oxidized phospholipids [75]. Lipid peroxidation is one of the major outcomes of free radical-mediated injury in neurological disorders [76]. Polyunsaturated fatty acid peroxidation triggers a devastating sequence of reactions in cell membranes. Once oxidative damage is initiated, ROS oxidize polyunsaturated fatty acids in the cell membrane in a self-propagating chain reaction. The cell membrane, which is composed of polyunsaturated fatty acids, is a primary target for ROS attack, leading to cell membrane damage. Increased ROS production is harmful, leading to adverse oxidative modifications to cell components, such as mitochondrial structures, which are sensitive targets of ROS-induced damage [77]. Polyunsaturated fatty acids can be further modified by cyclooxygenases to form prostaglandins, which are unstable and can be converted into various prostanoids depending on the cellular regulation of terminal prostanoid synthesis pathways [78]. On the other hand, LPC is a type of bioactive lysophospholipid that circulates in the body at high concentrations. LPC and LPE are highly abundant phospholipid components of PLDP that incorporate choline or phosphatidylethanolamine as their head group. PC hydrolysis at the sn-2 position by the superfamily of PLA_2 enzymes generates LPC [79]. The mechanisms of neuronal death in the disease remain unclear, although it has been postulated that cell death is due to apoptosis [80]. Reports have linked apoptosis to an increase in mitochondrial oxidative stress that causes cytochrome c release, subsequent caspase activation, and cell death [81–83]. A previous report suggested that LPC inhibits hydrogen peroxide-induced apoptosis in macrophages [84]. It has also been reported that LPE displays anti-inflammatory action when orally administered in zymosan-induced peritonitis, which is a model commonly used to study systemic inflammatory response syndrome [85]. LPE has been detected in human serum at concentrations of about several hundred nanograms per milliliter [86] and has been reported to function as an intercellular signaling molecule [87]. Numerous studies suggest that besides amyloid β-protein accumulation, dysregulation of intracellular Ca^{2+} homeostasis might act as an important progenitor of Alzheimer's disease. Reduced serum calcium levels are associated with the conversion of MCI to early Alzheimer's disease [88]. Many factors and signaling pathways that are activated by inflammation and oxidative stress are involved in the propagation of neurodegenerative diseases [89]. Our previous study suggested that 1-O-alkyl glycerophosphate (AGP), an ether-linked LPA, is present in the brain and spinal cord, and plays a crucial role during nervous system development. Tokumura described a phospholipase D (PLD) responsible for the degradation of lyso derivatives of platelet-activating factor (PAF) to AGP [90]. In addition, we found that AGP treatment increased the production of intracellular ROS and induced peroxisome proliferator-activated receptor γ (PPARγ) activation in microglial cells [91]. PPARγ is a member of the nuclear hormone receptor superfamily, many of which function as ligand-activated transcription factors. Intriguingly, AGP upregulated the expression levels of CD36 class B scavenger receptor, a high-affinity receptor for oxidized low-density lipoproteins (LDL). These findings suggest that AGP induces PPARγ activation, enhances CD36 expression, and increases the production of intracellular ROS in microglial cells. We showed that AGP strongly induced ROS-mediated microglial cell activation. ROS production in microglial cells was significantly increased upon treatment with AGP, and this production was attenuated by a synthetic irreversible PPARγ antagonist.

Additionally, PPARγ-induced and CD36-mediated microglial amyloid-β phagocytosis results in cognitive enhancement [91]. It is well known that inflammatory cytokines and signaling pathways play pivotal roles in microglial activation [92]. CD36-mediated ROS generation is an important factor that mediates AGP-induced cytokine signaling in microglial cells. These results indicate that inflammatory processes play a role in neurodegenerative disease progression and pathology, and that an extract of PLDP containing a mixture of physiologically and pharmacologically active phospholipids exerted potent anti-inflammatory and anti-oxidative effects against neurodegeneration underlying dementia. These studies suggest that lysophospholipids are of particular interest for their anti-inflammatory properties.

7. Conclusions and Future Perspectives

Accumulating evidence indicates that dementia is caused by damage to microglia–neuron communication [93]. Once activated, microglia can be potent immune effector cells that initiate both innate and adaptive immune responses and produce a number of cytokines, chemokines, and growth factors [94]. There has been increasing interest in the role of inflammation as a common mechanism of disease, including neurodegeneration. Common neurodegenerative diseases, including dementia, are associated with chronic neuroinflammation. This inflammation and subsequent tissue damage interfere with the ability of brain cells to communicate with each other. Signs and symptoms are linked to three stages of dementia: the early stage, middle stage, and late stage. A strong link has been observed between pro-inflammatory cytokines and neurodegeneration, both in clinical data and basic science research [95]. Recent evidence suggests that midlife risk factors for cardiovascular disease, including high cholesterol, hypertension, high homocysteine, and inflammation, are important risk factors for dementia in later years [96]. Furthermore, high cholesterol and hypertension have consistently displayed an association with increased risk of Alzheimer's disease and vascular dementia [97]. Vascular pathology plays a key role in the development of vascular dementia in addition to Alzheimer's disease [98]. An interesting report indicated that LPC and LPS attenuate the expression of inflammatory mediators in atherosclerosis [99]. Unfortunately, no treatment is currently available to cure dementia or to alter its progression. Numerous new treatments under investigation are in clinical trials. Currently, the principal goal of dementia care is early diagnosis, to promote early and optimal management. Although the exact mechanisms of action of PLDP are not fully understood, one possibility is a synergistic effect of phospholipid components in PLDP (Figure 1). Currently, LPC and LPE are the most attractive research targets in terms of biological activity and possible applications. Enzymatic digestion of LPC leads to the formation of various forms of bioactive lipids such as LPA and cPA, which are involved in modulating cardiovascular system physiology, wound healing, and carbohydrate metabolism, mediated by plasma membrane and nuclear receptors [15,100]. LPE is likely to have neuroprotective roles both in vivo and in vitro. We showed that media conditioned via exposure to LPE-treated microglia promoted morphological changes in a dose-dependent manner. Our study also indicated that LPC and LPE synergistically suppressed LPS-stimulated ROS production [39]. This finding is important given that microglia-mediated neuroinflammation is regarded as a pathological mechanism in many neurodegenerative diseases, such as dementia and Alzheimer's disease, and a key event in accelerating cognitive or functional decline. Thus, lysophospholipids a promising therapeutic candidate for the treatment of age-related cognitive impairments, including neurodegenerative diseases, such as dementia (Figure 2). The effect of PLDP and its component phospholipids on other mental diseases will be an interesting topic to explore. We aimed to identify a functional phospholipid contained within PLDP that has been confirmed to have clinical effects and to develop a new drug for treating dementia and Alzheimer's disease.

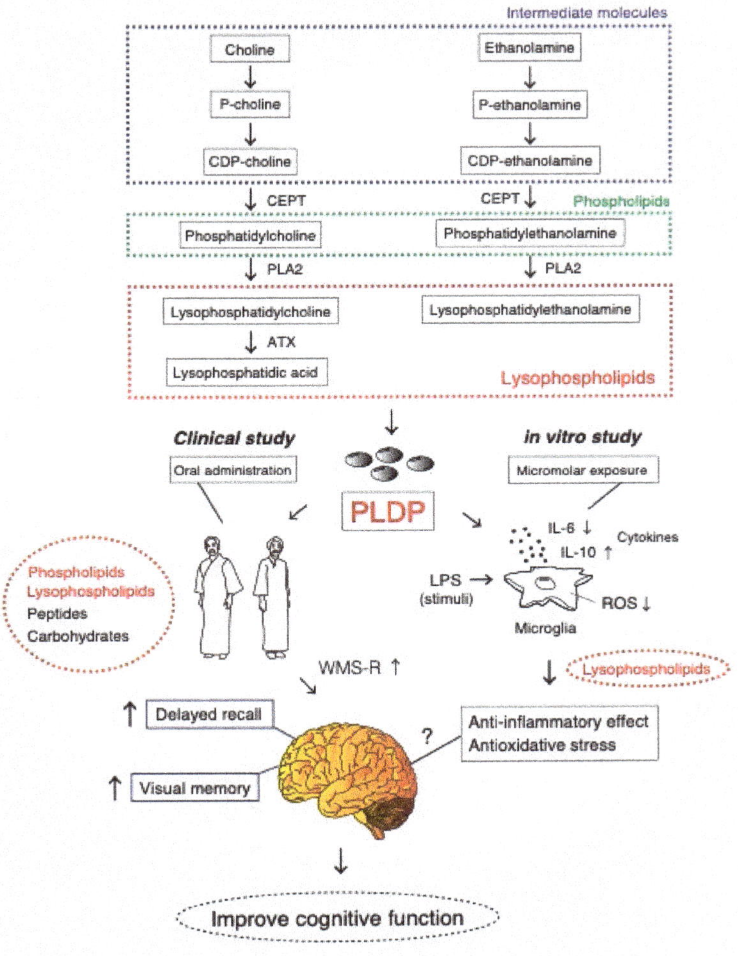

Figure 2. Effect of PLDP in vitro and in vivo. Oral administration of PLDP to healthy study participants (over 40 years of age) enhanced Visual Memory and Delayed Recall. Our primary focus was to identify a functional phospholipid contained within PLDP, confirm its clinical effects, and develop it as a new drug for treating neurodegenerative diseases, including dementia. PLDP: porcine liver decomposition product, CEPT: choline/ethanolamine phosphotransferase, PLA_2: Phospholipase A_2, ATX: Autotaxin, also known as ectonucleotide pyrophosphatase/phosphodiesterase family member 2, WMS-R: Wechsler Memory Scale.

Author Contributions: T.T., H.H., T.U., and Y.M. drafted the paper. T.T. produced the final draft. All authors have read and agreed to the published version of the manuscript.

Funding: This work was supported by the Japan Society for the Promotion of Science KAKENHI [grant number 20K09476 and 16K15660] to Hisao Haniu and Tamotsu Tsukahara, and by The Ito Foundation [grant number ken-1] to Tamotsu Tsukahara.

Conflicts of Interest: The authors declare no conflict of interest.

Abbreviations

PLDP	porcine liver decomposition product
MCI	mild cognitive impairment
LPA	lysophosphatidic acid
LPE	lysophosphatidylethanolamine
LPC	lysophosphatidylcholine
LPS	lipopolysaccharide
cPA	cyclic phosphatidic acid
ROS	reactive oxygen species
CNS	central nervous system

References

1. Eshkoor, S.A.; Hamid, T.A.; Mun, C.Y.; Ng, C.K. Mild cognitive impairment and its management in older people. *Clin. Interv. Aging* **2015**, *10*, 687–693. [CrossRef] [PubMed]
2. Kelley, B.J.; Petersen, R.C. Alzheimer's disease and mild cognitive impairment. *Neurol. Clin.* **2007**, *25*, 577–609. [CrossRef] [PubMed]
3. Wiesmann, M.; Kiliaan, A.J.; Claassen, J.A. Vascular aspects of cognitive impairment and dementia. *J. Cereb. Blood Flow Metab.* **2013**, *33*, 1696–1706. [CrossRef] [PubMed]
4. Bruce, K.D.; Zsombok, A.; Eckel, R.H. Lipid Processing in the Brain: A Key Regulator of Systemic Metabolism. *Front. Endocrinol.* **2017**, *8*, 60. [CrossRef]
5. Joensuu, M.; Wallis, T.P.; Saber, S.H.; Meunier, F.A. Phospholipases in neuronal function: A role in learning and memory? *J. Neurochem.* **2020**, *153*, 300–333. [CrossRef]
6. Birgbauer, E.; Chun, J. New developments in the biological functions of lysophospholipids. *Cell Mol. Life Sci.* **2006**, *63*, 2695–2701. [CrossRef]
7. Anliker, B.; Chun, J. Cell surface receptors in lysophospholipid signaling. *Semin. Cell Dev. Biol.* **2004**, *15*, 457–465. [CrossRef]
8. Lin, K.H.; Ho, Y.H.; Chiang, J.C.; Li, M.W.; Lin, S.H.; Chen, W.M.; Chiang, C.L.; Lin, Y.N.; Yang, Y.J.; Chen, C.N.; et al. Pharmacological activation of lysophosphatidic acid receptors regulates erythropoiesis. *Sci. Rep.* **2016**, *6*, 27050. [CrossRef]
9. Tigyi, G. Aiming drug discovery at lysophosphatidic acid targets. *Br. J. Pharmacol.* **2010**, *161*, 241–270. [CrossRef]
10. Zhang, C.; Baker, D.L.; Yasuda, S.; Makarova, N.; Balazs, L.; Johnson, L.R.; Marathe, G.K.; McIntyre, T.M.; Xu, Y.; Prestwich, G.D.; et al. Lysophosphatidic acid induces neointima formation through PPARgamma activation. *J. Exp. Med.* **2004**, *199*, 763–774. [CrossRef]
11. Fujiwara, Y.; Sebok, A.; Meakin, S.; Kobayashi, T.; Murakami-Murofushi, K.; Tigyi, G. Cyclic phosphatidic acid elicits neurotrophin-like actions in embryonic hippocampal neurons. *J. Neurochem.* **2003**, *87*, 1272–1283. [CrossRef]
12. Goetzl, E.J.; Tigyi, G. Lysophospholipids and their G protein-coupled receptors in biology and diseases. *J. Cell Biochem.* **2004**, *92*, 867–868. [CrossRef] [PubMed]
13. Wepy, J.A.; Galligan, J.J.; Kingsley, P.J.; Xu, S.; Goodman, M.C.; Tallman, K.A.; Rouzer, C.A.; Marnett, L.J. Lysophospholipases cooperate to mediate lipid homeostasis and lysophospholipid signaling. *J. Lipid Res.* **2019**, *60*, 360–374. [CrossRef] [PubMed]
14. Chan, P.; Suridjan, I.; Mohammad, D.; Herrmann, N.; Mazereeuw, G.; Hillyer, L.M.; Ma, D.W.L.; Oh, P.I.; Lanctot, K.L. Novel Phospholipid Signature of Depressive Symptoms in Patients With Coronary Artery Disease. *J. Am. Heart Assoc.* **2018**, *7*, e008278. [CrossRef] [PubMed]
15. Tsukahara, T.; Tsukahara, R.; Fujiwara, Y.; Yue, J.; Cheng, Y.; Guo, H.; Bolen, A.; Zhang, C.; Balazs, L.; Re, F.; et al. Phospholipase D2-dependent inhibition of the nuclear hormone receptor PPARgamma by cyclic phosphatidic acid. *Mol. Cell* **2010**, *39*, 421–432. [CrossRef] [PubMed]

16. Yamamoto, S.; Gotoh, M.; Kawamura, Y.; Yamashina, K.; Yagishita, S.; Awaji, T.; Tanaka, M.; Maruyama, K.; Murakami-Murofushi, K.; Yoshikawa, K. Cyclic phosphatidic acid treatment suppress cuprizone-induced demyelination and motor dysfunction in mice. *Eur. J. Pharmacol.* **2014**, *741*, 17–24. [CrossRef] [PubMed]
17. Hussain, R.; Zubair, H.; Pursell, S.; Shahab, M. Neurodegenerative Diseases: Regenerative Mechanisms and Novel Therapeutic Approaches. *Brain Sci.* **2018**, *8*, 177. [CrossRef]
18. Sweeney, P.; Park, H.; Baumann, M.; Dunlop, J.; Frydman, J.; Kopito, R.; McCampbell, A.; Leblanc, G.; Venkateswaran, A.; Nurmi, A.; et al. Protein misfolding in neurodegenerative diseases: Implications and strategies. *Transl. Neurodegener* **2017**, *6*, 6. [CrossRef]
19. McQuade, A.; Blurton-Jones, M. Microglia in Alzheimer's Disease: Exploring How Genetics and Phenotype Influence Risk. *J. Mol. Biol.* **2019**, *431*, 1805–1817. [CrossRef]
20. Aloni, E.; Oni-Biton, E.; Tsoory, M.; Moallem, D.H.; Segal, M. Synaptopodin Deficiency Ameliorates Symptoms in the 3xTg Mouse Model of Alzheimer's Disease. *J. Neurosci.* **2019**, *39*, 3983–3992. [CrossRef]
21. Ohm, D.T.; Fought, A.J.; Martersteck, A.; Coventry, C.; Sridhar, J.; Gefen, T.; Weintraub, S.; Bigio, E.; Mesulam, M.M.; Rogalski, E.; et al. Accumulation of neurofibrillary tangles and activated microglia is associated with lower neuron densities in the aphasic variant of Alzheimer's disease. *Brain Pathol.* **2020**. [CrossRef] [PubMed]
22. Chew, G.; Petretto, E. Transcriptional Networks of Microglia in Alzheimer's Disease and Insights into Pathogenesis. *Genes* **2019**, *10*, 798. [CrossRef] [PubMed]
23. Sierksma, A.; Lu, A.; Mancuso, R.; Fattorelli, N.; Thrupp, N.; Salta, E.; Zoco, J.; Blum, D.; Buee, L.; De Strooper, B.; et al. Novel Alzheimer risk genes determine the microglia response to amyloid-beta but not to TAU pathology. *EMBO Mol. Med.* **2020**, *12*, e10606. [CrossRef]
24. Vincenti, J.E.; Murphy, L.; Grabert, K.; McColl, B.W.; Cancellotti, E.; Freeman, T.C.; Manson, J.C. Defining the Microglia Response during the Time Course of Chronic Neurodegeneration. *J. Virol.* **2015**, *90*, 3003–3017. [CrossRef] [PubMed]
25. Wang, W.Y.; Tan, M.S.; Yu, J.T.; Tan, L. Role of pro-inflammatory cytokines released from microglia in Alzheimer's disease. *Ann. Transl Med.* **2015**, *3*, 136.
26. Pozzo, E.D.; Tremolanti, C.; Costa, B.; Giacomelli, C.; Milenkovic, V.M.; Bader, S.; Wetzel, C.H.; Rupprecht, R.; Taliani, S.; Settimo, F.D.; et al. Microglial Pro-Inflammatory and Anti-Inflammatory Phenotypes Are Modulated by Translocator Protein Activation. *Int. J. Mol. Sci* **2019**, *20*, 4467. [CrossRef]
27. Tjalkens, R.B.; Popichak, K.A.; Kirkley, K.A. Inflammatory Activation of Microglia and Astrocytes in Manganese Neurotoxicity. *Adv. Neurobiol.* **2017**, *18*, 159–181.
28. Patel, A.R.; Ritzel, R.; McCullough, L.D.; Liu, F. Microglia and ischemic stroke: A double-edged sword. *Int. J. Physiol. Pathophysiol. Pharmacol.* **2013**, *5*, 73–90.
29. Matsuda, Y.; Haniu, H.; Tsukahara, T.; Uemura, T.; Inoue, T.; Sako, K.I.; Kojima, J.; Mori, T.; Sato, K. Oral administration of porcine liver decomposition product for 4weeks enhances visual memory and delayed recall in healthy adults over 40years of age: A randomized, double-blind, placebo-controlled study. *Exp. Gerontol.* **2020**, *141*, 111064. [CrossRef]
30. Agrawal, I.; Jha, S. Mitochondrial Dysfunction and Alzheimer's Disease: Role of Microglia. *Front. Aging Neurosci.* **2020**, *12*, 252. [CrossRef]
31. Di Meo, S.; Reed, T.T.; Venditti, P.; Victor, V.M. Role of ROS and RNS Sources in Physiological and Pathological Conditions. *Oxid Med. Cell Longev.* **2016**, *2016*, 1245049. [CrossRef] [PubMed]
32. Picca, A.; Calvani, R.; Coelho-Junior, H.J.; Landi, F.; Bernabei, R.; Marzetti, E. Mitochondrial Dysfunction, Oxidative Stress, and Neuroinflammation: Intertwined Roads to Neurodegeneration. *Antioxidants* **2020**, *9*, 647. [CrossRef] [PubMed]
33. Ries, M.; Sastre, M. Mechanisms of Abeta Clearance and Degradation by Glial Cells. *Front. Aging Neurosci.* **2016**, *8*, 160. [CrossRef] [PubMed]
34. Gold, M.; El Khoury, J. beta-amyloid, microglia, and the inflammasome in Alzheimer's disease. *Semin. Immunopathol.* **2015**, *37*, 607–611. [CrossRef]
35. Guan, Y.; Han, F. Key Mechanisms and Potential Targets of the NLRP3 Inflammasome in Neurodegenerative Diseases. *Front. Integr. Neurosci.* **2020**, *14*, 37. [CrossRef]
36. Mora, L.; Gallego, M.; Toldra, F. ACEI-Inhibitory Peptides Naturally Generated in Meat and Meat Products and Their Health Relevance. *Nutrients* **2018**, *10*, 1259. [CrossRef]

37. Ristic-Medic, D.; Ristic, G.; Tepsic, V.; Ristic, G.N. Effects of different quantities of fat on serum and liver lipids, phospholipid class distribution and fatty acid composition in alcohol-treated rats. *J. Nutr. Sci. Vitaminol. (Tokyo)* **2003**, *49*, 367–374. [CrossRef]
38. Yu, H.C.; Hsu, J.L.; Chang, C.I.; Tan, F.J. Antioxidant properties of porcine liver proteins hydrolyzed using Monascus purpureus. *Food Sci. Biotechnol.* **2017**, *26*, 1217–1225. [CrossRef]
39. Tsukahara, T.; Haniu, H.; Uemura, T.; Matsuda, Y. Porcine liver decomposition product-derived lysophospholipids promote microglial activation in vitro. *Sci. Rep.* **2020**, *10*, 3748. [CrossRef]
40. Nicolson, G.L.; Ash, M.E. Membrane Lipid Replacement for chronic illnesses, aging and cancer using oral glycerolphospholipid formulations with fructooligosaccharides to restore phospholipid function in cellular membranes, organelles, cells and tissues. *Biochim. Biophys. Acta Biomembr.* **2017**, *1859 Pt B*, 1704–1724. [CrossRef]
41. Jove, M.; Pradas, I.; Dominguez-Gonzalez, M.; Ferrer, I.; Pamplona, R. Lipids and lipoxidation in human brain aging. Mitochondrial ATP-synthase as a key lipoxidation target. *Redox Biol.* **2019**, *23*, 101082. [CrossRef] [PubMed]
42. Choi, J.; Yin, T.; Shinozaki, K.; Lampe, J.W.; Stevens, J.F.; Becker, L.B.; Kim, J. Comprehensive analysis of phospholipids in the brain, heart, kidney, and liver: Brain phospholipids are least enriched with polyunsaturated fatty acids. *Mol. Cell Biochem.* **2018**, *442*, 187–201. [CrossRef]
43. Tigyi, G. New trends in lysophospholipid research. *Biochim. Biophys. Acta* **2013**, 1831. [CrossRef] [PubMed]
44. Hui, D.Y. Intestinal phospholipid and lysophospholipid metabolism in cardiometabolic disease. *Curr. Opin. Lipidol.* **2016**, *27*, 507–512. [CrossRef] [PubMed]
45. Escalante, J.; McQuade, R.M.; Stojanovska, V.; Nurgali, K. Impact of chemotherapy on gastrointestinal functions and the enteric nervous system. *Maturitas* **2017**, *105*, 23–29. [CrossRef]
46. Rein, M.J.; Renouf, M.; Cruz-Hernandez, C.; Actis-Goretta, L.; Thakkar, S.K.; da Silva Pinto, M. Bioavailability of bioactive food compounds: A challenging journey to bioefficacy. *Br. J. Clin. Pharmacol.* **2013**, *75*, 588–602. [CrossRef]
47. Schoeler, M.; Caesar, R. Dietary lipids, gut microbiota and lipid metabolism. *Rev. Endocr. Metab. Disord.* **2019**, *20*, 461–472. [CrossRef]
48. Sturm, A.; Dignass, A.U. Modulation of gastrointestinal wound repair and inflammation by phospholipids. *Biochim. Biophys. Acta* **2002**, *1582*, 282–288. [CrossRef]
49. Smith, J.A.; Das, A.; Ray, S.K.; Banik, N.L. Role of pro-inflammatory cytokines released from microglia in neurodegenerative diseases. *Brain Res. Bull.* **2012**, *87*, 10–20. [CrossRef]
50. Baenziger, J.E.; Henault, C.M.; Therien, J.P.; Sun, J. Nicotinic acetylcholine receptor-lipid interactions: Mechanistic insight and biological function. *Biochim. Biophys. Acta* **2015**, *1848*, 1806–1817. [CrossRef]
51. Tsukahara, T.; Matsuda, Y.; Haniu, H. Lysophospholipid-Related Diseases and PPARgamma Signaling Pathway. *Int. J. Mol. Sci* **2017**, *18*, 2730. [CrossRef] [PubMed]
52. Chen, L.; Deng, H.; Cui, H.; Fang, J.; Zuo, Z.; Deng, J.; Li, Y.; Wang, X.; Zhao, L. Inflammatory responses and inflammation-associated diseases in organs. *Oncotarget* **2018**, *9*, 7204–7218. [CrossRef] [PubMed]
53. Zhang, J.M.; An, J. Cytokines, inflammation, and pain. *Int. Anesthesiol. Clin.* **2007**, *45*, 27–37. [CrossRef]
54. Chen, W.W.; Zhang, X.; Huang, W.J. Role of neuroinflammation in neurodegenerative diseases (Review). *Mol. Med. Rep.* **2016**, *13*, 3391–3396. [CrossRef] [PubMed]
55. Kim, Y.S.; Joh, T.H. Microglia, major player in the brain inflammation: Their roles in the pathogenesis of Parkinson's disease. *Exp. Mol. Med.* **2006**, *38*, 333–347. [CrossRef] [PubMed]
56. Su, L.J.; Zhang, J.H.; Gomez, H.; Murugan, R.; Hong, X.; Xu, D.; Jiang, F.; Peng, Z.Y. Reactive Oxygen Species-Induced Lipid Peroxidation in Apoptosis, Autophagy, and Ferroptosis. *Oxid. Med. Cell Longev.* **2019**, *2019*, 5080843. [CrossRef]
57. Tayebati, S.K. Phospholipid and Lipid Derivatives as Potential Neuroprotective Compounds. *Molecules* **2018**, *23*, 2257. [CrossRef]
58. Ladron de Guevara-Miranda, D.; Moreno-Fernandez, R.D.; Gil-Rodriguez, S.; Rosell-Valle, C.; Estivill-Torrus, G.; Serrano, A.; Pavon, F.J.; Rodriguez de Fonseca, F.; Santin, L.J.; Castilla-Ortega, E. Lysophosphatidic acid-induced increase in adult hippocampal neurogenesis facilitates the forgetting of cocaine-contextual memory. *Addict. Biol.* **2019**, *24*, 458–470. [CrossRef]
59. Lin, D.A.; Boyce, J.A. Lysophospholipids as mediators of immunity. *Adv. Immunol.* **2006**, *89*, 141–167.

60. Teo, S.T.; Yung, Y.C.; Herr, D.R.; Chun, J. Lysophosphatidic acid in vascular development and disease. *IUBMB Life* **2009**, *61*, 791–799. [CrossRef]
61. Yan, J.J.; Jung, J.S.; Lee, J.E.; Lee, J.; Huh, S.O.; Kim, H.S.; Jung, K.C.; Cho, J.Y.; Nam, J.S.; Suh, H.W.; et al. Therapeutic effects of lysophosphatidylcholine in experimental sepsis. *Nat. Med.* **2004**, *10*, 161–167. [CrossRef]
62. Kany, S.; Vollrath, J.T.; Relja, B. Cytokines in Inflammatory Disease. *Int. J. Mol. Sci* **2019**, *20*, 6008. [CrossRef]
63. Erta, M.; Quintana, A.; Hidalgo, J. Interleukin-6, a major cytokine in the central nervous system. *Int. J. Biol. Sci.* **2012**, *8*, 1254–1266. [CrossRef] [PubMed]
64. Woodcock, T.; Morganti-Kossmann, M.C. The role of markers of inflammation in traumatic brain injury. *Front. Neurol.* **2013**, *4*, 18. [CrossRef]
65. Bobbo, V.C.D.; Jara, C.P.; Mendes, N.F.; Morari, J.; Velloso, L.A.; Araujo, E.P. Interleukin-6 Expression by Hypothalamic Microglia in Multiple Inflammatory Contexts: A Systematic Review. *Biomed. Res. Int.* **2019**, *2019*, 1365210. [CrossRef]
66. Zhu, Y.; Chen, X.; Liu, Z.; Peng, Y.P.; Qiu, Y.H. Interleukin-10 Protection against Lipopolysaccharide-Induced Neuro-Inflammation and Neurotoxicity in Ventral Mesencephalic Cultures. *Int. J. Mol. Sci.* **2015**, *17*, 25. [CrossRef] [PubMed]
67. Lively, S.; Schlichter, L.C. Microglia Responses to Pro-inflammatory Stimuli (LPS, IFNgamma+TNFalpha) and Reprogramming by Resolving Cytokines (IL-4, IL-10). *Front. Cell Neurosci.* **2018**, *12*, 215. [CrossRef]
68. Berlato, C.; Cassatella, M.A.; Kinjyo, I.; Gatto, L.; Yoshimura, A.; Bazzoni, F. Involvement of suppressor of cytokine signaling-3 as a mediator of the inhibitory effects of IL-10 on lipopolysaccharide-induced macrophage activation. *J. Immunol.* **2002**, *168*, 6404–6411. [CrossRef]
69. Laffer, B.; Bauer, D.; Wasmuth, S.; Busch, M.; Jalilvand, T.V.; Thanos, S.; Meyer Zu Horste, G.; Loser, K.; Langmann, T.; Heiligenhaus, A.; et al. Loss of IL-10 Promotes Differentiation of Microglia to a M1 Phenotype. *Front. Cell Neurosci.* **2019**, *13*, 430. [CrossRef] [PubMed]
70. Chitnis, T.; Weiner, H.L. CNS inflammation and neurodegeneration. *J. Clin. Invest.* **2017**, *127*, 3577–3587. [CrossRef]
71. Pizzino, G.; Irrera, N.; Cucinotta, M.; Pallio, G.; Mannino, F.; Arcoraci, V.; Squadrito, F.; Altavilla, D.; Bitto, A. Oxidative Stress: Harms and Benefits for Human Health. *Oxid. Med. Cell Longev.* **2017**, *2017*, 8416763. [CrossRef] [PubMed]
72. Sayre, L.M.; Perry, G.; Smith, M.A. Oxidative stress and neurotoxicity. *Chem. Res. Toxicol.* **2008**, *21*, 172–188. [CrossRef] [PubMed]
73. Luca, M.; Luca, A.; Calandra, C. The Role of Oxidative Damage in the Pathogenesis and Progression of Alzheimer's Disease and Vascular Dementia. *Oxid. Med. Cell Longev.* **2015**, *2015*, 504678. [CrossRef] [PubMed]
74. Chen, X.; Guo, C.; Kong, J. Oxidative stress in neurodegenerative diseases. *Neural Regen Res.* **2012**, *7*, 376–385.
75. Salim, S. Oxidative Stress and the Central Nervous System. *J. Pharmacol. Exp. Ther* **2017**, *360*, 201–205. [CrossRef]
76. Shichiri, M. The role of lipid peroxidation in neurological disorders. *J. Clin. Biochem. Nutr.* **2014**, *54*, 151–160. [CrossRef]
77. Teixeira, J.P.; de Castro, A.A.; Soares, F.V.; da Cunha, E.F.F.; Ramalho, T.C. Future Therapeutic Perspectives into the Alzheimer's Disease Targeting the Oxidative Stress Hypothesis. *Molecules* **2019**, *24*, 4410. [CrossRef]
78. Kanner, J. Dietary advanced lipid oxidation endproducts are risk factors to human health. *Mol. Nutr. Food Res.* **2007**, *51*, 1094–1101. [CrossRef]
79. Sato, H.; Taketomi, Y.; Murakami, M. Metabolic regulation by secreted phospholipase A2. *Inflamm. Regen* **2016**, *36*, 7. [CrossRef]
80. Fricker, M.; Tolkovsky, A.M.; Borutaite, V.; Coleman, M.; Brown, G.C. Neuronal Cell Death. *Physiol. Rev.* **2018**, *98*, 813–880. [CrossRef]
81. Barrera, G. Oxidative stress and lipid peroxidation products in cancer progression and therapy. *ISRN Oncol.* **2012**, *2012*, 137289. [CrossRef] [PubMed]
82. Cadenas, E. Mitochondrial free radical production and cell signaling. *Mol. Aspects Med.* **2004**, *25*, 17–26. [CrossRef] [PubMed]
83. Simon, H.U.; Haj-Yehia, A.; Levi-Schaffer, F. Role of reactive oxygen species (ROS) in apoptosis induction. *Apoptosis* **2000**, *5*, 415–418. [CrossRef]

84. Nishikawa, Y.; Furukawa, A.; Shiga, I.; Muroi, Y.; Ishii, T.; Hongo, Y.; Takahashi, S.; Sugawara, T.; Koshino, H.; Ohnishi, M. Cytoprotective Effects of Lysophospholipids from Sea Cucumber Holothuria atra. *PLoS ONE* **2015**, *10*, e0135701. [CrossRef]
85. Hung, N.D.; Kim, M.R.; Sok, D.E. 2-Polyunsaturated acyl lysophosphatidylethanolamine attenuates inflammatory response in zymosan A-induced peritonitis in mice. *Lipids* **2011**, *46*, 893–906. [CrossRef]
86. Makide, K.; Kitamura, H.; Sato, Y.; Okutani, M.; Aoki, J. Emerging lysophospholipid mediators, lysophosphatidylserine, lysophosphatidylthreonine, lysophosphatidylethanolamine and lysophosphatidylglycerol. *Prostaglandins Other Lipid Mediat* **2009**, *89*, 135–139. [CrossRef] [PubMed]
87. Lee, J.M.; Park, S.J.; Im, D.S. Calcium Signaling of Lysophosphatidylethanolamine through LPA1 in Human SH-SY5Y Neuroblastoma Cells. *Biomol. Ther. (Seoul)* **2017**, *25*, 194–201. [CrossRef]
88. Sato, K.; Mano, T.; Ihara, R.; Suzuki, K.; Tomita, N.; Arai, H.; Ishii, K.; Senda, M.; Ito, K.; Ikeuchi, T.; et al. Lower Serum Calcium as a Potentially Associated Factor for Conversion of Mild Cognitive Impairment to Early Alzheimer's Disease in the Japanese Alzheimer's Disease Neuroimaging Initiative. *J. Alzheimers Dis* **2019**, *68*, 777–788. [CrossRef]
89. Yang, Y.; Jiang, G.; Zhang, P.; Fan, J. Programmed cell death and its role in inflammation. *Mil. Med. Res.* **2015**, *2*, 12. [CrossRef] [PubMed]
90. Tokumura, A.; Harada, K.; Fukuzawa, K.; Tsukatani, H. Involvement of lysophospholipase D in the production of lysophosphatidic acid in rat plasma. *Biochim. Biophys. Acta* **1986**, *875*, 31–38.
91. Tsukahara, T. 1-O-alkyl glycerophosphate-induced CD36 expression drives oxidative stress in microglial cells. *Cell Signal.* **2020**, *65*, 109459. [CrossRef] [PubMed]
92. Subhramanyam, C.S.; Wang, C.; Hu, Q.; Dheen, S.T. Microglia-mediated neuroinflammation in neurodegenerative diseases. *Semin. Cell Dev. Biol.* **2019**, *94*, 112–120. [CrossRef] [PubMed]
93. Clayton, K.A.; Van Enoo, A.A.; Ikezu, T. Alzheimer's Disease: The Role of Microglia in Brain Homeostasis and Proteopathy. *Front. Neurosci.* **2017**, *11*, 680. [CrossRef] [PubMed]
94. Town, T.; Nikolic, V.; Tan, J. The microglial "activation" continuum: From innate to adaptive responses. *J. Neuroinflamm.* **2005**, *2*, 24. [CrossRef] [PubMed]
95. Alam, Q.; Alam, M.Z.; Mushtaq, G.; Damanhouri, G.A.; Rasool, M.; Kamal, M.A.; Haque, A. Inflammatory Process in Alzheimer's and Parkinson's Diseases: Central Role of Cytokines. *Curr. Pharm. Des.* **2016**, *22*, 541–548. [CrossRef] [PubMed]
96. de Bruijn, R.F.; Ikram, M.A. Cardiovascular risk factors and future risk of Alzheimer's disease. *BMC Med.* **2014**, *12*, 130. [CrossRef] [PubMed]
97. Duron, E.; Hanon, O. Vascular risk factors, cognitive decline, and dementia. *Vasc. Health Risk Manag.* **2008**, *4*, 363–381.
98. van Oijen, M.; de Jong, F.J.; Witteman, J.C.; Hofman, A.; Koudstaal, P.J.; Breteler, M.M. Atherosclerosis and risk for dementia. *Ann. Neurol.* **2007**, *61*, 403–410. [CrossRef]
99. Matsumoto, T.; Kobayashi, T.; Kamata, K. Role of lysophosphatidylcholine (LPC) in atherosclerosis. *Curr. Med. Chem.* **2007**, *14*, 3209–3220. [CrossRef]
100. Drzazga, A.; Sowinska, A.; Koziolkiewicz, M. Lysophosphatidylcholine and lysophosphatidylinosiol—novel promissing signaling molecules and their possible therapeutic activity. *Acta Pol. Pharm.* **2014**, *71*, 887–899.

biomedicines

MDPI

Review

The Anti-Inflammatory and Antioxidant Properties of n-3 PUFAs: Their Role in Cardiovascular Protection

Francesca Oppedisano [1], Roberta Macrì [1], Micaela Gliozzi [1], Vincenzo Musolino [1], Cristina Carresi [1], Jessica Maiuolo [1], Francesca Bosco [1], Saverio Nucera [1], Maria Caterina Zito [1], Lorenza Guarnieri [1], Federica Scarano [1], Caterina Nicita [1], Anna Rita Coppoletta [1], Stefano Ruga [1], Miriam Scicchitano [1], Rocco Mollace [1,2], Ernesto Palma [1] and Vincenzo Mollace [1,3,*]

1 Institute of Research for Food Safety and Health (IRC-FSH), Department of Health Sciences, University "Magna Graecia" of Catanzaro, 88100 Catanzaro, Italy; oppedisanof@libero.it (F.O.); robertamacri85@gmail.com (R.M.); gliozzi@unicz.it (M.G.); v.musolino@unicz.it (V.M.); carresi@unicz.it (C.C.); jessicamaiuolo@virgilio.it (J.M.); boscofrancescabf@libero.it (F.B.); saverio.nucera@hotmail.it (S.N.); mariacaterina.zito@libero.it (M.C.Z.); lorenzacz808@gmail.com (L.G.); federicascar87@gmail.com (F.S.); caterina.nicita@gmail.com (C.N.); annarita.coppoletta@libero.it (A.R.C.); rugast1@gmail.com (S.R.); miriam.scicchitano@hotmail.it (M.S.); rocco.mollace@gmail.com (R.M.); palma@unicz.it (E.P.)

2 Division of Cardiology, University Hospital Policlinico Tor Vergata, 00133 Rome, Italy

3 IRCCS San Raffaele Pisana, 00163 Roma, Italy

* Correspondence: mollace@unicz.it

Received: 25 June 2020; Accepted: 24 August 2020; Published: 25 August 2020

Abstract: Polyunsaturated fatty acids (n-3 PUFAs) are long-chain polyunsaturated fatty acids with 18, 20 or 22 carbon atoms, which have been found able to counteract cardiovascular diseases. Eicosapentaenoic acid (EPA) and docosahexaenoic acid (DHA), in particular, have been found to produce both vaso- and cardio-protective response via modulation of membrane phospholipids thereby improving cardiac mitochondrial functions and energy production. However, antioxidant properties of n-3 PUFAs, along with their anti-inflammatory effect in both blood vessels and cardiac cells, seem to exert beneficial effects in cardiovascular impairment. In fact, dietary supplementation with n-3 PUFAs has been demonstrated to reduce oxidative stress-related mitochondrial dysfunction and endothelial cell apoptosis, an effect occurring via an increased activity of endogenous antioxidant enzymes. On the other hand, n-3 PUFAs have been shown to counteract the release of pro-inflammatory cytokines in both vascular tissues and in the myocardium, thereby restoring vascular reactivity and myocardial performance. Here we summarize the molecular mechanisms underlying the anti-oxidant and anti-inflammatory effect of n-3 PUFAs in vascular and cardiac tissues and their implication in the prevention and treatment of cardiovascular disease.

Keywords: n-3 PUFAs; oxidative stress; endogenous antioxidants; anti-inflammatory response; cardiovascular diseases

1. Introduction

Nutraceutical supplementation is considered a viable approach for prophylaxis and treatment of heart diseases [1–4]. In particular, the efficacy of polyunsaturated fatty acids (PUFAs) in the treatment of various pathologies and, especially, of cardiovascular diseases is known since long time and a large body of clinical data on their protective effect has been collected over the last decades [5–8], though several pathophysiological implications on their use still remain unclear [9].

Humans and other mammals are not able to synthesize [10]. Therefore, linoleic acid (LA, 18:2, omega-6) and α-linolenic acid (ALA, 18:3, omega-3), denoted as essential fatty acids, must be included in the diet. Docosahexaenoic acid (DHA, 22:6 n-3) and eicosapentaenoic acid (EPA, 20:5 n-3) are members of n-3 PUFAs subfamily of PUFAs being obtained from the precursor ALA or dietary fish oils; ALA, in turn, can also be found in nuts and leafy vegetables. For the prevention of cardiovascular disease (CVD), a higher consumption of n-3 PUFAs is recommended. Indeed, many studies have shown that an increase in consumption of n-3 PUFAs leads to a decrease in cases of cardiovascular disease. In particular, it has been reported that eating fatty fish a few times a week halves coronary heart disease (CHD) deaths and reduces the probability of death from a heart attack by one third [11–14]. The beneficial effects of n-3 PUFAs are due to a set of various mechanisms of action. Indeed, they have an antiarrhythmic and antithrombotic action, reduce plasma triglyceride levels and resolve inflammatory states, regulate the expression of several genes and transcription factors, and act on membrane fluidity [15,16]. In many pathologies, free radicals (such as peroxynitrite) increase proinflammatory cytokines synthesis, regulate the cyclooxygenase (COX) pathway, and promote proinflammatory prostaglandin E2 (PGE_2) synthesis [17]. In the treatment of these diseases, n-3 PUFAs fatty acids (ω-3) have the same effects as many antioxidants, in fact, they protect endothelial cells and cardiomyocytes from damage and cell death [18]. In addition to the collected evidence, demonstrating the beneficial responses of dietary n-3 PUFAs supplementation on the cardiovascular system, some concerns have been expressed about their potential detrimental effects in different tissues due to their potential pro-oxidant effect [19]. In particular, oxidative stress and n-3 PUFAs are strongly correlated. Long- or very long-chain fatty acids have many "fragile" double bonds between carbon atoms. Therefore, the n-3 PUFAs undergo lipid peroxidation during oxidative stress, generating highly cytotoxic reactive products [20]. This is particularly dangerous in the central nervous system (CNS) [21]. In particular, it is not clear whether or not exogenously given PUFAs have a safety profile which would allow for their extensive use in the general population. Based on these concerns, the European Food Safety Authority (EFSA) expressed its opinion and claimed that, for any population group, there is not enough data to establish a tolerable upper intake level for n-3 LC PUFA (DHA, EPA and Docosapentaenoic acid (DPA), individually or combined). Indeed, for the adult population, the supplemental intakes of EPA and DHA combined at doses up to 5 g/day, and additional intakes of EPA alone up to 1.8 g/day, do not raise safety concerns. Furthermore, for the general population, the supplemental intakes of DHA alone up to 1 g/day do not raise safety concerns [22].

In this review, we summarize some of the recent advances regarding the potential antioxidant effects of n-3 PUFAs supplementation on the cardiovascular system along with their anti-inflammatory and cardioprotective effect in vitro and in vivo.

2. Antioxidant and Antinflammatory Properties of n-3 PUFAs

2.1. Mitochondrial Oxidative Stress and n-3 PUFAs

Molecular and cellular research shows that n-3 PUFAs have cardioprotective effects [23]. A diet rich in n-3 PUFAs has a beneficial effect on blood pressure, heart rate, left ventricular diastolic filling, and endothelial functions [24]. Therefore, n-3 PUFAs have a beneficial effect on cardiac hemodynamic factors [25]. In particular, PUFAs act as antioxidants when they are inserted into the cell membranes and regulate the antioxidant signalling pathways. Mitochondrial membranes of eukaryotic cells have a high DHA content indicating that DHA is a fundamental phospholipid for adenosine triphosphate (ATP) synthesis by oxidative phosphorylation. In mitochondria, DHA acts on many pathways; reducing oxidative stress and cytochrome c oxidase (complex IV) activity as well as increasing manganese-dependent superoxide dismutase (Mn-SOD) activity. Rats fed a high fish oil diet demonstrate a higher expression and activity of the antioxidant enzyme superoxide dismutase (SOD) and an inhibition of membrane peroxidation process as expressed by the reduced content of thio-barbituric acid (TBARS) products. The action of oxidized n-3 PUFAs is directed against Kelch-like ECH-associated protein 1 (Keap1), the negative regulator of the nuclear factor erythroid 2–related factor 2 (Nrf2). Dissociation of Keap1 from Cullin3 induces Nrf2-dependent antioxidant gene expression [26]. Additional antioxidant action of n-3 PUFAs reduces myocytes sensitivity to reactive oxygen species (ROS)-induced ischemia reperfusion (I/R) injury and increases SOD and glutathione peroxidase (GSH-Px) levels. Hypoxia condition decreases oxidative markers and increases antioxidant enzymes expression, whereas oxidized n-3 PUFAs act on sirtuin1 (SIRT1) and forkhead box (FOXO) protein, thereby increasing SOD levels. Furthermore, in human and rat studies, EPA and DHA determined F2-isoprostane reduction, an oxidative stress marker in urine [27,28].

Thus, n-3 PUFAs supplementation leads to substantial antioxidant response, an effect that occurs mainly via restoring imbalanced endogenous antioxidant moieties.

2.2. Nitric Oxide, Endothelial Dysfunction and n-3 PUFAs

An effect of n-3 PUFA fatty acids, which correlates with their antioxidant properties, is represented by counteraction of endothelial dysfunction, an effect which reduces arterial stiffness [29,30]. Endothelial dysfunction is determined by a reduction in endothelium-dependent vasodilation due to impaired nitric oxide (NO) bioavailability [31,32]. In fact, NO is the most important molecule for vasodilation, derived from the endothelium. In addition, NO has an anti-atherosclerotic action, reducing smooth muscle cell proliferation, platelet aggregation, and leukocyte adhesion [33]. It is known that an increase in oxidative stress induces endothelial dysfunction since ROS reduce NO bioavailability and increase synthesis of the most toxic species, i.e., peroxynitrite [34]. Changes in NO bioavailability cause procoagulable and prothrombotic conditions and vascular inflammation [35]. Important receptor-mediated cell signal transduction pathways, including the NO-cGMP pathway, are present in caveolae and lipid rafts of endothelial cell membranes [36]. n-3 PUFAs may regulate the caveolae composition resulting in increased NO production [37]. In particular, n-3 PUFA fatty acids stimulate endothelial nitric oxide synthase (eNOS) activity and expression [38]. Moreover, EPA determines a higher NO synthesis by increasing AMP-activated protein kinase (AMPK)-induced eNOS activation and eNOS dissociation from inhibitory scaffolding protein caveolin [39] (Figure 1). eNOS activity is also stimulated by DHA which favours the binding between eNOS and heat shock protein 90 (HSP-90), with activation of the PKB/AKt pathway. Thus, eNOS is phosphorylated and activated [18,40,41] and this represents the most relevant consequence of antioxidant-response elicited by supplementation with n-3 PUFAs.

2.3. Cell Membranes and Anti-Inflammatory Effects of n-3 PUFAs

Modulation of the cell membrane properties represents a supplemental molecular mechanism by which n-3 PUFAs lead to cardio-protective and vaso-protective response. In fact, linoleic acid and α-linolenic acid are fundamental constituents of cell membranes and are able to determine an impaired fluidity of membrane. Therefore, they determine and affect the behaviour of membrane-bound enzymes and receptors [42–44]. In particular, evidence has been collected showing that n-3 PUFAs inhibit both the interleukin (IL)-1, 2, 6 synthesis and the protein kinase C signalling pathway [45]. This correlates with studies showing that n-3 PUFAs interfere in various ways in inflammatory processes, inhibiting IkB phosphorylation and therefore the NF-kB signaling pathway, or through PPARα/γ, or through a ligand for GPR120, which reduces both TLR-4 and tumour necrosis factor alpha (TNF-α) signalling pathway [42,43]. Moreover, n-3 PUFAs regulate leukotrienes, prostaglandins and thromboxanes synthesis, through activation of cytosolic phospholipase A_2 ($cPLA_2$), cyclooxygenase 2, and production of PGE_2, as a $cPLA_2$ inhibitor, modify the metabolic pathway of arachidonic acid [17,18,46,47].

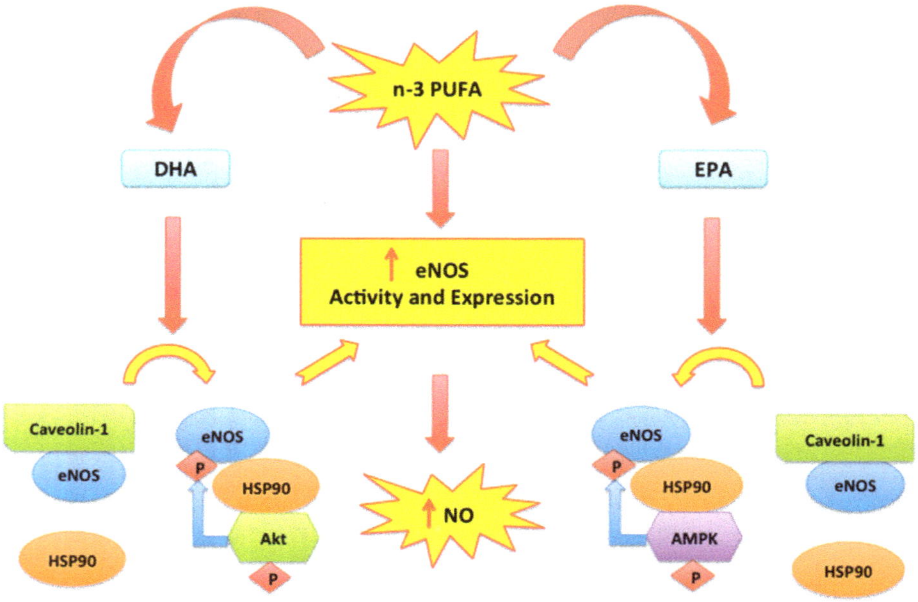

Figure 1. n-3 PUFA mediated eNOS modulation. n-3 PUFA (EPA and DHA) determine a higher NO synthesis by increasing eNOS activity and expression. The unbinding of eNOS/caveolin-1 complex and the recruitment of HSP-90 allow eNOS phosphorylation and activation mediated by Akt and AMPK [18,40,41].

2.4. N-3 PUFA-Derived Mediators

Maresins, protectins, and resolvins are called specialized pro-resolving mediators (SPMs). They derive from ω-3 and have anti-inflammatory properties [48].

It is known that atherosclerosis is an unresolved inflammatory pathology in which vascular wall damage occurs. This damage is likely to be caused by reduced synthesis of SPMs, therefore it is probable that an increase in SPMs could reduce the local inflammatory response and resolve the damage caused by atherosclerosis [49]. Numerous in vivo studies attest to the cardioprotective role of specialized pro-resolving mediators. Resolvin E series, such as RvE1, are synthesized from eicosapentaenoic acid and resolve acute inflammation states as they switch off leukocyte trafficking, favour the clearance of inflammatory cells and debris as well as inhibit cytokine synthesis [50–53]. In rats treated with RvE1, after I/R, myocardial infarct size was reduced by 70% compared to control group, when administered before reperfusion. In particular, the results demonstrate that RvE1 reduces heart damage by direct action on cardiomyocytes [54].

On the contrary, biosynthesis of D-series resolvin, maresins, and protectins starts with DHA. For example, PD1 protects against brain ischemia and renal I/R injury while Resolvin D1 (RvD1) is effective against I/R and atherosclerosis [55,56].

Even after an infarct, RvD1 administration resolves the acute inflammation as it stimulates the specialized pro-resolving mediator synthesis in the spleen and favours their transfer to the anti-inflammatory M2 macrophages in the left ventricle, preventing the onset of cardiac fibrosis and ensuring the normal heart function. Epoxides, such as epoxyeicosatetraenoic acids (EpETEs) and epoxydocosapentaenoic acids (EpDPAs), are obtained from EPA and DHA with reactions catalyzed by CYP450 monooxygenase and are termed lipid mediators. They perform an anti-inflammatory action in cardiovascular disease, dilate the pulmonary arteries, activate the smooth muscle of the coronary arteries, and provide an anti-arrhythmic action. For these reasons, studies have to be carried out regarding the inhibition of epoxide hydrolysis in order to render them stable and thus increasing their functionality in cardiovascular disease therapy [42,57,58] (Figure 2).

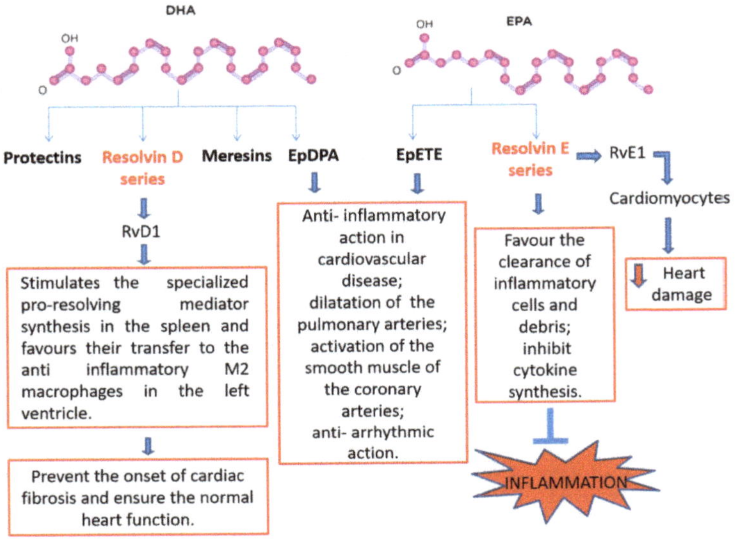

Figure 2. Beneficial effects and potential mechanisms of n-3 PUFA-derived mediators.

3. Vaso-Protective Activities of n-3 PUFAs

Arterial wall stiffness and endothelial dysfunction indicate a high probability that more or less fatal cardiovascular disease may arise. Overt atherosclerosis is caused by the concomitance of numerous alterations concerning the vessel wall anatomy, vascular endothelium, endothelial-derived factors, and circulating cytokines [35]. It has been shown that n-3 PUFAs have positive effects on numerous molecular and physiological pathways characteristic of the disease as they regulate arterial stiffness and endothelial dysfunction and therefore prevent atherosclerosis and cardiovascular diseases [59,60]. In vivo studies on mice have shown that n-3 PUFAs fatty acids inhibit atherogenesis as they reduce the lipid deposition in the arterial layers, thus inhibiting the Low Density Lipoproteins (LDL) uptake, favouring their removal from the aortic media and inhibiting the lipoprotein lipases synthesis [61].

A diet rich in ω-3 decreases the macrophages and pro-inflammatory markers favouring anti-atherogenic activity [62].

Furthermore, studies conducted in cell lines treated with EPA and DHA have shown a reduction in the proliferation of vascular smooth muscle cells when ω-3 are inserted into membrane phospholipids thereby slowing the progression of cell cycle [63,64]. Similar results were obtained by observing the coronary arteries of subjects who had taken fish oil supplementation. The n-3 PUFAs fatty acids act favourably on plaque stability and prevent breakage thus reducing the onset of thrombotic phenomena [64].

Arterial wall stiffness is determined by active and passive mechanisms of the arterial hemodynamics. Endothelium cells are controlled by molecular and cellular mechanisms which influence the elasticity and mechanical characteristics of the vessels [65].

EPA and DHA act on these mechanisms. A further beneficial effect of n-3 PUFAs intake on wall stiffness is blood pressure reduction. In vivo and clinical studies have documented that a high heart rate, directly related to the progression of arterial stiffness, increases the risk of cardiovascular events. In fact, intake of n-3 PUFAs decreases heart rate and promotes recovery after physical activity. It is also thought that the heart rate reduction is determined by direct effects on cardiac electrophysiology [64]. It is possible that EPA and DHA both modulate the balance between the parasympathetic and sympathetic systems as well as the aortic stiffness and muscle sympathetic nerve activity, thus favouring the neurogenic autonomic function of cardiovascular system [40,66,67].

3.1. N-3 PUFAs and Atherosclerosis

In vivo studies show that n-3 PUFAs have the capacity to reverse atherosclerosis, therefore a diet richer in ω-3 protects against coronary artery disease (CAD). It is known that EPA and DHA accumulate in adipose tissue. Thus, in this tissue, they could act on the altered endocrine function, reduce low-grade inflammation caused by obesity, and regulate adipokine gene expression [68]. In patients with stable coronary artery disease, n-3 PUFAs may be added to pharmacological and interventional therapy as they improve adipokine plasma levels. In particular, the plasma levels of adiponectin are enhanced while those of leptin are reduced after 1-month of ω-3 administration. This is especially important in patients with coronary artery disease and many risk factors, because the statins used in pharmacological treatment could influence adipokines plasma levels [22].

It was suggested that in white adipose tissue (WAT) n-3 PUFAs modulates the release of adipokine and cytokines. As key mediators n-3 PUFAs effect on adipose tissue was proposed the protein GPR120 and the receptor PPAR-Y [69]. It was proposed that this process involve the suppression of IKK complex activation and JNK phosphorylation, and the reduction of TNF-α secretion, or the formation of a complex between GPR120 and β-arrestin2 down-regulating inflammatory pathway. Further n-3 PUFAs reduce the levels of macrophage, IL-6, TNF-a, MCP-1, and inducible nitric oxide synthase (iNOS) in WAT. Meanwhile, n-3 PUFA PPAR-Y-binding promotes the production of anti-inflammatory and insulin-sensitizing adipocytokines [69].

About anti-atherosclerotic effect, n-3 PUFAs and its metabolites, SPMs, could be helpful in counteract atherosclerosis related inflammation [70]. It was proposed that this protective effect occurs through an increase of n-3 PUFAs metabolites (18-monohydroxy EPA, RvE1, RvD1) and a reduction of eicosanoids, such as thromboxane A2 or leukotriene B4, which are pro-inflammatory mediators. Both of these actions determines a reduction in adenosine diphosphate induction of platelet aggregation, coagulation and thrombosis, and a decrease of pro-inflammatory cytokines interleukin-6 (IL-6). Overall, these effects lead to higher plaque stability increasing thicker fibrous cap, reducing oxidized LDL uptake, migration of vascular smooth muscle cells, lesional oxidative stress and necrosis, reducing atherosclerotic lesions progression and vascular inflammation [71].

The actions on atherosclerotic plaque was observed in an animal model of hyperlipidemia where pre-treatment with EPA reduced lipid deposition, macrophage adhesion, VCAM-1, ICAM-1 and MCP-1 on endothelial cells and increase content of collagen and smooth muscle cells in atherosclerotic lesions [72].

Further, in a model of diet induced atherosclerosis, in ApoE * 3Leiden transgenic mouse, the endogenous oxidation product of the n-3 PUFA, eicosapentaenoic acid (EPA), RvE1, was administered alone or in combination with atorvastatin for 16 weeks, showing a reduction of atherosclerotic lesions in both type of treatment, more pronounced in co-treatment. Even the pathway of Interferon gamma and TNF-α were downregulated, suggesting an anti-inflammatory action of RvE1 in atherogenesis [73].

The beneficial effect of n-3 PUFAs on atherosclerotic lesions was also due to the modulation of cellular oxidative stress and of total antioxidant status, as have been demonstrated in apolipoprotein E knockout mice. ApoE (−/−) mice fed a diet rich in fish oil for 10 weeks showed an increase of antioxidant enzymes activities such as SOD and catalase (CAT) activities [74]. Fish oil rich diet in ApoE (−/−) mice also increased NO production and eNOS expression and lowered iNOS and reduce lipid peroxidation [75].

Also on vascular endothelial cells n-3 PUFA reduced oxidative stress- induced DNA damage. Under H_2O_2 stimulation in aortic endothelial cells, EPA and DHA reduced γ-H2AX foci formation and the activation of kinase ATM, suggesting a reduction of DNA damage response. Further, EPA and DHA also decrease intracellular reactive oxygen species and increase antioxidant defence (heme oxygenase-1, thioredoxin reductase 1, ferritin light chain, ferritin heavy chain and manganese superoxide dismutase) mediating upregulation of NRF2 result in cardiovascular protection [76].

Moreover, in a clinical retrospective analysis of 121 patients conducted in Japan, it was reported that the use of EPA in patients with CAD undergoing percutaneous coronary intervention decreased mean lipid index, macrophage grade and plaque instability [77].

3.2. The Effect of n-3 PUFAs in Platelet Function

It is known that n-3 PUFAs can inhibit normal platelet function, thus indicating platelet involvement in EPA and DHA mediated cardioprotection. In fact, numerous studies indicate that platelets treated with EPA and DHA show a reduction in the rate of thrombin formation and the exposure of platelet phosphatidylserine. This treatment reduces thrombus formation and modifies the processing of thrombin precursor proteins [78]. An additional result indicates that when whole blood is treated with ω-3, there is more occlusion time and less fibrin accumulation under flow conditions. Moreover, in vitro studies show that n-3 PUFAs reduce, without eliminating, the procoagulant ability of platelets; this represents one of the cardioprotective mechanisms of ω-3 in subjects with a diet rich in EPA and DHA [79,80].

Along with anti-coagulant action, PUFAs exert anti-platelet effect. Indeed, PUFAs are important constituent of platelet membrane. Free PUFAs were produced by cytoplasmic phospholipase A2 action and they are oxygenated by cyclooxygenase, lipoxygenase and CYP450 into oxylipins. These oxylipins are lipid mediators that regulate platelet function and thrombosus formation. It was proposed that n-3 PUFAs reduced platelet aggregation and thromboxane release through regulation of COX-1 and 12-LOX. In particular, EPA compete with arachidonic acid for platelet COX-1 inhibiting this pathway, reducing thromboxane A2 and increasing the release of other thromboxane, such as TXA3, and suppressing thromboxane receptor. Meanwhile, EPA can increase prostaglandins and NO synthesis in endothelial cells [81,82].

Moreover, it was found that higher levels of platelet phospholipis n-3 PUFA were related to reduced mortality for CVD [83], and that n-3 PUFA supplements is helpful in reduction of platelet aggregation with reduction in ADP-induced platelet aggregation in patients with cardiovascular diseases even if this effect was not proven in healthy patients [84].

It was proposed that anti-platelet effect of n-3 PUFA could depend on gender. EPA seems to have more effectiveness in male while DHA in female as observed by an inverse correlation between testosterone levels and platelet aggregation after EPA administration and the observation of the higher levels of serum DHA in women independently from diet presence of DHA [85].

3.3. N-3 PUFAs Index and Coronary Artery Disease (CAD)

The N-3 PUFAs index represents the EPA + DHA percentage contained in the erythrocyte membranes [86]. It has been shown that the fatty acid content in the red blood cell membrane is related to their content in the myocardium. Furthermore, the fatty acids composition of red blood cells is more stable than that of plasma. For this reason, the fatty acid content in the heart can be estimated by measuring the fatty acid content in the erythrocyte membrane. Since it is known that variations in fatty acid content can influence cardiovascular events, it is essential to measure their contents in the erythrocytes membrane in addition to measuring the n-3 PUFAs index. These parameters vary with the diet, therefore they are measured in clinical studies to verify n-3 PUFAs effects as it is known that a higher consumption of n-3 PUFAs causes changes in fatty acids composition in red blood cell membranes, with an increase of the ω-3 index and the lowering of oleic acid. This is very important because this condition reduces the risk of Coronary Artery Disease in the general population [87].

The ratio of serum EPA/arachidonic acid (AA) was considered as a marker of the potential risk of CAD [88]. In a retrospective clinical trials (TREAT-CAD study) of 149 CAD patients who had taken EPA as dietary supplement or not and CAD patients with an EPA/AA ratio > 0.4 taken as cut off,

EPA reduced the cumulative incidence of cardiovascular death and improve the long-term prognosis in CAD patients with an EPA/AA ratio ≤ 0.4 [89].

Analysis of serum n-3 PUFAs levels in Chinese in-patients ($n = 460$) with multiple cardiovascular risk factors or an established diagnosis of CAD, concluded that these levels were lower in patients with CAD than those with cardiovascular risk factors and that high serum n-3 PUFAs concentration is associated with decreased CAD proportion at a relatively younger age [90].

When taken with an anti-atherosclerotic drug, such as statin, EPA modulate high-density lipoprotein particle size (HDL) in stable CAD patients. In particular, EPA reduced serum levels of HDL3, with an increase of the EPA/AA ratio and of the HDL2/HDL3 ratio. It meant that EPA promoted the conversion of HDL3, with low levels of lipid content, in to large HDL particles that contain more lipid, suggesting a beneficial therapeutic effect of EPA supplementation in statin therapy in counteract coronary artery disease [88].

4. The Cardio-Protective Response of n-3 PUFAs Supplementation

As previously described, the n-3 PUFAs have a beneficial role in cardiovascular health; they reduce triglyceride levels enhance high-density lipoprotein levels, and reduce platelet aggregation by preventing coronary arteries occlusion [59,60]. Moreover, they promote a normal heart rhythm, increase arterial compliance, reduce atherosclerosis, and have an anti-inflammatory action [12]. In the Gruppo Italiano per lo Studio della Sopravvivenza nell'Infarto Miocardico (GISSI) trial, the group supplemented with n-3 PUFAs showed a significant reduction in cardiovascular, coronary and sudden cardiac death. The American Heart Association (AHA) recommends the dose of >1 g/day of EPA + DHA dosage defined in the GISSI-Prevenzione study to patients suffering from CAD. This dose lowers triglyceride levels, preserves cardiac function, and decreases the risk of coronary heart disease. In fact, numerous clinical studies report the anti-hypertensive and anti-hyperlipidemic action of n-3 PUFAs [91–95].

They reduce hyperlipidemia because they control gene expression, simultaneously inhibiting lipogenesis and activating lipolysis, and increasing fatty acid β-oxidation. n-3 PUFA therapy has shown promising results in primary and in secondary prevention of cardiovascular diseases [11,42,57,87].

4.1. The Effects of n-3 PUFAs in Myocardial Ischemia and Reperfusion

Many studies show that the heart undergoes oxidative stress following myocardial I/R [96,97]. This condition increases ROS synthesis, while at the same time decreasing antioxidant synthesis, thus generating the oxidation of biomolecules and consequent cellular damage [98]. Increased intake of EPA and DHA changes the fatty acid content of myocardial membrane phospholipids providing a higher percentage of DHA and an increase in peroxidisability index values. Nevertheless, there is a reduction in oxidative damage following I/R. In fact, in the I/R condition and greater DHA availability, documentation shows both an increase in myocardial peroxidation with greater basal fatty acid peroxidation and a greater chronic activity of endogenous antioxidant enzyme Mn-SOD together with a decrease in lipid oxidation due to I/R and consequent reduction of heart attack cases. Therefore, during ischemic preconditioning (IPC), ROS have a dual function; generating cellular damage and activating protective signalling processes at the same time. In this context, EPA and DHA intake is linked to both reduction in the ROS levels through lipid peroxidation and increased endogenous antioxidants availability. ROS and endogenous antioxidants are considered, respectively, triggers and mediators of delayed phase ischemic preconditioning. Therefore, the addition of fish oil in the diet is fundamental for the role of n-3 PUFAs in the form of the delayed phase IPC and also because a constant intake of n-3 PUFAs inserted into the membrane phospholipids guarantees constant resistance to damage caused by I/R. For this reason, ischemic protection by n-3 PUFAs is called "nutritional preconditioning" [44,99]. In the heart, n-3 PUFAs act mainly at the mitochondrial level, in fact, they increase the expression of the mitochondrial antioxidant enzyme Mn-SOD; leaving the expression of the other antioxidants such as copper zinc superoxide dismutase (CuZnSOD) and GSx unchanged. Experiments conducted in vivo on mice show that increased Mn-SOD activity resulted in sustained cardioprotection due to heat stress and in the delayed window of ischemic preconditioning. Instead, in the heart, increased expression of Mn-SOD reduces frequency, improves efficiency of oxygen consumption, and ameliorates contractile function. These properties are common to fish oil when taken as a dietary source. In addition, research conducted in rats shows that some fish oil properties, such as lower oxygen consumption in the heart, less sensitivity to I/R damage, and arrhythmias, are due to changes in mitochondrial Ca^{2+}. In order for the n-3 PUFAs to carry out their cardioprotective action, they must enter and remain in the myocardium constantly for at least seven days, while their action can last for months, thanks to their lasting insertion in the membrane [28,44].

It has been shown, therefore, that the presence of fish oil in the diet increases the percentage of n-3 PUFAs content in the myocardium membrane, thus increasing the basal peroxidation of cellular fatty acids and consequently increasing Mn-SOD activity. In hearts subjected to acute regional I/R, there is a reduction in stimulated lipid oxidation and myocardial damage. The constant physiological stress generated by this intake, called "oxidative shielding", if also generated by minimum and regular fish oil doses, could confirm its cardioprotective effect [44]. Beneficial effects result in a reduction in myocardial oxygen consumption and heart rate, with an increase in coronary reserve. Consequently, n-3 PUFAs generates protective preconditioning effects on the damage caused by I/R; thereby improving post-ischemic recovery [28]. In addition to EPA and DHA, alpha linolenic acid (ALA), present in plant foods, can also have cardioprotective effects, particularly during an ischemic attack. This statement derives from data obtained in experiments conducted on cardiomyocytes isolated from adult rats. Cultured cardiomyocytes were pre-treated with ALA for 24 h and subsequently subjected to three different conditions; a group of control cells exposed to non-ischemic conditions, a group exposed to simulated ischemia (ISCH) and another to simulated I/R. It has been shown that in pretreated cardiomyocytes, ALA is incorporated into phosphatidylcholine, thus generating a protective effect on cardiomyocytes subjected to ischemia or I/R. It is likely that ALA has this effect by inhibiting DNA fragmentation during the apoptotic process. Furthermore, ALA inhibits the synthesis of two pro-apoptotic oxidized phosphatidylcholine (OxPC) species that increase significantly during ischemia and I/R, thus resulting in the impairment of apoptosis [7].

4.2. The Potential for n-3 PUFAs Supplementation in Heart Failure

In recent years, numerous studies have been conducted concerning the heterogeneous and complex syndrome known as heart failure (HF). In particular, heart failure with reduced ejection fraction (EF) and heart failure with preserved ejection fraction (HFpEF) were defined [100–103]. The majority of the population is affected by heart failure with preserved ejection fraction, prevalent in the ageing population. Moreover, the common therapies for heart failure are ineffective in cases of heart failure with preserved ejection fraction. Numerous clinical studies document the lower rates of mortality and hospitalization for CHD associated with higher blood levels of n-3 PUFAs fatty acids. Many meta-analyses confirm these data indicating that the risk of CHD and consequently that of sudden death are reduced in the presence of n-3 PUFAs [87,104]. In literature, few studies are reported regarding the effect of n-3 PUFAs on heart failure in vivo and in vitro. Furthermore, no animal model is able to reproduce the phenotypic change and the complex pathophysiology of heart failure with preserved ejection fraction. Therefore, a surgical model of after load induced heart failure, defined as transverse aortic constriction (TAC), has been recreated, which causes some effects of remodelling heart failure with preserved ejection fraction such as: hypertrophy, interstitial cardiac fibrosis, and diastolic dysfunction. In this TAC model, it has been proved that a diet rich in n-3 PUFAs prevents the interstitial fibrosis onset and diastolic heart dysfunction. Furthermore, a direct effect of n-3 PUFAs on cardiac fibroblasts has been reported which prevents the onset of fibrosis. Such evidence suggests that a diet rich in n-3 PUFAs may represent a new therapy for heart failure with preserved ejection fraction [105] Important data indicate that EPA prevents fibrosis by a particular mechanism of action, in fact, it does not accumulate in cardiac myocytes or in fibroblasts. Furthermore, the FFA receptor 4 (FFAR4), a G protein-coupled receptor (GPR) for long chain fatty acids such as EPA and DHA, has proven effective in the prevention of fibrotic signalling in adult cardiac fibroblasts cultures. Studies to define the link between the FFA4 receptor and the n-3 PUFAs were conducted on FFAR4 knockout mice, indicating that in macrophages these fatty acids activate the receptor-mediated anti-inflammatory signalling. Recently, a meta-analysis reported that in the blood of patients treated with a fixed dose of EPA + DHA significantly different levels of these fatty acids were recorded and, moreover, higher values of these were correlated with a lower incidence of CHD risk [8,105,106]. DHA may have a particular cardioprotective role in heart failure conditions caused by pressure overload. These properties are linked to the ease with which DHA is inserted into cardiac fibroblasts and myocytes membranes, modifying their elasticity, fluidity, ion permeability, phase behaviour, fusion, and protein function. Furthermore, DHA inhibits the opening of the mitochondrial transition pores as reported in data obtained in the transverse aortic constriction surgical model. When DHA and EPA are present in the diet together, lower levels of EPA are needed to have the same decrease in fibrosis, indicating that DHA could potentiate the effect of EPA on fibrosis inhibition [105].

5. Adverse Effects of PUFAs in Cardiovascular Risk Factors

As mentioned above, n-3 PUFAs are a widely used dietary supplements. However, besides their antioxidant and anti-inflammatory properties, which ascribe to the cardiovascular and vasoprotective actions, n-3 PUFAs are also responsible of side effects [20]. These side effects could be related both to high intake of n-3 PUFAs or to oxidative reactions [63].

Oxidation of n-3 PUFAs could develop following bad storage condition and usage, temperature, light, bad processing conditions, fish cooking, refining process or presence of molecular oxygen responsible of cytotoxicity, genotoxic effects reducing nutritional values of n-3 PUFAs [19,20].

Indeed, n-3 PUFAs is prone to undergo oxidation leading to peroxyl radical formation initiating radical reactions with any hydrogen-donating substance [107].

The progression of lipid peroxidation determines the formation of secondary reactions products, overall leading to the formation of fatty acid peroxides, aldehydes, alcohols, isoprostanes and neuroprostanes [20,107].

It was observed that a dietary oxidized n-3 PUFAs, in particular intestinal absorption of an oxidized n-3 PUFAs end-product such as 4-hydroxy-2-hexenal (4-HHE), induce oxidative stress and inflammation [19]. Mice fed high fat diet, containing lipid mixture of oxidized n-3 PUFAs (EPA and DHA, both in form of triacylglycerols or phospholipids) for eight weeks, showed increased plasma levels of 4-HHE, IL-6 and MCP-1. Further, oxidized n-3 PUFAs, enhance inflammatory response through the activation of NF-kB pathway in small intestine tissue, and enhance levels of glutathione peroxidase and GRP78 as signals of redox stress and an effort to counteract inflammation and oxidative stress [19].

In a single blind clinical trial, 52 women take omega-3 fatty acid supplements in capsules, which were at different levels of oxidation, less oxidized oil pills, highly oxidized oil pills or no capsules, and a rich fish diet for all groups for 30 days. The analysis of total cholesterols, triglycerides and glucose at the beginning and the end of the trial, showed a reduction in triglyceride and cholesterol levels taking less oxidative omega-3 capsules rather than high oxidative omega-3 capsules, which revert the effect on lipid profile. Further, the diastolic and systolic pressure levels decrease in less oxidized n-3 capsules, while no differences were present in highly n-3 oxidized capsules, overall demonstrating the importance of oxidative levels of n-3 supplements [108].

Although beneficial anti-platelet effects [52,53], it was proposed that an high intake of fish oil could increase bleeding time [109–113] and that the consumption of 3-4 g/die of EPA and DHA (helpful in patients with hypertriglyceridemia), moderately increase bleeding times, suggesting that particular attention is needed in patients with anticoagulant drugs therapy [63,113–115]. On the other hand, several studies suggest n-3 PUFA are not bleeding risk factor [116,117].

Even if it was proposed that PUFAs affects glucose regulation in obese individuals, probably enhancing hepatic gluconeogenesis, mediating hepatic fatty acid oxidation [118], an increase in fasting glucose and HbA1c after intake of fish or fish oil, was observed in a few study [119].

Further, the high presence of methylmercury, dioxins and polychlorinated biphenyls as contaminants in fish, is debated. Indeed, the high presence of these food pollutants determines adverse effects on CAD [120,121], counteracting cardiovascular benefits of EPA and DHA in accordance on environmental levels. Diets, in which fish represent the major source of contaminants, as observed in several European countries, as well as in Canada and Israel, determined a reduction of the cardio-protective effects of n-3 PUFAs versus myocardial infarction due to the presence of methyl mercury [121,122] or polychlorinated biphenyls [123].

Finally, it was reported that, in patients with chronic heart failure of New York Heart Association class II–IV, the administration of 1 g n-3 PUFA (850–882 mg eicosapentaenoic acid and docosahexaenoic acid as ethyl esters in the average ratio of 1:1·2) determines gastrointestinal adverse effect of minor clinical relevance. However, the rate of patients that discontinued n-3 PUFA because of this side effect were the same in both placebo and n-3 PUFA group [124].

6. Conclusions

The use of supplementation with n-3 PUFA has demonstrated, in recent years, to produce both vaso- and cardio-protective responses, which have widely been demonstrated under both in vitro and in vivo settings. These data have been confirmed in patients suggesting their use, along with current therapy, in atherosclerosis prevention, vascular disease management and, finally for heart failure treatment. Many pathophysiological factors seem to contribute on their beneficial effect on vascular system. However, emerging evidence suggest that antioxidant and anti-inflammatory properties of n-3 PUFA seem to play a key role on their efficacy in patients undergoing cardiovascular pathologies (Figure 3). Further studies in larger cohort of patients are required to confirm their extensive use in general population for reducing the risk of severe cardiovascular diseases.

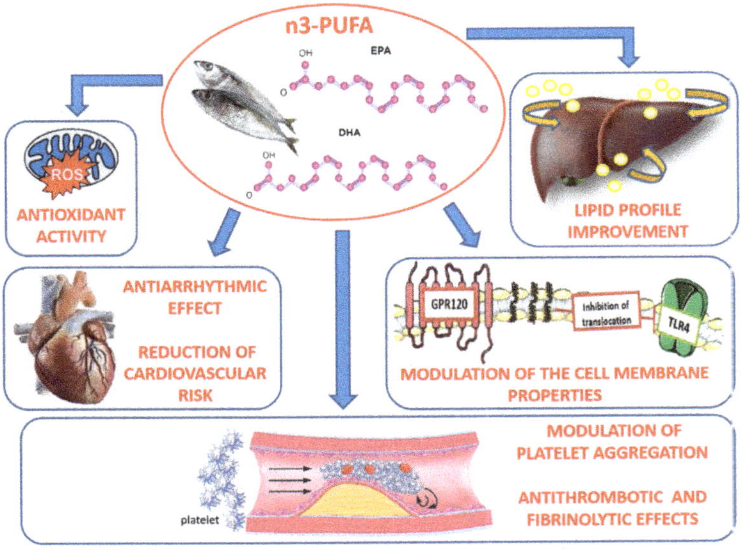

Figure 3. Summary of multifactorial activities of n-3 PUFAs to reduce cardiovascular risk. The n-3 PUFAs (EPA and DHA) improve lipid profile, systemic inflammation and platelet aggregation; furthermore, they have antiarrhythmic, antithrombotic, fibrinolytic effects and antioxidant activity, which concur to reduce heart disease risk.

Author Contributions: V.M. (Vincenzo Mollace) conceptualized and designed the review. F.O., V.M. (Vincenzo Mollace) wrote the manuscript. V.M. (Vincenzo Musolino), M.G., M.S. proofread the manuscript. R.M. (Roberta Macrì), C.C., J.M., F.B., S.N., M.C.Z., L.G., F.S., C.N., A.R.C., S.R., R.M. (Rocco Mollace), V.M. (Vincenzo Mollace), E.P. participated in drafting the article and revising it critically. The manuscript has been read and approved by all named authors. All authors have read and agreed to the published version of the manuscript.

Funding: This research was funded by Programma Operativo Nazionale, PON MIUR 03PE_00078_1 and 03PE_00078_2 (Nutramed).

Acknowledgments: We thank Yavette Shupe for language editing and proofreading.

Conflicts of Interest: The authors declare no conflict of interest.

References

1. Sosnowska, B.; Penson, P.; Banach, M. The Role of Nutraceuticals in the Prevention of Cardiovascular Disease. *Cardiovasc. Diagn. Ther.* **2017**, *7*, S21–S31. [CrossRef]
2. Rivellese, A.A.; Ciciola, P.; Costabile, G.; Vetrani, C.; Vitale, M. The Possible Role of Nutraceuticals in the Prevention of Cardiovascular Disease. *High Blood Press. Cardiovasc. Prev.* **2019**, *26*, 101–111. [CrossRef] [PubMed]
3. Carresi, C.; Musolino, V.; Gliozzi, M.; Maiuolo, J.; Mollace, R.; Nucera, S.; Maretta, A.; Sergi, D.; Muscoli, S.; Gratteri, S.; et al. Anti-oxidant effect of bergamot polyphenolic fraction counteracts doxorubicin-induced cardiomyopathy: Role of autophagy and c-kitposCD45negCD31neg cardiac stem cell activation. *J. Mol. Cell. Cardiol.* **2018**, *119*, 10–18. [CrossRef] [PubMed]
4. Mollace, V.; Ragusa, S.; Sacco, I.; Muscoli, C.; Sculco, F.; Visalli, V.; Palma, E.; Muscoli, S.; Mondello, L.; Dugo, P.; et al. The protective effect of bergamot oil extract on lecitine-like oxyLDL receptor-1 expression in balloon injury-related neointima formation. *J. Cardiovasc. Pharmacol. Ther.* **2008**, *13*, 120–129. [CrossRef]
5. Siscovick, D.S.; Barringer, T.A.; Fretts, A.M.; Wu, J.H.; Lichtenstein, A.H.; Costello, R.B.; Kris-Etherton, P.M.; Jacobson, T.A.; Engler, M.B.; Alger, H.M.; et al. N-3 PUFAs Polyunsaturated Fatty Acid (Fish Oil) Supplementation and the Prevention of Clinical Cardiovascular Disease: A Science Advisory From the American Heart Association. *Circulation* **2017**, *1*, e867–e884. [CrossRef]
6. Aung, T.; Halsey, J.; Kromhout, D.; Gerstein, H.C.; Marchioli, R.; Tavazzi, L.; Gelejinse, J.M.; Rauch, B.; Ness, A.; Galan, P.; et al. Associations of N-3 PUFAs Fatty Acid Supplement Use With Cardiovascular Disease Risks. *JAMA Cardiol.* **2018**, *1*, 225–234. [CrossRef] [PubMed]
7. Ganguly, R.; Hasanally, D.; Stamenkovic, A.; Maddaford, T.G.; Chaudhary, R.; Pierce, G.N.; Ravandi, A. Alpha linolenic acid decreases apoptosis and oxidized phospholipids in cardiomyocytes during ischemia/reperfusion. *Mol. Cell. Biochem.* **2017**. [CrossRef] [PubMed]
8. Oppedisano, F.; Maiuolo, J.; Gliozzi, M.; Musolino, V.; Carresi, C.; Nucera, S.; Scicchitano, M.; Scarano, F.; Bosco, F.; Macrì, R.; et al. The Potential for Natural Antioxidant Supplementation in the Early Stages of Neurodegenerative Disorders. *Int. J. Mol. Sci.* **2020**, *21*, 2618. [CrossRef] [PubMed]
9. Sokoła-Wysoczańska, E.; Wysoczański, T.; Wagner, J.; Czyż, K.; Bodkowski, R.; Lochyński, S.; Patkowska-Sokoła, B. Polyunsaturated Fatty Acids and Their Potential Therapeutic Role in Cardiovascular System Disorders—A Review. *Nutrients* **2018**, *10*, 1561. [CrossRef]
10. Lee, J.M.; Lee, H.; Kang, S.; Park, W.J. Fatty Acid Desaturases, Polyunsaturated Fatty Acid Regulation, and Biotechnological Advances. *Nutrients* **2016**, *8*, 23. [CrossRef]
11. Cao, Y.; Lu, L.; Liang, J.; Liu, M.; Li, X.; Sun, R.; Zheng, Y.; Zhang, P. N-3 PUFAs Fatty Acids and Primary and Secondary Prevention of Cardiovascular Disease. *Cell Biochem. Biophys.* **2015**, *72*, 77–81. [CrossRef] [PubMed]
12. Chaddha, A.; Eagle, K.A. Cardiology Patient Page. N-3 PUFAs Fatty Acids and Heart Health. *Circulation* **2015**, *132*, e350ULATIe352. [CrossRef] [PubMed]
13. Kris-Etherton, P.M.; Fleming, J.A. Emerging nutrition science on fatty acids and cardiovascular disease: Nutritionists' perspectives. *Adv. Nutr.* **2015**, *6*, 326S–337S. [CrossRef] [PubMed]
14. O'Connell, T.D.; Block, R.C.; Huang, S.P.; Shearer, G.C. ω3-Polyunsaturated fatty acids for heart failure: Effects of dose on efficacy and novel signaling through free fatty acid receptor 4. *J. Mol. Cell. Cardiol.* **2017**, *103*, 74–92. [CrossRef]

15. Adkins, Y.; Kelley, D.S. Mechanisms underlying the cardioprotective effects of n-3 PUFAs polyunsaturated fatty acids. *J. Nutr. Biochem.* **2010**, *21*, 781–792. [CrossRef]
16. Tortosa-Caparros, E.; Navas-Carrillo, D.; Marin, F.; Orenes-Pinero, E. Anti-inflammatory Effects of Omega 3 and Omega 6 Polyunsaturated Fatty Acids in Cardiovascular Disease and Metabolic Syndrome. *Crit. Rev. Food Sci. Nutr.* **2017**, *2*, 3421–3429. [CrossRef]
17. Mollace, V.; Muscoli, C.; Masini, E.; Cuzzocrea, S.; Salvemini, D. Modulation of prostaglandin synthesis by nitric oxide and nitric oxide donors. *Pharmacol. Rev.* **2005**, *57*, 217–252. [CrossRef]
18. Mollace, V.; Gliozzi, M.; Carresi, C.; Musolino, V.; Oppedisano, F. Re-assessing the mechanism of action of n-3 PUFAs. *Int. J. Cardiol.* **2013**, *170*, S8–S11. [CrossRef]
19. Awada, M.; Soulage, C.O.; Mevnier, A.; Debard, C.; Plaisancié, P.; Benoit, B.; Picard, G.; Loizon, E.; Estienne, M.; Peretti, N.; et al. Dietary oxidized *n*-3 PUFA induce oxidative stress and inflammation: Role of intestinal absorption of 4-HHE and reactivity in intestinal cells. *J. Lipid Res.* **2012**, *53*, 2069–2080. [CrossRef]
20. Wang, W.; Yang, H.; Johnson, D.; Gensler, C.; Decker, E.; Zhang, G. Chemistry and Biology of ω-3 PUFA Peroxidation-Derived Compounds. *Prostaglandins Other Lipid Mediat.* **2017**, *132*, 84–91. [CrossRef]
21. Yang, B.; Li, R.; Greenlief, C.M.; Fritsche, K.L.; Gu, Z.; Cui, J.; Lee, J.C.; Beversdorf, D.Q.; Sun, G.Y. Unveiling Anti-Oxidative and Anti-Inflammatory Effects of Docosahexaenoic Acid and Its Lipid Peroxidation Product on Lipopolysaccharide-Stimulated BV-2 Microglial Cells. *J. Neuroinflammation* **2018**, *9*, 202. [CrossRef] [PubMed]
22. Mostowik, M.; Gajos, G.; Zalewski, J.; Nessler, J.; Undas, A. N-3 PUFAs polyunsaturated fatty acids increase plasma adiponectin to leptin ratio in stable coronary artery disease. *Cardiovasc. Drugs Ther.* **2013**, *27*, 289–295. [CrossRef] [PubMed]
23. Roy, J.; Le Guennec, J.Y. Cardioprotective Effects of Omega 3 Fatty Acids: Origin of the Variability. *J. Muscle Res. Cell Motil.* **2017**, *38*, 25–30. [CrossRef] [PubMed]
24. Chrysohoou, C.; Metallinos, G.; Georgiopoulos, G.; Mendrinos, D.; Papanikolaou, A.; Magkas, N.; Pitsavos, C.; Vyssoulis, G.; Stefanadis, C.; Tousoulis, D. Short Term n-3 PUFAs Polyunsaturated Fatty Acid Supplementation Induces Favorable Changes in Right Ventricle Function and Diastolic Filling Pressure in Patients With Chronic Heart Failure; A Randomized Clinical Trial. *Vasc. Pharmacol.* **2016**, *79*, 43–50. [CrossRef] [PubMed]
25. Mozaffarian, D. Fish, n-3 Fatty Acids, and Cardiovascular Haemodynamics. *J. Cardiovasc. Med.* **2007**, *8*, S23–S26. [CrossRef]
26. Li, R.; Jia, Z.; Zhu, H. Regulation of Nrf2 Signaling. *React. Oxyg. Species (Apex)* **2019**, *8*, 312–322. [CrossRef]
27. Rodrigo, R.; Prieto, J.C.; Castillo, R. Cardioprotection against ischaemia/reperfusion by vitamins C and E plus n-3 fatty acids: Molecular mechanisms and potential clinical applications. *Clin. Sci.* **2013**, *124*, 1–15. [CrossRef]
28. Herrera, E.A.; Farías, J.G.; González-Candia, A.; Short, S.E.; Carrasco-Pozo, C.; Castillo, R.L. Ω3 Supplementation and intermittent hypobaric hypoxia induce cardioprotection enhancing antioxidant mechanisms in adult rats. *Mar. Drugs* **2015**, *13*, 838–860. [CrossRef]
29. Mozaffarian, D.; Wu, J.H.Y. N-3 PUFAs fatty acids and cardiovascular disease: Effects on risk factors, molecular pathways, and clinical events. *J. Am. Coll. Cardiol.* **2011**, *58*, 2047–2067. [CrossRef]
30. Cabo, J.; Alonso, R.; Mata, P. N-3 PUFAs fatty acids and blood pressure. *Br. J. Nutr.* **2012**, *107*, S195–S200. [CrossRef]
31. Gross, S.S.; Wolin, M.S. Nitric Oxide: Pathophysiological Mechanisms. *Annu. Rev. Physiother.* **1995**, *57*, 737–769. [CrossRef] [PubMed]
32. Moncada, S.; Higgs, E.A. Endogenous nitric oxide: Physiology, pathology and clinical relevance. *Eur. J. Clin. Investig.* **1991**, *21*, 361–374. [CrossRef] [PubMed]
33. Versari, D.; Daghini, E.; Virdis, A.; Ghiadoni, L.; Taddei, S. Endothelial Dysfunction as a Target for Prevention of Cardiovascular Disease. *Diabetes Care* **2009**, *32*, S314–S321. [CrossRef] [PubMed]
34. Münzel, T.; Camici, G.G.; Maack, C.; Bonetti, N.R.; Fuster, V.; Kovacic, J.C. Impact of Oxidative Stress on the Heart and Vasculature Part 2 of a 3-Part Series. *J. Am. Coll. Cardiol.* **2017**, *70*, 212–229. [CrossRef] [PubMed]
35. Gliozzi, M.; Scicchitano, M.; Bosco, F.; Musolino, V.; Carresi, C.; Scarano, F.; Maiuolo, J.; Nucera, S.; Maretta, A.; Paone, S.; et al. Modulation of Nitric Oxide Synthases by Oxidized LDLs: Role in Vascular Inflammation and Atherosclerosis Development. *Int. J. Mol. Sci.* **2019**, *4*, 3294. [CrossRef]

36. Maiuolo, J.; Gliozzi, M.; Musolino, V.; Carresi, C.; Nucera, S.; Macrì, R.; Scicchitano, M.; Bosco, F.; Scarano, F.; Ruga, S.; et al. The Role of Endothelial Dysfunction in Peripheral Blood Nerve Barrier: Molecular Mechanisms and Pathophysiological Implications. *Int. J. Mol. Sci.* **2019**, *20*, 3022. [CrossRef]
37. Li, Q.; Zhang, Q.; Wang, M.; Zhao, S.; Ma, J.; Luo, N.; Li, N.; Li, Y.; Xu, G.; Li, J. Eicosapentaenoic acid modifies lipid composition in caveolae and induces translocation of endothelial nitric oxide synthase. *Biochimie* **2007**, *89*, 169–177. [CrossRef]
38. Gousset-Dupont, A.; Robert, V.; Grynberg, A.; Lacour, B.; Tardivel, S. The effect of n-3 PUFA on eNOS activity and expression in Ea hy 926 cells. *Prostaglandins Leukot. Essent. Fat. Acids* **2007**, *76*, 131–139. [CrossRef]
39. Wu, Y.; Zhang, C.; Dong, Y.; Wang, S.; Song, P.; Viollet, B.; Zou, M.H. Activation of the AMP-Activated Protein Kinase by Eicosapentaenoic Acid (EPA, 20:5 n-3) Improves Endothelial Function In Vivo. *PLoS ONE* **2012**, *7*, e35508. [CrossRef]
40. Zanetti, M.; Grillo, A.; Losurdo, P.; Panizon, E.; Mearelli, F.; Cattin, L.; Barazzoni, R.; Carretta, R. N-3 PUFAs Polyunsaturated Fatty Acids: Structural and Functional Effects on the Vascular Wall. *BioMed Res. Int.* **2015**, *2015*, 791978. [CrossRef]
41. Lamoke, F.; Mazzone, V.; Persichini, T.; Maraschi, A.; Harris, M.B.; Venema, R.C.; Colasanti, M.; Gliozzi, M.; Muscoli, C.; Bartoli, M.; et al. Amyloid β peptide-induced inhibition of endothelial nitric oxide production involves oxidative stress-mediated constitutive eNOS/HSP90 interaction and disruption of agonist-mediated Akt activation. *J. Neuroinflammation.* **2015**, *3*, 12–84. [CrossRef]
42. Endo, J.; Arita, M. Cardioprotective mechanism of n-3 PUFAs polyunsaturated fatty acids. *J. Cardiol.* **2016**, *67*, 22–27. [CrossRef]
43. Alzoubi, M.R.; Aldomi Al-Domi, H. Could n-3 PUFAs fatty acids a therapeutic treatment of the immune-metabolic consequence of intermittent hypoxia in obstructive sleep apnea? *Diabetes Metab. Syndr.* **2017**, *11*. [CrossRef] [PubMed]
44. Abdukeyum, G.G.; Owen, A.J.; Larkin, T.A.; McLennan, P.L. Up-Regulation of Mitochondrial Antioxidant Superoxide Dismutase Underpins Persistent Cardiac Nutritional-Preconditioning by Long Chain n-3 Polyunsaturated Fatty Acids in the Rat. *J. Clin. Med.* **2016**, *5*, 32. [CrossRef] [PubMed]
45. Kim, W.; Khan, N.A.; McMurray, D.N.; Prior, I.A.; Wang, N.; Chapkin, R.S. Regulatory Activity of Polyunsaturated Fatty Acids in T-Cell Signaling. *Prog. Lipid Res.* **2010**, *49*, 250–261. [CrossRef] [PubMed]
46. Kakoti, B.B.; Hernandez-Ontiveros, D.G.; Kataki, M.S.; Shah, K.; Pathak, Y.; Panguluri, S.K. Resveratrol and N-3 PUFAs Fatty Acid: Its Implications in Cardiovascular Diseases. *Front. Cardiovasc. Med.* **2015**, *2*, 38. [CrossRef] [PubMed]
47. Jiang, J.; Li, K.; Wang, F.; Yang, B.; Fu, Y.; Zheng, J.; Li, D. Effect of Marine-Derived n-3 Polyunsaturated Fatty. *PLoS ONE* **2016**, *25*, e0147351. [CrossRef]
48. Recchiuti, A.; Serhan, C.N. Pro-Resolving Lipid Mediators (SPMs) and Their Actions in Regulating miRNA in Novel Resolution Circuits in Inflammation. *Front. Immunol.* **2012**, *22*, 298. [CrossRef] [PubMed]
49. Fredman, G.; Tabas, I. Boosting Inflammation Resolution in Atherosclerosis. *Am. J. Pathol.* **2017**, *187*, 1211–1221. [CrossRef]
50. Serhan, C.N. Pro-resolving lipid mediators are leads for resolution physiology. *Nature* **2014**, *510*, 92–101. [CrossRef] [PubMed]
51. Cash, J.L.; Norling, L.V.; Perretti, M. Resolution of inflammation: Targeting GPCRs that interact with lipids and peptides. *Drug Discov. Today* **2014**, *19*, 1186–1192. [CrossRef] [PubMed]
52. Spite, M.; Clària, J.; Serhan, C.N. Resolvins, specialized proresolving lipid mediators, and their potential roles in metabolic diseases. *Cell Metab.* **2014**, *19*, 21–36. [CrossRef] [PubMed]
53. Herrera, B.S.; Hasturk, H.; Kantarci, A.; Freire, M.O.; Nguyen, O.; Kansal, S.; Van Dyke, T.E. Impact of resolvin E1 on murine neutrophil phagocytosis in type 2 diabetes. *Infect. Immun.* **2015**, *83*, 792–801. [CrossRef] [PubMed]
54. Keyes, K.T.; Ye, Y.; Lin, Y.; Zhang, C.; Perez-Polo, J.R.; Gjorstrup, P.; Birnbaum, Y. Resolvin E1 protects the rat heart against reperfusion injury. *Am. J. Physiol. Heart Circ. Physiol.* **2010**, *299*, H153–H164. [CrossRef]
55. Kain, V.; Ingle, K.A.; Colas, R.A.; Dalli, J.; Prabhu, S.D.; Serhan, C.N.; Joshi, M.; Halade, G.V. Resolvin D1 activates the inflammation resolving response at splenic and ventricular site following myocardial infarction leading to improved ventricular function. *J. Mol. Cell. Cardiol.* **2015**, *84*, 24–35. [CrossRef]
56. Duffield, J.S.; Hong, S.; Vaidya, V.S.; Lu, Y.; Fredman, G.; Serhan, C.N.; Bonventre, J.V. Resolvin D series and protectin D1 mitigate acute kidney injury. *J. Immunol.* **2006**, *177*, 5902–5911. [CrossRef]

57. Fischer, R.; Konkel, A.; Mehling, H.; Blossey, K.; Gapelyuk, A.; Wessel, N.; von Schacky, C.; Dechend, R.; Muller, D.N.; Rothe, M.; et al. Dietary n-3 PUFAs fatty acids modulate the eicosanoid profile in man primarily via the CYP-epoxygenase pathway. *J. Lipid Res.* **2014**, *55*, 1150–1164. [CrossRef]
58. Gilbert, K.; Malick, M.; Madingou, N.; Touchette, C.; Bourque-Riel, V.; Tomaro, L.; Rousseau, G. Metabolites derived from n-3 PUFAs polyunsaturated fatty acids are important for cardioprotection. *Eur. J. Pharmacol.* **2015**, *769*, 147–153. [CrossRef]
59. Massaro, M.; Scoditti, E.; Carluccio, M.A.; De Caterina, R. Nutraceuticals and Prevention of Atherosclerosis: Focus on ω-3 Polyunsaturated Fatty Acids and Mediterranean Diet Polyphenols. *Cardiovasc. Ther.* **2010**, *28*, e13–e19. [CrossRef]
60. Gliozzi, M.; Maiuolo, J.; Oppedisano, F.; Mollace, V. The effect of bergamot polyphenolic fraction in patients with non alcoholic liver steato-hepatitis and metabolic syndrome. *PharmaNutrition* **2016**, *4S*, S27–S31. [CrossRef]
61. Chuchun, L.; Chang, T.S.; Matsuzaki, M.; Worgall, T.S.; Deckelbaum, R.J. n-3 Fatty Acids Reduce Arterial LDL-Cholesterol Delivery and Arterial Lipoprotein Lipase Levels and Lipase Distribution. *Arter. Thromb. Vasc. Biol.* **2009**, *29*, 555–561.
62. Chang, C.L.; Seo, T.; Du, C.B.; Accili, D.; Deckelbaum, R.J. n-3 Fatty acids decrease arterial low-density lipoprotein cholesterol delivery and lipoprotein lipase levels in insulin-resistant mice. *Arter. Thromb. Vasc. Biol.* **2010**, *30*, 2510–2517. [CrossRef]
63. Ander, B.P.; Dupasquier, C.M.; Prociuk, M.A.; Pierce, G.N. Polyunsaturated fatty acids and their effects on cardiovascular disease. *Exp. Clin. Cardiol.* **2003**, *8*, 164–172. [PubMed]
64. Colussi, G.; Catena, C.; Novello, M.; Bertin, N.; Sechi, L.A. Impact of omega-3 polyunsaturated fatty acids on vascular function and blood pressure: Relevance for cardiovascular outcomes. *Nutr. Metab. Cardiovas.* **2017**, *27*, 191–200. [CrossRef] [PubMed]
65. Lacolley, P.; Regnault, V.; Segers, P.; Laurent, S. Vascular Smooth Muscle Cells and Arterial Stiffening: Relevance in Development, Aging, and Disease. *Physiol. Rev.* **2017**, *97*, 1555–1617. [CrossRef] [PubMed]
66. Nelson, J.R.; Wani, O.; May, H.T.; Budoff, M. Potential benefits of eicosapentaenoic acid on atherosclerotic plaques. *Vascul. Pharmacol.* **2017**, *91*, 1–9. [CrossRef] [PubMed]
67. Limbu, R.; Cottrell, G.S.; McNeish, A.J. Characterisation of the vasodilation effects of DHA and EPA, n-3 PUFAs (fish oils), in rat aorta and mesenteric resistance arteries. *PLoS ONE* **2018**, *13*, e0192484. [CrossRef]
68. Liddle, D.M.; Hutchinson, A.L.; Wellings, H.R.; Power, K.A.; Robinson, L.E.; Monk, J.M. Integrated Immunomodulatory Mechanisms through which Long-Chain n-3 Polyunsaturated Fatty Acids Attenuate Obese Adipose Tissue Dysfunction. *Nutrients* **2017**, *9*, 1289. [CrossRef]
69. Brown, L.H.; Mutch, D.M. Mechanisms underlying N3-PUFA regulation of white adipose tissue endocrine function. *Curr. Opin. Pharmacol.* **2020**, *52*, 40–46. [CrossRef]
70. Bäck, M.; Hansson, G.K. Omega-3 fatty acids, cardiovascular risk, and the resolution of inflammation. *FASEB J.* **2019**, *33*, 1536–1539. [CrossRef]
71. Simonetto, M.; Infante, M.; Sacco, R.L.; Rundek, T.; Della-Morte, D. A Novel Anti-Inflammatory Role of Omega-3 PUFAs in Prevention and Treatment of Atherosclerosis and Vascular Cognitive Impairment and Dementia. *Nutrients* **2019**, *11*, 2279. [CrossRef]
72. Matsumoto, M.; Sata, M.; Fukuda, D.; Tanaka, K.; Soma, M.; Hirata, Y.; Nagai, R. Orally administered eicosapentaenoic acid reduces and stabilizes atherosclerotic lesions in ApoE-deficient mice. *Atherosclerosis* **2008**, *197*, 524–533. [CrossRef] [PubMed]
73. Salic, K.; Morrison, M.C.; Verschuren, L.; Wielinga, P.Y.; Wu, L.; Kleemann, R.; Gjorstrup, P.; Kooistra, T. Resolvin E1 attenuates atherosclerosis in absence of cholesterol-lowering effects and on top of atorvastatin. *Atherosclerosis* **2016**, *250*, 158–165. [CrossRef] [PubMed]
74. Wang, H.H.; Hung, T.M.; Wei, J.; Chiang, A. Fish oil increases antioxidant enzyme activities in macrophages and reduces atherosclerotic lesions in apoE-knockout mice. *Cardiovasc. Res.* **2004**, *61*, 169–176. [CrossRef]
75. Casós, K.; Zaragozá, M.C.; Zarkovic, N.; Zarkovic, K.; Andrisic, L.; Portero-Otín, M.; Cacabelos, D.; Mitjavila, M.T. A fish-oil-rich diet reduces vascular oxidative stress in apoE(-/-) mice. *Free Radic. Res.* **2010**, *44*, 821–829. [CrossRef] [PubMed]
76. Sakai, C.; Ishida, M.; Ohba, H.; Yamashita, H.; Uchida, H.; Yoshizumi, M.; Ishida, T. Fish oil omega-3 polyunsaturated fatty acids attenuate oxidative stress-induced DNA damage in vascular endothelial cells. *PLoS ONE* **2017**, *12*, e0187934. [CrossRef]

77. Konishi, T.; Sunaga, D.; Funayama, N.; Yamamoto, T.; Murakami, H.; Hotta, D.; Nojima, M.; Tanaka, S. Eicosapentaenoic acid therapy is associated with decreased coronary plaque instability assessed using optical frequency domain imaging. *Clin. Cardiol.* **2019**, *42*, 618–628. [CrossRef]
78. Larson, M.K.; Tormoen, G.W.; Weaver, L.J.; Luepke, K.J.; Patel, I.A.; Hjelmen, C.E.; Ensz, N.M.; McComas, L.S.; McCarty, O.J.T. Exogenous modification of platelet membranes with the omega-3 fatty acids EPA and DHA reduces platelet procoagulant activity and thrombus formation. *Am. J. Physiol. Cell Physiol.* **2013**, *304*, C273–C279. [CrossRef]
79. Larson, M.K.; Shearer, G.C.; Ashmore, J.H.; Anderson-Daniels, J.M.; Graslie, E.L.; Tholen, J.T.; Vogelaar, J.L.; Korth, A.J.; Nareddy, V.; Sprehe, M.; et al. Omega-3 fatty acids modulate collagen signaling in human platelets. *Prostaglandins Leukot Essent Fatty Acids.* **2011**, *84*, 93–98. [CrossRef]
80. Croset, M.; Lagarde, M. In vitro incorporation and metabolism of icosapentaenoic and docosahexaenoic acids in human platelets–effect on aggregation. *Thromb Haemost* **1986**, *56*, 57–62. [CrossRef]
81. Adili, R.; Hawley, M.; Holinstata, M. Regulation of platelet function and thrombosis by omega-3 and omega-6 polyunsaturated fatty acids. *Prostaglandins Other Lipid Mediat.* **2018**, *139*, 10–18. [CrossRef]
82. Sheikh, O.; Vande Hei, A.G.; Battisha, A.; Hammad, T.; Pham, S.; Chilton, R. Cardiovascular, electrophysiologic, and hematologic effects of omega-3 fatty acids beyond reducing hypertriglyceridemia: As it pertains to the recently published REDUCE-IT trial. *Cardiovasc. Diabetol.* **2019**, *18*, 84. [CrossRef]
83. Li, D.; Zhang, H.; Hsu-Hage, B.H.H.; Wahlqvist, M.L.; Sinclair, A.J. Original Communication The influence of fish, meat and polyunsaturated fat intakes on platelet phospholipid polyunsaturated fatty acids in male Melbourne Chinese and Caucasian. *Eur. J. Clin. Nutr.* **2001**, *55*, 1036–1042. [CrossRef] [PubMed]
84. Gao, L.; Cao, J.; Mao, Q.; Lu, X.; Zhou, X.; Fan, L. Influence of omega-3 polyunsaturated fatty acid-supplementation on platelet aggregation in humans: A meta-analysis of randomized controlled trials. *Atherosclerosis* **2013**, *226*, 328–334. [CrossRef] [PubMed]
85. Gasperi, V.; Catani, M.V.; Savini, I. Platelet Responses in Cardiovascular Disease: Sex-Related Differences in Nutritional and Pharmacological Interventions. *Cardiovasc. Ther.* **2020**, *2020*, 2342837. [CrossRef] [PubMed]
86. Von Schacky, C. N-3 PUFAs Index and Cardiovascular Health. *Nutrients* **2014**, *6*, 799–814. [CrossRef] [PubMed]
87. Lee, S.M.; An, W.S. Cardioprotective effects of ω-3 PUFAs in chronic kidney disease. *BioMed Res. Int.* **2013**, *2013*, 712949. [CrossRef]
88. Tani, S.; Matsuo, R.; Yagi, T.; Matsumoto, N. Administration of eicosapentaenoic acid may alter high-density lipoprotein heterogeneity in statin-treated patients with stable coronary artery disease: A 6-month randomized trial. *J. Cardiol.* **2020**, *75*, 282–288. [CrossRef]
89. Abe, S.; Sugimura, H.; Watanabe, S.; Murakami, Y.; Ebisawa, K.; Ioka, T.; Takahashi, T.; Ando, T.; Kono, K.; Inoue, T. Eicosapantaenoic acid treatment based on the EPA/AA ratio in patients with coronary artery disease: Follow-up data from the Tochigi Ryomo EPA/AA Trial in Coronary Artery Disease (TREAT-CAD) study. *Hypertens. Res.* **2018**. [CrossRef]
90. Liu, W.; Xie, X.; Liu, M.; Zhang, J.; Liang, W.; Chen, W. Serum ω-3 Polyunsaturated Fatty Acids and Potential Influence Factors in Elderly Patients with Multiple Cardiovascular Risk Factors. *Sci. Rep.* **2018**, *8*, 1102. [CrossRef]
91. Marchioli, R.; Barzi, F.; Bomba, E.; Chieffo, C.; Di Gregorio, D.; Di Mascio, R.; Franzosi, M.G.; Geraci, E.; Levantesi, G.; Maggioni, A.P.; et al. Early protection against sudden death by n-3 polyunsaturated fatty acids after myocardial infarction: Time-course analysis of the results of the Gruppo Italiano per lo Studio della Sopravvivenza nell'Infarto Miocardico (GISSI)-Prevenzione. *Circulation* **2002**, *105*, 1897–1903. [CrossRef]
92. Yagi, S.; Fukuda, D.; Aihara, K.I.; Akaike, M.; Shimabukuro, M.; Sata, M. n-3 Polyunsaturated Fatty Acids: Promising Nutrients for Preventing Cardiovascular Disease. *J. Atheroscler. Thromb.* **2017**, *24*, 999–1010. [CrossRef]
93. Shantakumari, N.; Eldeeb, R.A.; Ibrahim, S.A.M.; Sreedharan, J.; Otoum, S. Effect of PUFA on patients with hypertension: A hospital based study. *Indian Heart J.* **2014**, *66*, 408–414. [CrossRef] [PubMed]
94. Kelley, D.S.; Siegel, D.; Vemuri, M.; Mackey, B.E. Docosahexaenoic acid supplementation improves fasting and postprandial lipid profiles in hypertriglyceridemic men. *Am. J. Clin. Nutr.* **2007**, *86*, 324–333. [CrossRef] [PubMed]

95. Skulas-Ray, A.C.; Wilson, P.W.F.; Harris, W.S.; Brinton, E.A.; Kris-Etherton, P.M.; Richter, C.K.; Jacobson, T.A.; Engler, M.B.; Miller, M.; Robinson, J.G.; et al. Omega-3 Fatty Acids for the Management of Hypertriglyceridemia: A Science Advisory From the American Heart Association. *Circulation* **2019**, *140*, e673–e691. [CrossRef]
96. Gonzàlez_Montero, J.; Brito, R.; Gajardo, A.J.; Rodrigo, R. Myocardial reperfusion injury and oxidative stress: Therapeutic opportunities. *World J. Cardiol.* **2018**, *26*, 74–86. [CrossRef] [PubMed]
97. Sinning, C.; Westermann, D.; Clemmensen, P. Oxidative stress in ischemia and reperfusion: Current concepts, novel ideas and future perspectives. *Biomark. Med.* **2017**, *11*, 11031–11040. [CrossRef] [PubMed]
98. Granger, D.N.; Kvietys, P.R. Reperfusion injury and reactive oxygen species: The evolution of a concept. *Redox Biol.* **2015**, *6*, 524–551. [CrossRef] [PubMed]
99. Bird, J.K.; Calder, P.C. The Role of n-3 Long Chain Polyunsaturated Fatty Acids in Cardiovascular Disease Prevention, and Interactions with Statins. *Nutrients* **2018**, *10*, 775. [CrossRef]
100. Chen, Y.T.; Wong, L.L.; Liew, O.W.; Richards, A.M. Heart Failure with Reduced Ejection Fraction (HFrEF) and Preserved Ejection Fraction (HFpEF): The Diagnostic Value of Circulating MicroRNAs. *Cells* **2019**, *8*, 1651. [CrossRef]
101. Bishu, K.; Deswal, A.; Chen, H.H.; LeWinter, M.M.; Lewis, G.D.; Semigran, M.J.; Borlaug, B.A.; McNulty, S.; Hernandez, A.F.; Braunwald, E.; et al. Biomarkers in acutely decompensated heart failure with preserved or reduced ejection fraction. *Am. Heart J.* **2012**, *164*, 763–770.e3. [CrossRef] [PubMed]
102. Steinmann, E.; Brunner-La Rocca, H.P.; Maeder, M.T.; Kaufmann, B.A.; Pfisterer, M.; Rickenbacher, P. Is the clinical presentation of chronic heart failure different in elderly versus younger patients and those with preserved versus reduced ejection fraction? *Eur. J. Intern. Med.* **2018**, *57*, 61–69. [CrossRef] [PubMed]
103. Zhang, L.; Liebelt, J.J.; Madan, N.; Shan, J.; Taub, C.C. Comparison of Predictors of Heart Failure with Preserved Versus Reduced Ejection Fraction in a Multiracial Cohort of Preclinical Left Ventricular Diastolic Dysfunction. *Am. J. Cardiol.* **2017**, *119*, 1815–1820. [CrossRef] [PubMed]
104. Wang, C.; Xiong, B.; Huang, J. The Role of Omega-3 Polyunsaturated Fatty Acids in Heart Failure: A Meta-Analysis of Randomised Controlled Trials. *Nutrients* **2017**, *9*, 18. [CrossRef]
105. Eclov, J.A.; Qian, Q.; Redetzke, R.; Chen, Q.; Wu, S.C.; Healy, C.L.; Ortmeier, S.B.; Harmon, E.; Shearer, G.C.; O'Connell, T.D. EPA, not DHA, prevents fibrosis in pressure overload-induced heart failure: Potential role of free fatty acid receptor 4. *J. Lipid Res.* **2015**, *56*, 2297–2308. [CrossRef]
106. Zhang, P.Y. Role of ω-3 Fatty Acids in Cardiovascular Disease. *Cell Biochem. Biophys.* **2015**, *72*, 869–875. [CrossRef]
107. Bannenberg, G.; Mallon, C.; Edwards, H.; Yeadon, D.; Yan, K.; Johnson, H.; Ismail, A. Omega-3 Long-Chain Polyunsaturated Fatty Acid Content and Oxidation State of Fish Oil Supplements in New Zealand. *Sci. Rep.* **2017**, *7*, 1488. [CrossRef]
108. García-Hernández, V.M.; Gallar, M.; Sánchez-Soriano, J.; Micol, V.; Roche, E.; García-García, E. Effect of omega-3 dietary supplements with different oxidation levels in the lipidic profile of women: A randomized controlled trial. *Int. J. Food Sci. Nutr.* **2013**, *64*, 993–1000. [CrossRef]
109. Berliner, A.R.; Fine, D.M. There's something fishy about this bleeding. *NDT Plus* **2011**, *4*, 270–272. [CrossRef]
110. Stupin, M.; Kibel, A.; Stupin, A.; Selthofer-Relatić, K.; Matić, A.; Mihalj, M.; Mihaljević, Z.; Jukić, I.; Drenjančević, I. The Physiological Effect of n-3 Polyunsaturated Fatty Acids (n-3 PUFAs) Intake and Exercise on Hemorheology, Microvascular Function, and Physical Performance in Health and Cardiovascular Diseases; Is There an Interaction of Exercise and Dietary n-3 PUFA Intake? *Front. Physiol.* **2019**, *10*, 112.
111. Hansen, J.B.; Lyngmo, V.; Svensson, B.; Nordøy, A. Inhibition of exercise-induced shortening of bleeding time by fish oil in familial hypercholesterolemia (type IIa). *Arterioscler. Thromb.* **1993**, *13*, 98–104. [CrossRef] [PubMed]
112. Sanders, T.A.; Roshanai, F. The influence of different types of omega 3 polyunsaturated fatty acids on blood lipids and platelet function in healthy volunteers. *Clin. Sci.* **1983**, *64*, 91–99. [CrossRef]
113. Holub, B.J. Clinical nutrition: 4. Omega-3 fatty acids in cardiovascular care. *CMAJ* **2002**, *166*, 608–615. [PubMed]
114. Munk Begtrup, K.M.; Krag, A.E.; Hvas, A.M. No impact of fish oil supplements on bleeding risk: A systematic review. *Dan. Med. J.* **2017**, *64*, A5366.
115. Kris-Etherton, P.M. Omega-3 Fatty Acids and Cardiovascular Disease: New Recommendations from the American Heart Association. *Arterioscler. Thromb. Vasc. Biol.* **2003**, *23*, 151–152. [CrossRef] [PubMed]

116. Akrami, A.; Makiabadi, E.; Askarpour, M.; Zamani, K.; Hadi, A.; Mokari-Yamchi, A.; Babajafari, S.; Faghih, S.; Hojhabrimanesh, A. A Comparative Study of the Effect of Flaxseed Oil and Sunflower Oil on the Coagulation Score, Selected Oxidative and Inflammatory Parameters in Metabolic Syndrome Patients. *Clin. Nutr. Res.* **2020**, *9*, 63–72. [CrossRef] [PubMed]
117. Jeansen, S.; Renger, F.W.; Garthoff, J.A.; van Helvoort, A.; Calder, P.C. Fish oil LC-PUFAs do not affect blood coagulation parameters and bleeding manifestations: Analysis of 8 clinical studies with selected patient groups on omega-3-enriched medical nutrition. *Clin. Nutr.* **2018**, *37*, 948–957. [CrossRef] [PubMed]
118. Leonhardt, M.; Langhans, W. Lipid metabolism: Its role in energy regulation and obesity. In *Novel Food Ingredients for Weight Control*; Woodhead Publishing Series in Food Science, Technology and Nutrition: ETH Zürich, Switzerland, 2007; pp. 3–27. [CrossRef]
119. Telle-Hansen, V.H.; Gaundal, L.; Myhrstad, M.C.W. Polyunsaturated Fatty Acids and Glycemic Control in Type 2 Diabetes. *Nutrients* **2019**, *11*, 1067. [CrossRef]
120. Landmark, K.; Aursnes, I. Mercury, fish, fish oil and the risk of cardiovascular disease. *Tidsskr Nor Laegeforen.* **2004**, *124*, 198–200. [CrossRef]
121. Hu, X.F.; Laird, B.D.; Chan, H. Mercury diminishes the cardiovascular protective effect of omega-3 polyunsaturated fatty acids in the modern diet of Inuit in Canada. *Environ. Res.* **2017**, *152*, 470–477. [CrossRef]
122. Guallar, E.; Sanz-Gallardo, M.I.; Veer, P.V.T.; Bode, P.; Aro, A.; Gómez-Aracena, J.; Kark, J.D.; Riemersma, R.A.; Martín-Moreno, J.M.; Kok, F.J. Mercury, Fish Oils, and the Risk of Myocardial Infarction. *N. Engl. J. Med.* **2002**, *347*, 1747–1754. [CrossRef] [PubMed]
123. Bergkvist, C.; Berglund, M.; Glynn, A.; Julin, B.; Wolk, A.; Åkesson, A. Dietary exposure to polychlorinated biphenyls and risk of myocardial infarction in men—A population-based prospective cohort study. *Environ. Int.* **2016**, *88*, 9–14. [CrossRef] [PubMed]
124. Luigi Tavazzi, L.; Aldo, P.; Maggioni, A.P.; Roberto Marchioli, R.; Simona Barlera, S.; Maria Grazia Franzosi, M.G.; Roberto Latini, R.; Donata Lucci, D.; Gian Luigi Nicolosi, G.L.; Porcu, M.; et al. Effect of n-3 polyunsaturated fatty acids in patients with chronic heart failure (the GISSI-HF trial): A randomised, double-blind, placebo-controlled trial. *Randomized Control. Trial Lancet* **2008**, *372*, 1223–1230. [CrossRef]

biomedicines

MDPI

Review

Relationship between Diet, Microbiota, and Healthy Aging

Elisa Sanchez-Morate [1], Lucia Gimeno-Mallench [1,2], Kristine Stromsnes [1], Jorge Sanz-Ros [1], Aurora Román-Domínguez [1], Sergi Parejo-Pedrajas [1], Marta Inglés [3], Gloria Olaso [1], Juan Gambini [1,*] and Cristina Mas-Bargues [1]

1 Freshage Research Group, Department of Physiology, Faculty of Medicine, University of Valencia, CIBERFES-ISCIII, INCLIVA, 46010 Valencia, Spain; isanes@alumni.uv.es (E.S.-M.); lucia.gimeno@uv.es (L.G.-M.); krisbaks@alumni.uv.es (K.S.); sanzros@alumni.uv.es (J.S.-R.); aurodo@alumni.uv.es (A.R.-D.); sergi_spp_95@hotmail.com (S.P.-P.); gloria.olaso@uv.es (G.O.); cristina.mas@uv.es (C.M.-B.)

2 Department of Biomedical Sciences, Faculty of Health Sciences, Cardenal Herrera CEU University, 46115 Valencia, Spain

3 Freshage Research Group, Department of Physiotherapy, Faculty of Physiotherapy, University of Valencia, CIBERFES-ISCIII, INCLIVA, 46010 Valencia, Spain; marta.ingles@uv.es

* Correspondence: juan.gambini@uv.es

Received: 21 July 2020; Accepted: 6 August 2020; Published: 14 August 2020

Abstract: Due to medical advances and lifestyle changes, population life expectancy has increased. For this reason, it is important to achieve healthy aging by reducing the risk factors causing damage and pathologies associated with age. Through nutrition, one of the pillars of health, we are able to modify these factors through modulation of the intestinal microbiota. The Mediterranean and Oriental diets are proof of this, as well as the components present in them, such as fiber and polyphenols. These generate beneficial effects on the body thanks, in part, to their interaction with intestinal bacteria. Likewise, the low consumption of products with high fat content favors the state of the microbiota, contributing to the maintenance of good health.

Keywords: Mediterranean diet; Oriental diet; nutrition; polyphenols; microbiota; aging; health

---

1. Introduction

One of the most significant changes in today's society is that the population is aging more slowly than in the past. We live longer; the majority of the population has a life expectancy of 60 years or more. According to data from the World Health Organization (WHO), the percentage of people over 60 years will be duplicated on a worldwide scale before 2050 [1]. In 2020 the number of people of more than 60 years of age has been reported to be higher than those under five years, and by 2050 the number of elderly adults requiring help with daily tasks will quadruplicate [2].

Advances in medicine and public health care, as well as lifestyle changes, have had positive effects on life expectancy, mortality rates, and chronic disease prevalence, thereby causing an aging of the population [3].

Whether or not the impact of these factors on society is positive depends on the health status of the elderly. Therefore, it is important to prevent diseases associated with age, such as diabetes and cardiovascular diseases, to promote an active aging of the population and maintain social, mental, and physical wellbeing. In this regard, three pillars of active aging have been postulated: Participation, health and security [4,5]. We will focus our study around health.

It is important to keep in mind that the risk factors causing age related diseases can be modified. One of the factors that can act upon the health pillar is nutrition [6]. What, when, and how much we eat affects the quality of life. A well-balanced diet can modulate the proliferation of specific bacteria within the gut microbiota, which has been related to an improved health status for the elderly.

Microbiota

In this century, research related to microbiota has increased due to two primary advances: The holobiont theory of evolution, and metagenomics. The former one plays an important role in the physiology of superior organisms, and the latter one allows for the identification of microorganisms without a need for cultivation. As a result of these advances and of the increasing interest in this field of study, the concept of the "intestinal–brain axis" was created, with a tight relation between the intestinal microbiota and neurodegenerative diseases such as Parkinson, Alzheimer, stroke, and epilepsy [7]. Actually, a study performed in mice proved the presence of bacteria in the brain of these mice [8]. Furthermore, Roberts et al. obtained a micrography of a human brain where bacteria were visible in all the cerebral blood vessels, proving the existence of a brain microbiota [9]. Further supporting the idea of the presence of bacteria in the brain, a study using epilepsy patients demonstrated a reduction of convulsion frequency by antibiotic treatment [10]. All these data suggest that there might be a brain microbiota, and by extrapolation a whole organism microbiota.

The gastrointestinal tract is colonized by a set of microorganisms that include not only bacteria but also viruses, fungi, and protozoa. Unlike other microorganisms, these are not identified as pathogens by our immune system, but rather coexist symbiotically with the enterocytes [11]. So far, it is known that its composition contains a total of 52 different phyla and up to 35,000 different bacterial species [12], the large majority being Firmicutes, Bacteroidetes, Actinobacteria, and Proteobacteria (Figure 1).

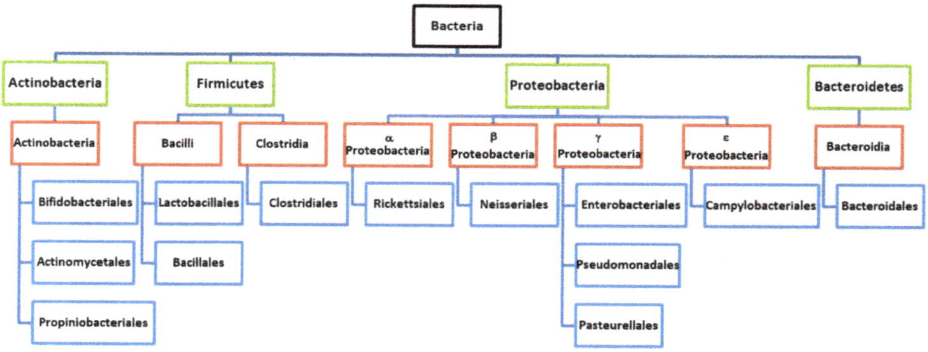

Figure 1. Taxonomy of microbiota. Black: Kingdom; green: Phylum; red: Class; blue: Order. Adapted from Unger et al., Pediatr. Res. 2015 [13]. Copyright © International Pediatric Research Foundation, Inc. 2015.

It is worth mentioning that there are differences in composition and number depending on the location along the gastrointestinal tract such that at the stomach level they are estimated at a density of 10^2 bacteria/mL and in the colon at around 10^{11} bacteria/mL [14].

Originally, the intestinal microbiota is formed in the placenta, where there are low levels of non-pathogenic bacteria, the majority being *Firmicutes* and *Bacteroidetes*. After birth, the child's intestine becomes rapidly colonized by the microbiota. Several studies show that this could already happen at the level of the uterus. Depending on whether the delivery is vaginal or by caesarean section, the intestine of the infant will be colonized by organisms from the maternal vagina or from the maternal skin flora. Another factor that influences the acquired microorganism is the type of diet the infant receives, breast milk or formula foods [11]. During the first three years of life, the child's microbiota is unstable and has little diversity. After the third year it acquires a milieu similar to that of the adult stage. In the case of older adults (>65 years), the microbiota is characterized by a decrease in Firmicutes and Bifidobacterium, with diversity in the patterns of abundance for Clostridium [15]. In relation to centenarians, differences in the composition of the microbiota are also evident, especially at the level of the Firmicutes subgroups, with a decrease in Clostridium and an increase in Bacilli. In addition, it is enriched by the edge Proteobacteria. Thus, as we age, progressive changes are produced in the morphology and function of the microbiota. This could alter its diversity and provoke inflammatory and metabolic disruption, causing inflammatory diseases in the intestine, such as irritable bowel, obesity, etc. [16]. The relation Firmicutes/Bacteroidetes is altered when the Firmicutes proportion is augmented over Bacteroides and generates consequences such as those found in obesity. However, this association is still polemic and under investigation [17,18]. While, on a global level, the Firmicutes and Bacteroidetes seem to decrease, Clostridium is increased in elderly adults [19]. In the last years, bacteria of the Clostridium genera have provoked a big interest for their impact on morbidity and mortality in the older generation [20]. They can act as opportunistic pathogens and cause diseases like intoxication through alimentation, necrotizing enterocolitis, or necrotic enteritis [21]. Furthermore, their incidence is increasing, and they have become the most frequent cause for nosocomial diarrhea, which can lead to the production of toxic megacolon and sepsis, and even to death [22].

However, through nutrition we can modify the microbiota to maintain intestinal health by stimulating beneficial bacteria, such as the Bacteroidetes and Firmicutes in balanced proportions, and diminishing prejudicial bacteria like Clostridium [16,23]. Additionally, maintaining a healthy diet throughout a lifespan might be beneficial for healthy aging.

2. Interplay between Aging and Microbiota

The composition and function of the microbiota changes in individuals of advanced age (>65 years), as has been mentioned earlier. Between physiological changes and lifestyles associated with aging, we find a decrease in dentures, a reduction in digestion and absorption, changes in appetite due to medication, and changes in living conditions such as hospitalization or elderly residences [24]. These factors might be responsible for changes in alimentation habits, and thereby nutrition.

The mechanism by which the microbiota changes with age is not yet fully understood. Lifestyle changes, and particularly diet, play an important role. As aging is often accompanied by a reduction in quantity and variety of aliments containing fiber, it often leads to a risk of malnourishment [25].

Additionally, the microbiota can modulate changes in aging related to innate immunity, sarcopenia, and cognitive function, which are essential components of the frailty syndrome [26]. This syndrome, was defined for the first time by Linda Fried in 2004 as "the physiological state characterized by an increase in vulnerability to external aggressors, as the result of a decrease or deregulation of the physiological reserves of multiple systems, which causes difficulties in maintaining homeostasis" [27]. Recent studies have suggested that the loss of intestinal microbiota is more related to age associated frailty than to chronological age [28]. In this context, elderly people can experience comorbidity affecting the intestine and its bacteria.

In 2007, a study performed by the ELDERMET group in Cork, Ireland, proved the existence of a correlation between diet, the microbiota, and health in elderly volunteers. The microbiota in relation to aging was studied in both community and long-stay residential care elderly subjects. The first group showed a loss in bacterial diversity due to a higher intake of medication, and a recuperation of microbial diversity when reducing antibiotics, whereas the second group showed a loss in microbial components associated with bad health, and a gain in microbiota associated with aging. Therefore, the previous correlation can be used to measure the difference between elderly that live in elderly homes or rehabilitation centers and those who live by themselves in the long run [29]. Claesson et al. supported these findings on the relation between diet, microbiota, and health status. Through analysis of separated fecal microbiota composition, they showed that in 178 subjects of advanced age a change in diet associated with that found when moving to a care facility generated a change in the composition of intestinal bacteria significantly correlated with measures of frailty, comorbidity, nutritional status, and inflammatory markers [15].

The most noticeable changes in the intestinal microbiota are produced during the transition from adult to elderly. In comparison to younger individuals, a decrease in microbial diversity is observed, specifically in Bifidobacterium, Firmicutes, and Clostridium [15]. These changes in the microbiota associated to age are a factor of high relevance in several diseases, such as chronic inflammation, neurodegeneration, cognitive deterioration, frailty, and diabetes types 1 and 2 [30]. In regard to extreme longevity, the microbiota of centenarians differs from that of elderly adults. Bacteroidetes and Firmicutes dominate their intestinal microbiota, making up more than 93% of the overall bacteria flora. However, comparing to younger adults, specific changes in the subgroups of Firmicutes are observed: Clostridium is decreased, and Bacilli augmented. Moreover, the intestinal microbiota of centenarians in enriched in Proteobacteria, a group containing bacteria recently redefined as "pathobionts", benign endogenous microbes which in dysbiosis can lead to pathologies [31,32].

Taken together, intestinal microbiota is subjected to constant changes throughout life and continues to change in old age and is closely linked to diet and health status, suggesting the possibility that microbial profiling may serve as a clinically useful biomarker in geriatric care. Predomination of one type of bacteria, or the over proliferation of bad bacteria upon good bacteria will have negative consequences. Thus, maintaining intestinal microbiota diversity seems to be a key point when seeking geriatric health [33]. Figure 2 shows microbiota evolution through aging.

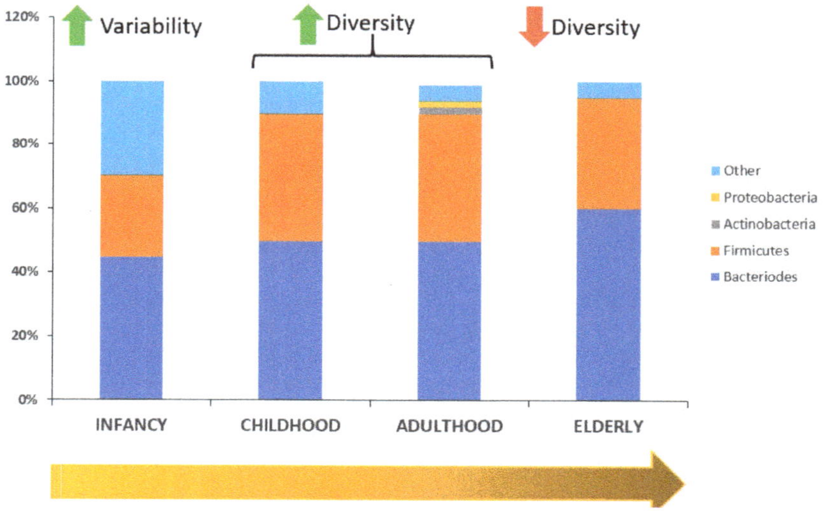

Figure 2. Intestinal microbiota changes through life.Green arrows signify increase. Red arrows signify decrease.

3. The Influence of Nutrition on the Microbiota and Aging

In this paragraph, we will comment on the two diets that are the most associated with healthy aging: the Mediterranean and the Oriental diets.

3.1. *The Mediterranean Diet*

The Mediterranean diet (MD) is characterized by a high daily consumption of fruits and vegetables, whole grains and legumes, and a lower consumption of meat, fish, and lactose-rich products. Additionally, it is also associated with olive oil as the major source of fats, and moderate intake of red wine [34–36].

It has been shown that following an MD can have multiple benefits as it delays the appearance of chronic diseases associated with age such as cancer, diabetes type 2, and neurodegenerative diseases [36–38]. Furthermore, recent data suggest that the MD promotes beneficial effects on the intestinal microbiota, favoring the diversity of the colon microbiota by increasing Bacteroidetes and Firmicutes and reducing Clostridium [37]. Another study carried out on 27 healthy subjects, who were monitored for MD compounds, showed how MD eating habits modified the composition and diversity of the microbiota. More specifically, they observed an increase in Bacteroidetes and a higher Bacteroidetes/Firmicutes ratio. This modification of the different microbiota populations has proven to exert anti-inflammatory effects. Accordingly, how MD can decrease the transcription factor E2F1 in colon cancer cells in order to decrease the proliferation of these cells has been studied. Additionally, it activates factors with protective effects against oxidative stress such as the transcription factor NRF2 [39,40].

Other studies support the beneficial effects of MD on cardiovascular diseases [39,41–44]. In one of these, low levels of triglycerides, high HDL cholesterol levels, and lower arterial pressures were found in those following the MD in comparison to a control group consuming a low-fat diet [43]. In the "Lyon Diet Study", the risk of severe cardiovascular events was reduced by 76% in the MD group. Additionally, a multicenter randomized study in Spain obtained similar results [44]. Moreover, how the risk of several types of cancer is decreased has also been studied, although the underlying mechanisms are still not clear [45,46]. This is reflected in the 605 patient cohort participating in the Lyon Heart Study, where the cancer risk decreased by 61% in the MD group in comparison to the control group [47]. One of the components of the MD is hydroxityrosol, a compound present in olive oil with antioxidant properties. It has been demonstrated that it reduces proliferation and induces apoptosis of certain cancer cells in the colon [48,49], prostate [50], and pancreas [51]. Furthermore, a clinical trial performed in Spain showed that the combination of the nutrients related to MD reduced pain and the inflammatory marker C-reactive in patients with breast cancer [52,53]. Likewise, various studies have analyzed the correlation between MD and diabetes type 2. MD has been seen to attenuate the augmentation of postprandial glycemia, reduce high peaks of insulin secretion, as well as diminish hyperlipidemia in patients with type 2 diabetes [54]. The PREDIMEM study "Prevention with the Mediterranean Diet" found that a bigger adherence to MD was inversely associated with the incidence of type 2 diabetes, which was reduced by 52% in the MD group compared to the control group [55]. In relation to neurodegenerative diseases, a high adherence to MD has been associated with improved cognitive function and lower risk of dementia [56–59]. However, many of these studies are observational, and can therefore not display a cause–effect relation. Moreover, other studies confirm the improvement in cognitive function in comparison to low-fat diet groups [47,60,61].

As we have previously described, MD reduces the risk of several diseases associated with aging. Furthermore, many studies demonstrate that MD promotes changes in the intestinal microbiota associated with healthy beneficial bacteria [34,37,39]. Consequently, the manipulation of the microbiota through MD should improve or benefit the treatment of these diseases [62–65]. However, the mechanisms through which MD promotes healthy changes on the intestinal microbiota are still not completely known.

3.2. *The Oriental Diet*

The Oriental Diet (OD) is well known for its health benefits. It has been demonstrated that the population following this diet has a longer lifespan, to the point where Japan has become one of the countries with the highest life expectancy rate. In addition to the long lifespan, the diet is also associated with a long health span. In the OD, one of the most common aliments is soy.

It is known that soy consumption has positive effects on the organism due to its ability to increase intestinal bacteria diversity. Tamura et al. divided rats in three groups based on diet for a two week period. The different diets were enriched either with casein protein, soy protein, or soy protein and high fat. After studying the microbiota through genes of 16S rRNA of feces, they were able to see how soy protein induced a bigger variety in intestinal bacteria, which is associated with a healthy microflora. Specifically, they observed an increase in Bacteroidetes and Proteobacteria, as well as in

Bifidobacterium and Enterococcus. On the other hand, they also addressed a decrease in Firmicutes and Lactococcus [66].

Soy contains a variety of polyphenols, genistein being one of them. Of all groups of polyphenols (stilbene, ligand, alcoholic polyphenols, etc.), genistein is an isoflavone, the structure of which is similar to that of estrogen, and is therefore also classified as a phytoestrogen [67]. Genistein is found almost exclusively in legumes, such as chickpeas and peas, and majorly in soy and its derivatives [68].

It has been observed that genistein consumption can have multiple benefits, within these the promotion of cardiovascular health, and thereby flexibility of blood vessels and reduction in cholesterol concentration [69]. As with many polyphenols, it is transformed and modified by the microbiota to enable its actions in the organism. It interacts with estrogenic receptors to alleviate symptoms associated with menopause, hot flashes, and osteoporosis, as well as exerting antiaromatase activity, which is key in the protection against breast cancer [70]. Several studies performed on rats have shown how the administration of genistein at early age counteracts dysbiosis in the intestinal microbiota provoked by a high fat diet [71]. These data are supported by research by Zhou et al. where they observed beneficial bacteria proliferation through perinatal supplementation [72]. López et al. also found that genistein can regulate the intestinal microbiota by reducing metabolic endotoxemia and the neuroinflammatory response to a high fat diet [73]. Additionally, genistein has antioxidative effects, as it blocks the formation of free radicals, hydrogen peroxide, and superoxide anion, and by overexpressing antioxidant enzymes [74]. Through these effects, it also has protective effects against ischemic stroke and neuroprotective effects against Alzheimer Disease by reducing the hyperphosphorylation of Tau protein [75,76]. Lastly, it has anti-inflammatory and antitumoral effects through its ability to inhibit key enzymes in the appearance and progression of tumors. It also regulates the tumoral microenvironment, causing a higher sensitivity to therapies by modulating the production of cytokines and chemokines, and activating immune cells [77,78].

Another polyphenol present in soy is daidzein; similarly to genistein, it is modified and transformed by the microbiota to equol, a compound with anti-inflammatory and anticarcinogenic properties. This has been demonstrated in several studies where it has been shown how daidzein inhibits the production of IL-2 and how the proliferation of tumoral cells in breast cancer is regulated by the blockage of PI3K/AKT [79]. Furthermore, it has been determined that equol protects β-pancreatic cells against streptozotocin-induced diabetes in rats [80].

Curcumin, a polyphenol found in turmeric root, is also abundantly present in OD. It has proven to be capable of exerting anti-inflammatory and anti-tumor effects, among others [81,82]. Regarding its role in the microbiota, it has been seen to directly modify it. Since its absorption and bioavailability is low, it can be found in significant amounts in the gastrointestinal tract after its consumption. In fact, curcumin administration considerably changed the relationship between beneficial and pathogenic bacteria by increasing the abundance of Bifidobacteria and Lactobacili and reducing the loads of Prevotellaceae, Choriobacteria, Enterobacteriaceae, and Enterococci [83].

Thereby, the OD reduces the risk of several diseases associated with aging. Additionally, numerous studies have shown how following an OD has positive effects on the microbiota by increasing the number of beneficial bacteria. However, as with the MD, the mechanisms by which this diet promotes healthy changes in the intestinal microbiota are still not fully known.

3.3. *Effects on the Microbiota by Compounds Present in Diet: Fiber, Fats, and Polyphenols*

As we have previously described, Mediterranean and Oriental diets have modulatory effects on intestinal microbiota. These diets include a wide variety of nutrients in balanced proportions that promote gut bacteria diversification and thus a healthy microflora. While practically all compounds we ingest through diet can have effects on the microbiota, in this review we will only focus on food compounds that are similar in the two diets, which include a high consumption of polyphenols and fibers, and a higher proportion of unsaturated fats (Table 1).

Table 1. Summaries of the main effects of each compound on the intestinal bacteria and the health consequences. Upward arrows signify increase. Downward arrows signify decrease.

Diet Compound	Microbiota Modification	Health Consequences
Fibers	↑Bifidobacterium ↑ Lactobacillus ↓ Pathogens	↓ Inflammation ↓ Hypertension ↓ Obesity
Saturated fats	↓ Bacteroides ↑ Firmicutes ↑ Proteobacteria	↑ Obesity ↑ Hypertension ↑ Atherosclerosis
Polyphenols	↑ Bifidobacterium ↓ Firmicutes ↓ Clostridium	↓ Inflammation ↑ Antioxidants

In the upcoming paragraphs, we will discuss in depth the beneficial effects of each one of these compounds.

3.3.1. Fibers

Diets rich in fibers such as, β-glucan, arabinoxylan, galactomannan, and pectines facilitate weight control, decrease systemic inflammation, and are fundamental in the maintenance of intestinal health by supplementing substrates for the health promoting bacteria (Bifidobacterium and Lactobacillus) [84].

Studies have shown that a diet rich in fiber generates beneficial effects for elderly adults, especially on the cardiovascular system. Fiber-rich diets reduce the risks for cardiovascular disease, such as obesity, diabetes, and hypertension. The inverse correlation between high consumption of fiber and weight gain risk has been demonstrated [38]. Additionally, fiber seems to have a positive impact on the composition of the intestinal microbiota, augmenting the number of beneficial bacteria, inhibiting the growth of pathogens, and reducing atherogenic serum cholesterol in the microbiome. Furthermore, it prohibits the intolerance to glucose by reducing postprandial hyperglycemia through the formation of a viscous layer around the small intestine, thereby slowing down the chyme transition. This in turn augments the thickness of the aqueous layer where solutes must pass to reach the enterocytic membrane, causing a decrease in glucose, lipids, and amino acid absorption. As a result, less biliary acids are absorbed, and in turn cholesterol levels are decreased, which employs the synthesis of new biliary acids [85].

In this manner, a high consumption of soluble and insoluble fibers is associated with lower risk of stroke, as shown in a study performed over 12 years [86]. Another study demonstrated that the ingestion of total fiber, cereal fiber, and vegetable fiber was associated with a lower risk of hypertension [87]. Not only that, a study about the association between ingested fiber in the diet per 1000 kcal and leucocyte telomere length showed that adults consuming high quantities of fiber had longer telomeres, which suggests that biological aging was significatively lower [88].

In conclusion, a diet rich in fiber facilitates the presence of beneficial intestinal bacteria, and thereby lowers the risk of diseases in elderly adults, leading to healthy aging.

3.3.2. Fats

Classic epidemiologic studies have demonstrated the relation between diets with a high content of saturated fats, and a higher risk of age-related diseases [89,90].

Studies with animals have shown that a high fat diet can determine the microbiome composition and affect the proportion of various families of bacteria in the intestine. In particular, rats that received a high fat diet showed a lower number of Bacteroidetes and a higher number of Firmicutes and Proteobacteria, which is a characteristic of obesity [91]. This change in the microbiota composition could occur rapidly. For example, the change from a diet poor in saturated fats and rich in vegetal polysaccharides to a diet high in fats and sugars changes the structure of the microbiota in one single day. Additionally, a diet high in saturated fats is related to increased risk of chronic diseases, such as metabolic syndrome, hypertension, and atherosclerosis due to the alterations of the microbiota [92–94].

More importantly, if we compare humans with two different diets, it is clear that the microbiome diversity in our intestines is affected by what we eat. An example of this is the proportion of Bacteroidetes/Firmicutes which was much higher in African children compared to Italian, as they follow a diet of less fats and sugars [95]. This is further confirmed in a study by Wan et al. where they showed that healthy young adults consuming high quantities of fats had adverse effects on the intestinal microbiota, fecal metabolites, and plasmatic proinflammatory factors derived from the intestine, which could serve as potential factors to modify long term health [96].

In conclusion, it is clear that fiber has a protective effect in the elderly, especially at the cardiovascular level, and can contribute to healthier biological aging, whereas a diet high in fats induces a dysbiosis which can trigger metabolic alterations associated with chronic diseases and those related to age. Additionally, it has also been shown to have protective effects in younger individuals.

3.3.3. Polyphenols

Polyphenols, which have been mentioned earlier in this review, can reach the intestinal microbiota and thereby modify the molecule itself, the metabolism of the bacteria, and the intestinal flora population. This seems to have beneficial effects, including anticarcinogen, anti-inflammatory, and antioxidant properties [97].

For example, ellagitannins are polyphenols present in walnuts, pomegranates, and raspberries, which, when in the intestine, are modified by the microbiota and transformed into different compounds. Urolithin is one of the most widely studied products, and it has been demonstrated that it can be absorbed through enterohepatic circulation and that it can be transported in blood, and thereby be distributed to different tissues and exert diverse actions. It possesses anticancer effects through the inhibition of the Wnt signalization pathway, which could have a protective effect against colon cancer [98]. It has also been attributed anti-inflammatory properties as it inhibits the formation of proinflammatory compounds, such as cyclooxygenase-2 (COX-2), prostaglandin synthase E (PGSE), and prostaglandin E2 (PGE2) [99]. An important finding in this regard was made by Selma MV et al. in 2014, when they discovered a new species of bacteria in the microbiota responsible for the synthesis of urolithin from ellagic acid, which is formed in the stomach, that they denominated *Gordonibacter urolithinfaciens* [100]. However, the metabolites obtained from polyphenols through diet vary between individuals depending on the microbiota. In fact, certain individuals do not synthesize urolithin at all after the ingestion of its precursors [100].

Other polyphenols, such as resveratrol and curcumin, exert specific changes on the intestinal microflora. Concretely, in a study where rats were administrated these two polyphenols, they observed alterations in the bacteria groups Bacteroidetes and Clostridium. This in turn provided metabolic benefits in these individuals such as glycemic control [101].

On the other hand, there are polyphenols, such as quercetin, caffeic acid, and rutin, that affect the fermentation balance between the principal groups of intestinal bacteria that influence health by proliferating Bifidobacterium and diminishing Bacteroidetes and Firmicutes. Additionally, these polyphenols stimulate the production of short chain fatty acids through these bacteria [102].

These findings indicate that there are specific populations of bacteria capable of synthesizing final products such as urolithin and equol. The population of these bacteria in individuals is heterogenous, meaning the bacteria population present in the microbiota in each individual is a personal characteristic trait.

4. Conclusions

Life expectancy is increasing considerably, directing us towards a model of an aging society, and it is therefore necessary to expand our knowledge on the effects of aging. Taking into account all repercussions on the intestinal microbiota, to study the role of the microbiota is an interesting path, as well as the potential benefits that can be achieved through diet. Through dietary interventions many diseases associated with age such as cardiovascular and neurodegenerative diseases, diabetes, chronic inflammation, and cancer risk could be prevented.

Therefore, it is important to continue researching different nutritional approaches to fight physiological damages that are produced in an organism by aging. In particular, chronic factors present in advanced stages of life, such as inflammation and oxidative stress, must be considered, as these factors can be diminished or augmented depending on the consumed diet.

Author Contributions: Conceptualization, J.G., E.S.-M. and C.M.-B.; methodology, L.G.-M., J.S.-R. and A.R.-D. software, S.P.-P. and M.I.; formal analysis, K.S. and J.G.; investigation, G.O., K.S., C.M.-B. and L.G.-M.; resources, J.G.; writing—original draft preparation, J.G., K.S. and C.M.-B.; writing—review and editing, E.S -M., M.I., K.S. and J.G.; visualization, J.G., G.O. and L.G.-M.; supervision, J.G. and C.M.-B.; All authors have read and agreed to the published version of the manuscript

Funding: This work was supported by FEDER [PIE15/00013], SAF2016-75508-R (Ministerio de 281 Economía y Competitividad), CB16/10/00435 (CIBERFES-ISCIII), PROMETEOII2014/056 282 (Conselleria de Educación, Investigación, Cultura y Deporte), The FRAILOMIC Initiative 283 (FP7-HEALTH-2012-Proposal no. 305483-2), ADVANTAGE-724099 (HP-JA) – DIALBFRAIL284 LATAM (825546 H2020-SC1-BHC) and GV/2019/092 from "Conselleria d'Educació, Cultura i Esport de la Generalitat Valenciana" to C.M.-B. Finally, Dr. C.M.-B. is recipient of a postdoctoral grant financed by Generalitat Valenciana (APOSTD/2018/230) and FSE (European Social Fund).

Conflicts of Interest: The authors declare no conflict of interest. The funders had no role in the design of the study; in the collection, analyses or interpretation of data; in the writing of the manuscript or in the decision to publish the results.

References

1. World Health Organization. 10 Datos Sobre el Envejecimiento y la Salud. Available online: https://www.who.int/features/factfiles/ageing/es/ (accessed on 6 November 2019).
2. World Health Organization. Envejecimiento y Salud. Available online: https://www.who.int/es/news-room/fact-sheets/detail/envejecimiento-y-salud (accessed on 6 November 2019).
3. Arc-Chagnaud, C.; Millan, F.; Salvador-Pascual, A.; Correas, A.G.; Olaso-Gonzalez, G.; De la Rosa, A.; Carretero, A.; Gomez-Cabrera, M.C.; Viña, J. Reversal of age-associated frailty by controlled physical exercise: The pre-clinical and clinical evidences. *Sports Med. Health Sci.* **2019**, *1*, 33–39. [CrossRef]
4. Limón-Mendizábal, M.R.; Ortega Navas, M.C. Envejecimiento activo y mejora de la calidad de vida en adultos mayores. *Rev. Psicol. Educ.* **2011**, *1*, 225–238.
5. Caballero-García, J.C. Aspectos generales de envejecimiento normal y patológico. In *Terapia Ocupacional en Geriatría: Principios y Práctica*; Elsevier Masson: Paris, France, 2010; pp. 41–60.
6. Vaiserman, A.M.; Koliada, A.K.; Marotta, F. Gut microbiota: A player in aging and a target for anti-aging intervention. *Ageing Res. Rev.* **2017**, *35*, 36–45. [CrossRef] [PubMed]
7. Castillo-Álvarez, F.; Marzo-Sola, M.E. Role of the gut microbiota in the development of various neurological diseases. *Neurologia* **2019**. [CrossRef]
8. Graham, F. Daily briefing: Hints of a microbiome in the brain. Gut bacteria might also live in our brain, new technique that turns mice transparent and mental-health first aid in the lab. *Nature Briefing*, 13 November 2018. Available online: https://www.nature.com/articles/d41586-018-07416-8 (accessed on 6 November 2019).
9. Servick, K. Do gut bacteria make a second home in our brains? *Science* **2018**. [CrossRef]
10. Braakman, H.M.H.; van Ingen, J. Can epilepsy be treated by antibiotics? *J. Neurol.* **2018**, *265*, 1934–1936. [CrossRef]
11. Jandhyala, S.M.; Talukdar, R.; Subramanyam, C.; Vuyyuru, H.; Sasikala, M.; Nageshwar Reddy, D. Role of the normal gut microbiota. *World J. Gastroenterol.* **2015**, *21*, 8787–8803. [CrossRef]
12. Frank, D.N.; St Amand, A.L.; Feldman, R.A.; Boedeker, E.C.; Harpaz, N.; Pace, N.R. Molecular-phylogenetic characterization of microbial community imbalances in human inflammatory bowel diseases. *Proc. Natl. Acad. Sci. USA* **2007**, *104*, 13780–13785. [CrossRef]
13. Unger, S.; Stintzi, A.; Shah, P.; Mack, D.; O'Connor, D.L. Gut microbiota of the very-low-birth-weight infant. *Pediatr. Res.* **2015**, *77*, 205–213. [CrossRef]
14. Tsai, Y.L.; Lin, T.L.; Chang, C.J.; Wu, T.R.; Lai, W.F.; Lu, C.C.; Lai, H.C. Probiotics, prebiotics and amelioration of diseases. *J. Biomed. Sci.* **2019**, *26*, 3. [CrossRef]

15. Claesson, M.J.; Cusack, S.; O'Sullivan, O.; Greene-Diniz, R.; de Weerd, H.; Flannery, E.; Marchesi, J.R.; Falush, D.; Dinan, T.; Fitzgerald, G.; et al. Composition, variability, and temporal stability of the intestinal microbiota of the elderly. *Proc. Natl. Acad. Sci. USA* **2011**, *108*, 4586–4591. [CrossRef] [PubMed]
16. Power, S.E.; O'Toole, P.W.; Stanton, C.; Ross, R.P.; Fitzgerald, G.F. Intestinal microbiota, diet and health. *Br. J. Nutr.* **2014**, *111*, 387–402. [CrossRef]
17. Cigarran Guldris, S.; González Parra, E.; Cases Amenós, A. Gut microbiota in chronic kidney disease. *Nefrologia* **2017**, *37*, 9–19. [CrossRef] [PubMed]
18. Arias, A.; Mach, N. Efecto de los probióticos en el control de la obesidad en humanos: Hipótesis no demostradas. *Rev. Española Nutr. Hum. Dietética* **2012**, *16*, 100–107. [CrossRef]
19. Ribera Casado, J.M. Intestinal microbiota and ageing: A new intervention route? *Rev. Esp. Geriatr. Gerontol.* **2016**, *51*, 290–295. [CrossRef] [PubMed]
20. Morosini, M.I.; Cercenado, E.; Ardanuy, C.; Torres, C. Phenotypic detection of resistance mechanisms in gram-positive bacteria. *Enferm. Infecc. Microbiol. Clin.* **2012**, *30*, 325–332. [CrossRef]
21. Morris, W.E.; Fernández-Miyakawa, M.E. Toxins of Clostridium perfringens. *Rev. Argent. Microbiol.* **2009**, *41*, 251–260.
22. Monge, D.; Morosini, M.; Millán, I.; Pérez Canosa, C.; Manso, M.; Guzman, M.F.; Asensio, A. Risk factors for Clostridium difficile infections in hospitalized patients. *Med. Clin.* **2011**, *137*, 575–580. [CrossRef]
23. Cardona, F.; Andrés-Lacueva, C.; Tulipani, S.; Tinahones, F.J.; Queipo-Ortuño, M.I. Benefits of polyphenols on gut microbiota and implications in human health. *J. Nutr. Biochem.* **2013**, *24*, 1415–1422. [CrossRef]
24. O'Toole, P.W.; Jeffery, I.B. Gut microbiota and aging. *Science* **2015**, *350*, 1214–1215. [CrossRef]
25. Alang, N.; Kelly, C.R. Weight gain after fecal microbiota transplantation. *Open Forum Infect. Dis.* **2015**, *2*. [CrossRef] [PubMed]
26. Mills, S.; Stanton, C.; Lane, J.A.; Smith, G.J.; Ross, R.P. Precision Nutrition and the Microbiome, Part I: Current State of the Science. *Nutrients* **2019**, *11*, 923. [CrossRef] [PubMed]
27. Fried, L.P.; Ferrucci, L.; Darer, J.; Williamson, J.D.; Anderson, G. Untangling the concepts of disability, frailty, and comorbidity: Implications for improved targeting and care. *J. Gerontol. A Biol. Sci. Med. Sci.* **2004**, *59*, 255–263. [CrossRef] [PubMed]
28. Rondanelli, M.; Giacosa, A.; Faliva, M.A.; Perna, S.; Allieri, F.; Castellazzi, A.M. Review on microbiota and effectiveness of probiotics use in older. *World J. Clin. Cases* **2015**, *3*, 156–162. [CrossRef]
29. Jeffery, I.B.; Lynch, D.B.; O'Toole, P.W. Composition and temporal stability of the gut microbiota in older persons. *ISME J.* **2016**, *10*, 170–182. [CrossRef] [PubMed]
30. Claesson, M.J.; Jeffery, I.B.; Conde, S.; Power, S.E.; O'Connor, E.M.; Cusack, S.; Harris, H.M.; Coakley, M.; Lakshminarayanan, B.; O'Sullivan, O.; et al. Gut microbiota composition correlates with diet and health in the elderly. *Nature* **2012**, *488*, 178–184. [CrossRef] [PubMed]
31. Nagpal, R.; Mainali, R.; Ahmadi, S.; Wang, S.; Singh, R.; Kavanagh, K.; Kitzman, D.W.; Kushugulova, A.; Marotta, F.; Yadav, H. Gut microbiome and aging: Physiological and mechanistic insights. *Nutr. Healthy Aging* **2018**, *4*, 267–285. [CrossRef]
32. Sebastián Domingo, J.J.; Sánchez Sánchez, C. From the intestinal flora to the microbiome. *Rev. Esp. Enferm. Dig.* **2018**, *110*, 51–56. [CrossRef]
33. Kostic, A.D.; Howitt, M.R.; Garrett, W.S. Exploring host-microbiota interactions in animal models and humans. *Genes Dev.* **2013**, *27*, 701–718. [CrossRef]
34. Biagi, E.; Nylund, L.; Candela, M.; Ostan, R.; Bucci, L.; Pini, E.; Nikkïla, J.; Monti, D.; Satokari, R.; Franceschi, C.; et al. Through ageing, and beyond: Gut microbiota and inflammatory status in seniors and centenarians. *PLoS ONE* **2010**, *5*, e10667. [CrossRef]
35. Del Chierico, F.; Vernocchi, P.; Dallapiccola, B.; Putignani, L. Mediterranean diet and health: Food effects on gut microbiota and disease control. *Int. J. Mol. Sci.* **2014**, *15*, 11678–11699. [CrossRef]
36. Huhn, S.; Kharabian Masouleh, S.; Stumvoll, M.; Villringer, A.; Witte, A.V. Components of a Mediterranean diet and their impact on cognitive functions in aging. *Front. Aging Neurosci.* **2015**, *7*, 132. [CrossRef]
37. Tosti, V.; Bertozzi, B.; Fontana, L. Health Benefits of the Mediterranean Diet: Metabolic and Molecular Mechanisms. *J. Gerontol. A Biol. Sci. Med. Sci.* **2018**, *73*, 318–326. [CrossRef]
38. Franceschi, C.; Ostan, R.; Santoro, A. Nutrition and Inflammation: Are Centenarians Similar to Individuals on Calorie-Restricted Diets? *Annu. Rev. Nutr.* **2018**, *38*, 329–356. [CrossRef]

39. De Pablos, R.M.; Espinosa-Oliva, A.M.; Hornedo-Ortega, R.; Cano, M.; Arguelles, S. Hydroxytyrosol protects from aging process via AMPK and autophagy; a review of its effects on cancer, metabolic syndrome, osteoporosis, immune-mediated and neurodegenerative diseases. *Pharmacol. Res.* **2019**, *143*, 58–72. [CrossRef]
40. Ortega, R.M.; Aparicio Vizuete, A.; Jiménez Ortega, A.I.; Rodríguez Rodríguez, E. Wholegrain cereals and sanitary benefits. *Nutr. Hosp.* **2015**, *32*, 25–31. [CrossRef]
41. De Filippis, F.; Pellegrini, N.; Vannini, L.; Jeffery, I.B.; La Storia, A.; Laghi, L.; Serrazanetti, D.I.; Di Cagno, R.; Ferrocino, I.; Lazzi, C.; et al. High-level adherence to a Mediterranean diet beneficially impacts the gut microbiota and associated metabolome. *Gut* **2016**, *65*, 1812–1821. [CrossRef]
42. Estruch, R.; Ros, E.; Salas-Salvadó, J.; Covas, M.I.; Corella, D.; Arós, F.; Gómez-Gracia, E.; Ruiz-Gutiérrez, V.; Fiol, M.; Lapetra, J.; et al. Primary Prevention of Cardiovascular Disease with a Mediterranean Diet Supplemented with Extra-Virgin Olive Oil or Nuts. *N. Engl. J. Med.* **2018**, *378*, e34. [CrossRef]
43. De Lorgeril, M.; Salen, P.; Martin, J.L.; Monjaud, I.; Delaye, J.; Mamelle, N. Mediterranean diet, traditional risk factors, and the rate of cardiovascular complications after myocardial infarction: Final report of the Lyon Diet Heart Study. *Circulation* **1999**, *99*, 779–785. [CrossRef]
44. Wade, A.T.; Davis, C.R.; Dyer, K.A.; Hodgson, J.M.; Woodman, R.J.; Keage, H.A.D.; Murphy, K.J. A Mediterranean Diet with Fresh, Lean Pork Improves Processing Speed and Mood: Cognitive Findings from the MedPork Randomised Controlled Trial. *Nutrients* **2019**, *11*, 1521. [CrossRef]
45. De Lorgeril, M.; Salen, P.; Martin, J.L.; Mamelle, N.; Monjaud, I.; Touboul, P.; Delaye, J. Effect of a mediterranean type of diet on the rate of cardiovascular complications in patients with coronary artery disease. Insights into the cardioprotective effect of certain nutriments. *J. Am. Coll. Cardiol.* **1996**, *28*, 1103–1108. [CrossRef]
46. Ostan, R.; Lanzarini, C.; Pini, E.; Scurti, M.; Vianello, D.; Bertarelli, C.; Fabbri, C.; Izzi, M.; Palmas, G.; Biondi, F.; et al. Inflammaging and cancer: A challenge for the Mediterranean diet. *Nutrients* **2015**, *7*, 2589–2621. [CrossRef]
47. Willis, A.; Greene, M.; Braxton-lloyd, K. An Experimental Study of a Mediterranean-style Diet Supplemented with Nuts and Extra-virgin Olive Oil for Cardiovascular Disease Risk Reduction: The Healthy Hearts Program (P12-021-19). *Curr. Dev. Nutr.* **2019**, *3*. [CrossRef]
48. Tyrovolas, S.; Panagiotakos, D.B. The role of Mediterranean type of diet on the development of cancer and cardiovascular disease, in the elderly: A systematic review. *Maturitas* **2010**, *65*, 122–130. [CrossRef]
49. Sun, L.; Luo, C.; Liu, J. Hydroxytyrosol induces apoptosis in human colon cancer cells through ROS generation. *Food Funct.* **2014**, *5*, 1909–1914. [CrossRef]
50. Luo, C.; Li, Y.; Wang, H.; Cui, Y.; Feng, Z.; Li, H.; Wang, Y.; Wurtz, K.; Weber, P.; Long, J.; et al. Hydroxytyrosol promotes superoxide production and defects in autophagy leading to anti-proliferation and apoptosis on human prostate cancer cells. *Curr. Cancer Drug Targets* **2013**, *13*, 625–639. [CrossRef]
51. Goldsmith, C.D.; Bond, D.R.; Jankowski, H.; Weidenhofer, J.; Stathopoulos, C.E.; Roach, P.D.; Scarlett, C.J. The Olive Biophenols Oleuropein and Hydroxytyrosol Selectively Reduce Proliferation, Influence the Cell Cycle, and Induce Apoptosis in Pancreatic Cancer Cells. *Int. J. Mol. Sci.* **2018**, *19*, 1937. [CrossRef]
52. Cruz-Lozano, M.; González-González, A.; Marchal, J.A.; Muñoz-Muela, E.; Molina, M.P.; Cara, F.E.; Brown, A.M.; García-Rivas, G.; Hernández-Brenes, C.; Lorente, J.A.; et al. Hydroxytyrosol inhibits cancer stem cells and the metastatic capacity of triple-negative breast cancer cell lines by the simultaneous targeting of epithelial-to-mesenchymal transition, Wnt/β-catenin and TGFβ signaling pathways. *Eur. J. Nutr.* **2019**, *58*, 3207–3219. [CrossRef]
53. Sirianni, R.; Chimento, A.; De Luca, A.; Casaburi, I.; Rizza, P.; Onofrio, A.; Iacopetta, D.; Puoci, F.; Andò, S.; Maggiolini, M.; et al. Oleuropein and hydroxytyrosol inhibit MCF-7 breast cancer cell proliferation interfering with ERK1/2 activation. *Mol. Nutr. Food Res.* **2010**, *54*, 833–840. [CrossRef]
54. Martínez, N.; Herrera, M.; Frías, L.; Provencio, M.; Pérez-Carrión, R.; Díaz, V.; Morse, M.; Crespo, M.C. A combination of hydroxytyrosol, omega-3 fatty acids and curcumin improves pain and inflammation among early stage breast cancer patients receiving adjuvant hormonal therapy: Results of a pilot study. *Clin. Transl. Oncol.* **2019**, *21*, 489–498. [CrossRef]

55. Gomez-Marin, B.; Gomez-Delgado, F.; Lopez-Moreno, J.; Alcala-Diaz, J.F.; Jimenez-Lucena, R.; Torres-Peña, J.D.; Garcia-Rios, A.; Ortiz-Morales, A.M.; Yubero-Serrano, E.M.; Del Mar Malagon, M.; et al. Long-term consumption of a Mediterranean diet improves postprandial lipemia in patients with type 2 diabetes: The Cordioprev randomized trial. *Am. J. Clin. Nutr.* **2018**, *108*, 963–970. [CrossRef]
56. Prattichizzo, F.; De Nigris, V.; Spiga, R.; Mancuso, E.; La Sala, L.; Antonicelli, R.; Testa, R.; Procopio, A.D.; Olivieri, F.; Ceriello, A. Inflammageing and metaflammation: The yin and yang of type 2 diabetes. *Ageing Res. Rev.* **2018**, *41*, 1–17. [CrossRef]
57. Caracciolo, B.; Xu, W.; Collins, S.; Fratiglioni, L. Cognitive decline, dietary factors and gut-brain interactions. *Mech. Ageing Dev.* **2014**, *136-137*, 59–69. [CrossRef]
58. Féart, C.; Samieri, C.; Allès, B.; Barberger-Gateau, P. Potential benefits of adherence to the Mediterranean diet on cognitive health. *Proc. Nutr. Soc.* **2013**, *72*, 140–152. [CrossRef]
59. Lange, K.W.; Guo, J.; Kanaya, S.; Lange, K.M.; Nakamura, Y.; Li, S. Medical foods in Alzheimer's disease. *Food Sci. Hum. Wellness* **2019**, *8*, 1–7. [CrossRef]
60. Shannon, O.M.; Stephan, B.C.M.; Granic, A.; Lentjes, M.; Hayat, S.; Mulligan, A.; Brayne, C.; Khaw, K.T.; Bundy, R.; Aldred, S.; et al. Mediterranean diet adherence and cognitive function in older UK adults: The European Prospective Investigation into Cancer and Nutrition-Norfolk (EPIC-Norfolk) Study. *Am. J. Clin. Nutr.* **2019**, *110*, 938–948. [CrossRef]
61. Martínez-Lapiscina, E.H.; Clavero, P.; Toledo, E.; Estruch, R.; Salas-Salvadó, J.; San Julián, B.; Sanchez-Tainta, A.; Ros, E.; Valls-Pedret, C.; Martinez-Gonzalez, M. Mediterranean diet improves cognition: The PREDIMED-NAVARRA randomised trial. *J. Neurol. Neurosurg. Psychiatry* **2013**, *84*, 1318–1325. [CrossRef]
62. Valls-Pedret, C.; Sala-Vila, A.; Serra-Mir, M.; Corella, D.; de la Torre, R.; Martínez-González, M.; Martínez-Lapiscina, E.H.; Fitó, M.; Pérez-Heras, A.; Salas-Salvadó, J.; et al. Mediterranean Diet and Age-Related Cognitive Decline: A Randomized Clinical Trial. *JAMA Intern. Med.* **2015**, *175*, 1094–1103. [CrossRef]
63. Bhatt, A.P.; Redinbo, M.R.; Bultman, S.J. The role of the microbiome in cancer development and therapy. *CA Cancer J. Clin.* **2017**, *67*, 326–344. [CrossRef]
64. Esteve, E.; Ricart, W.; Fernández-Real, J.M. Gut microbiota interactions with obesity, insulin resistance and type 2 diabetes: Did gut microbiote co-evolve with insulin resistance? *Curr. Opin. Clin. Nutr. Metab. Care* **2011**, *14*, 483–490. [CrossRef]
65. Tang, W.H.; Wang, Z.; Levison, B.S.; Koeth, R.A.; Britt, E.B.; Fu, X.; Wu, Y.; Hazen, S.L. Intestinal microbial metabolism of phosphatidylcholine and cardiovascular risk. *N. Engl. J. Med.* **2013**, *368*, 1575–1584. [CrossRef]
66. Tamura, K.; Sasaki, H.; Shiga, K.; Miyakawa, H.; Shibata, S. The Timing Effects of Soy Protein Intake on Mice Gut Microbiota. *Nutrients* **2019**, *12*, 87. [CrossRef]
67. Kuiper, G.G.; Lemmen, J.G.; Carlsson, B.; Corton, J.C.; Safe, S.H.; van der Saag, P.T.; van der Burg, B.; Gustafsson, J.A. Interaction of estrogenic chemicals and phytoestrogens with estrogen receptor beta. *Endocrinology* **1998**, *139*, 4252–4263. [CrossRef]
68. Liggins, J.; Bluck, L.J.; Runswick, S.; Atkinson, C.; Coward, W.A.; Bingham, S.A. Daidzein and genistein content of fruits and nuts. *J. Nutr. Biochem.* **2000**, *11*, 326–331. [CrossRef]
69. Bäckhed, F.; Ding, H.; Wang, T.; Hooper, L.V.; Koh, G.Y.; Nagy, A.; Semenkovich, C.F.; Gordon, J.I. The gut microbiota as an environmental factor that regulates fat storage. *Proc. Natl. Acad. Sci. USA* **2004**, *101*, 15718–15723. [CrossRef]
70. Schwiertz, A.; Taras, D.; Schäfer, K.; Beijer, S.; Bos, N.A.; Donus, C.; Hardt, P.D. Microbiota and SCFA in lean and overweight healthy subjects. *Obesity (Silver Spring)* **2010**, *18*, 190–195. [CrossRef]
71. Zhou, L.; Xiao, X.; Zhang, Q.; Zheng, J.; Deng, M. Maternal Genistein Intake Mitigates the Deleterious Effects of High-Fat Diet on Glucose and Lipid Metabolism and Modulates Gut Microbiota in Adult Life of Male Mice. *Front. Physiol.* **2019**, *10*, 985. [CrossRef]
72. Zhou, L.; Xiao, X.; Zhang, Q.; Zheng, J.; Li, M.; Wang, X.; Deng, M.; Zhai, X.; Liu, J. Gut microbiota might be a crucial factor in deciphering the metabolic benefits of perinatal genistein consumption in dams and adult female offspring. *Food Funct.* **2019**, *10*, 4505–4521. [CrossRef]
73. López, P.; Sánchez, M.; Perez-Cruz, C.; Velázquez-Villegas, L.A.; Syeda, T.; Aguilar-López, M.; Rocha-Viggiano, A.K.; Del Carmen Silva-Lucero, M.; Torre-Villalvazo, I.; Noriega, L.G.; et al. Long-Term Genistein Consumption Modifies Gut Microbiota, Improving Glucose Metabolism, Metabolic Endotoxemia, and Cognitive Function in Mice Fed a High-Fat Diet. *Mol. Nutr. Food Res.* **2018**, *62*, e1800313. [CrossRef]

74. Borras, C.; Gambini, J.; Gomez-Cabrera, M.C.; Sastre, J.; Pallardo, F.V.; Mann, G.E.; Vina, J. Genistein, a soy isoflavone, up-regulates expression of antioxidant genes: Involvement of estrogen receptors, ERK1/2, and NFkappaB. *FASEB J.* **2006**, *20*, 2136–2138. [CrossRef]
75. Pryde, S.E.; Duncan, S.H.; Hold, G.L.; Stewart, C.S.; Flint, H.J. The microbiology of butyrate formation in the human colon. *FEMS Microbiol. Lett.* **2002**, *217*, 133–139. [CrossRef] [PubMed]
76. David, L.A.; Materna, A.C.; Friedman, J.; Campos-Baptista, M.I.; Blackburn, M.C.; Perrotta, A.; Erdman, S.E.; Alm, E.J. Host lifestyle affects human microbiota on daily timescales. *Genome Biol.* **2014**, *15*, R89. [CrossRef] [PubMed]
77. Hamilton, M.J.; Weingarden, A.R.; Sadowsky, M.J.; Khoruts, A. Standardized frozen preparation for transplantation of fecal microbiota for recurrent Clostridium difficile infection. *Am. J. Gastroenterol.* **2012**, *107*, 761–767. [CrossRef]
78. Aroniadis, O.C.; Brandt, L.J. Intestinal microbiota and the efficacy of fecal microbiota transplantation in gastrointestinal disease. *Gastroenterol. Hepatol.* **2014**, *10*, 230–237.
79. Zhang, J.; Ren, L.; Yu, M.; Liu, X.; Ma, W.; Huang, L.; Li, X.; Ye, X. S-equol inhibits proliferation and promotes apoptosis of human breast cancer MCF-7 cells via regulating miR-10a-5p and PI3K/AKT pathway. *Arch. Biochem. Biophys.* **2019**, *672*, 108064. [CrossRef] [PubMed]
80. Horiuchi, H.; Usami, A.; Shirai, R.; Harada, N.; Ikushiro, S.; Sakaki, T.; Nakano, Y.; Inui, H.; Yamaji, R. S-Equol Activates cAMP Signaling at the Plasma Membrane of INS-1 Pancreatic β-Cells and Protects against Streptozotocin-Induced Hyperglycemia by Increasing β-Cell Function in Male Mice. *J. Nutr.* **2017**, *147*, 1631–1639. [CrossRef] [PubMed]
81. Bielak-Zmijewska, A.; Grabowska, W.; Ciolko, A.; Bojko, A.; Mosieniak, G.; Bijoch, Ł.; Sikora, E. The Role of Curcumin in the Modulation of Ageing. *Int. J. Mol. Sci.* **2019**, *20*, 1239. [CrossRef] [PubMed]
82. Skyvalidas, D.; Mavropoulos, A.; Tsiogkas, S.; Dardiotis, E.; Liaskos, C.; Mamuris, Z.; Roussaki-Schulze, A.; Sakkas, L.I.; Zafiriou, E.; Bogdanos, D.P. Curcumin mediates attenuation of pro-inflammatory interferon γ and interleukin 17 cytokine responses in psoriatic disease, strengthening its role as a dietary immunosuppressant. *Nutr. Res.* **2020**, *75*, 95–108. [CrossRef] [PubMed]
83. Di Meo, F.; Margarucci, S.; Galderisi, U.; Crispi, S.; Peluso, G. Curcumin, Gut Microbiota, and Neuroprotection. *Nutrients* **2019**, *11*, 2426. [CrossRef]
84. Ticinesi, A.; Tana, C.; Nouvenne, A.; Prati, B.; Lauretani, F.; Meschi, T. Gut microbiota, cognitive frailty and dementia in older individuals: A systematic review. *Clin. Interv. Aging* **2018**, *13*, 1497–1511. [CrossRef]
85. Arana Cañedo-Argüelles, C. Fibra dietética. *Rev. Pediatría Atención Primaria* **2006**, *8* (Suppl. 1), 83–97.
86. Pascual, V.; Perez Martinez, P.; Fernández, J.M.; Solá, R.; Pallarés, V.; Romero Secín, A.; Pérez Jiménez, F.; Ros, E. SEA/SEMERGEN consensus document 2019: Dietary recommendations in the prevention of cardiovascular disease. *Semergen* **2019**, *45*, 333–348. [CrossRef] [PubMed]
87. Casiglia, E.; Tikhonoff, V.; Caffi, S.; Boschetti, G.; Grasselli, C.; Saugo, M.; Giordano, N.; Rapisarda, V.; Spinella, P.; Palatini, P. High dietary fiber intake prevents stroke at a population level. *Clin. Nutr.* **2013**, *32*, 811–818. [CrossRef] [PubMed]
88. Larsson, S.C.; Wolk, A. Dietary fiber intake is inversely associated with stroke incidence in healthy Swedish adults. *J. Nutr.* **2014**, *144*, 1952–1955. [CrossRef] [PubMed]
89. Tucker, L.A. Dietary Fiber and Telomere Length in 5674 U.S. Adults: An NHANES Study of Biological Aging. *Nutrients* **2018**, *10*, 400. [CrossRef]
90. Kuller, L.H. Dietary fat and chronic diseases: Epidemiologic overview. *J. Am. Diet. Assoc.* **1997**, *97*, S9–S15. [CrossRef]
91. Everitt, A.V.; Hilmer, S.N.; Brand-Miller, J.C.; Jamieson, H.A.; Truswell, A.S.; Sharma, A.P.; Mason, R.S.; Morris, B.J.; Le Couteur, D.G. Dietary approaches that delay age-related diseases. *Clin. Interv. Aging* **2006**, *1*, 11–31. [CrossRef]
92. Turnbaugh, P.J.; Ridaura, V.K.; Faith, J.J.; Rey, F.E.; Knight, R.; Gordon, J.I. The effect of diet on the human gut microbiome: A metagenomic analysis in humanized gnotobiotic mice. *Sci. Transl. Med.* **2009**, *1*, 6ra14. [CrossRef]
93. Ma, J.; Li, H. The Role of Gut Microbiota in Atherosclerosis and Hypertension. *Front. Pharmacol.* **2018**, *9*, 1082. [CrossRef]

94. Zhang, C.; Zhang, M.; Wang, S.; Han, R.; Cao, Y.; Hua, W.; Mao, Y.; Zhang, X.; Pang, X.; Wei, C.; et al. Interactions between gut microbiota, host genetics and diet relevant to development of metabolic syndromes in mice. *ISME J.* **2010**, *4*, 232–241. [CrossRef]
95. Brandsma, E.; Kloosterhuis, N.J.; Koster, M.; Dekker, D.C.; Gijbels, M.J.J.; van der Velden, S.; Ríos-Morales, M.; van Faassen, M.J.R.; Loreti, M.G.; de Bruin, A.; et al. A Proinflammatory Gut Microbiota Increases Systemic Inflammation and Accelerates Atherosclerosis. *Circ. Res.* **2019**, *124*, 94–100. [CrossRef] [PubMed]
96. De Filippo, C.; Cavalieri, D.; Di Paola, M.; Ramazzotti, M.; Poullet, J.B.; Massart, S.; Collini, S.; Pieraccini, G.; Lionetti, P. Impact of diet in shaping gut microbiota revealed by a comparative study in children from Europe and rural Africa. *Proc. Natl. Acad. Sci. USA* **2010**, *107*, 14691–14696. [CrossRef] [PubMed]
97. Larrosa, M.; Luceri, C.; Vivoli, E.; Pagliuca, C.; Lodovici, M.; Moneti, G.; Dolara, P. Polyphenol metabolites from colonic microbiota exert anti-inflammatory activity on different inflammation models. *Mol. Nutr. Food Res.* **2009**, *53*, 1044–1054. [CrossRef] [PubMed]
98. Handy, D.E.; Castro, R.; Loscalzo, J. Epigenetic modifications: Basic mechanisms and role in cardiovascular disease. *Circulation* **2011**, *123*, 2145–2156. [CrossRef] [PubMed]
99. Larrosa, M.; González-Sarrías, A.; Yáñez-Gascón, M.J.; Selma, M.V.; Azorín-Ortuño, M.; Toti, S.; Tomás-Barberán, F.; Dolara, P.; Espín, J.C. Anti-inflammatory properties of a pomegranate extract and its metabolite urolithin-A in a colitis rat model and the effect of colon inflammation on phenolic metabolism. *J. Nutr. Biochem.* **2010**, *21*, 717–725. [CrossRef]
100. Selma, M.V.; Tomás-Barberán, F.A.; Beltrán, D.; García-Villalba, R.; Espín, J.C. Gordonibacter urolithinfaciens sp. nov., a urolithin-producing bacterium isolated from the human gut. *Int. J. Syst. Evol. Microbiol.* **2014**, *64*, 2346–2352. [CrossRef]
101. Sreng, N.; Champion, S.; Martin, J.C.; Khelaifia, S.; Christensen, J.E.; Padmanabhan, R.; Azalbert, V.; Blasco-Baque, V.; Loubieres, P.; Pechere, L.; et al. Resveratrol-mediated glycemic regulation is blunted by curcumin and is associated to modulation of gut microbiota. *J. Nutr. Biochem.* **2019**, *72*, 108218. [CrossRef]
102. Parkar, S.G.; Trower, T.M.; Stevenson, D.E. Fecal microbial metabolism of polyphenols and its effects on human gut microbiota. *Anaerobe* **2013**, *23*, 12–19. [CrossRef]

biomedicines

MDPI

Review

Antiplatelet Therapy for Acute Respiratory Distress Syndrome

Chuan-Mu Chen [1,2,†], Hsiao-Ching Lu [3,†], Yu-Tang Tung [4,5,6,*] and Wei Chen [1,7,*]

1. Department of Life Sciences, National Chung Hsing University, 145 Xingda Road, Taichung 402, Taiwan; chchen1@dragon.nchu.edu.tw
2. The iEGG and Animal Biotechnology Center, and the Rong Hsing Research Center for Translational Medicine, National Chung Hsing University, Taichung 402, Taiwan
3. Division of Respiratory Therapy, Chia-Yi Christian Hospital, Chiayi 60002, Taiwan; 00614@cych.org.tw
4. Graduate Institute of Metabolism and Obesity Sciences, Taipei Medical University, Taipei 110, Taiwan
5. Nutrition Research Center, Taipei Medical University Hospital, Taipei City 110, Taiwan
6. Cell Physiology and Molecular Image Research Center, Wan Fang Hospital, Taipei Medical University, Taipei 110, Taiwan
7. Division of Pulmonary and Critical Care Medicine, Chia-Yi Christian Hospital, Chiayi 60002, Taiwan

* Correspondence: f91625059@tmu.edu.tw (Y.-T.T.); peteralfa2004@gmail.com (W.C.); Tel.: +886-227361661 (Y.-T.T.); +886-5-2779365 (ext. 6172) (W.C.)

† These authors contributed equally to this work.

Received: 11 June 2020; Accepted: 18 July 2020; Published: 21 July 2020

Abstract: Acute respiratory distress syndrome (ARDS) is a common and devastating syndrome that contributes to serious morbidities and mortality in critically ill patients. No known pharmacologic therapy is beneficial in the treatment of ARDS, and the only effective management is through a protective lung strategy. Platelets play a crucial role in the pathogenesis of ARDS, and antiplatelet therapy may be a potential medication for ARDS. In this review, we introduce the overall pathogenesis of ARDS, and then focus on platelet-related mechanisms underlying the development of ARDS, including platelet adhesion to the injured vessel wall, platelet-leukocyte-endothelium interactions, platelet-related lipid mediators, and neutrophil extracellular traps. We further summarize antiplatelet therapy, including aspirin, glycoprotein IIb/IIIa receptor antagonists, and P2Y12 inhibitors for ARDS in experimental and clinical studies and a meta-analysis. Novel aspirin-derived agents, aspirin-triggered lipoxin, and aspirin-triggered resolvin D1 are also described here. In this narrative review, we summarize the current knowledge of the role of platelets in the pathogenesis of ARDS, and the potential benefits of antiplatelet therapy for the prevention and treatment of ARDS.

Keywords: acute respiratory distress syndrome; antiplatelet; aspirin; therapy

1. Introduction

1.1. Definition and Epidemiology of ARDS

Acute respiratory distress syndrome (ARDS), or acute lung injury, is a devastating syndrome that contributes to serious morbidities and mortality in critically ill patients. The definition of this syndrome includes the acute onset of respiratory failure, bilateral infiltrates observed on chest radiographs, hypoxemia with a PaO_2/FiO_2 ratio ≤ 300 mmHg with at least positive end-expiratory pressure of 5 cmH_2O, and no evidence of left atrial hypertension [1,2]. A variety of clinical disorders are associated with the development of ARDS, including direct lung injury, such as bacterial pneumonia, aspiration of gastric contents, or indirect lung injury, such as sepsis, trauma, and transfusion of blood product [3]. The crude incidence of ARDS was around 15 to 80 per 100,000 people per year worldwide [4,5], and the mortality rate is high (approaching 40%) [4]. The only effective management to date to improve the survival rate of this syndrome is a protective lung strategy, with lower tidal volume ventilation [6]. Although numerous promising therapies have been effective in the prevention of ARDS in experimental models, the successful translation to clinical application is still lacking [7–9]. In addition, in those who survive the illness, ARDS caused a substantial social burden, such as reduced exercise stamina and health-related quality of life, and increased costs and use of health care services [4,10–15]. Therefore, the discovery of medications to prevent the development of ARDS is crucial.

1.2. Pathogenesis of ARDS

The pathological features of ARDS are best described at three time points: acute, subacute, and chronic phases [16–18]. The acute or exudative phase (the first 1–6 days) is characterized by the influx of protein-rich edema fluid, accompanied by the accumulation of neutrophils, macrophages, exosomes [19], and red blood cells (polymorphonuclear leukocyte [PMN] predominant) into the air spaces as a consequence of the increased permeability of the alveolar–capillary barrier [20,21], as shown in Figure 1. As a result of both endothelial and epithelial injury, denuding of the alveolar epithelium and prominent hyaline membranes can be seen [3,22]. The robust inflammatory response is due to the release of oxidants, proteases, and other potentially toxic agents from activated leukocytes [23,24]. In the air space, alveolar macrophages secrete cytokines, interleukin (IL)-1, -6, -8, and -10, and tumor necrosis factor-α (TNF-α), which act locally to stimulate chemotaxis and activate neutrophils. Macrophages also secrete other cytokines, including IL-1, -6, and -10. IL-1 can also stimulate the production of extracellular matrix by fibroblasts. Neutrophils can release oxidants, proteases, leukotrienes, and other pro-inflammatory molecules, such as platelet-activating factor (PAF). An imbalance between pro-inflammatory and anti-inflammatory mediators can be found in ARDS. A number of anti-inflammatory mediators are also present in the alveolar milieu, including IL-1–receptor antagonist, club cell protein 16 [25], soluble tumor necrosis factor receptor, autoantibodies against IL-8, and cytokines such as IL-10 and -11 [3]. In the subacute or proliferative phase (the next 7–14 days), some edema has usually been reabsorbed, and is often accompanied by interstitial fibrosis, a proliferation of type 2 alveolar cells, and the disruption of capillary function, due to microvascular thrombus formation. Infiltration of fibroblasts and collagen deposition may also be observed. Some experts view ARDS as a vascular microthombotic disease, and its pathogenesis is based on a novel "two-path unifying theory" of hemostasis and "two-activation theory of the endothelium", promoting molecular pathogenesis [26]. Some patients have a rapid resolution of the disorder [27], but others have progression to fibrotic lung injury, which is called the chronic or fibrotic phase (usually after 14 days). In the chronic phase, there is a resolution of the acute neutrophilic infiltrate with more mononuclear cells and alveolar macrophages in the alveoli, and often more fibrosis, with ongoing evidence of alveolar epithelial repair [17].

Overall, dysregulated inflammation [28,29], the inappropriate accumulation and activity of leukocytes and platelets [30], uncontrolled activation of coagulation pathways, and altered permeability of alveolar endothelial and epithelial barriers are pathophysiological hallmarks of ARDS [3,31,32]. Of note, endotheliopathy activates two independent molecular pathways: inflammatory and microthrombotic. The inflammatory pathway initiates inflammation, but the microthrombotic pathway more seriously produces "microthrombi strings" composed of platelet- von Willebrand factor multimer complexes, which become anchored on injured endothelial cells and causes disseminated intravascular microthrombosis [26]. Activated neutrophils affect surrounding lung tissue via several potentially pathogenic cellular mechanisms, including the release of lysosomal proteolytic enzymes [33], the production of prostanoids [34], and the generation of highly reactive oxygen radicals and intermediates [35]. All these mechanisms lead to tissue damage, increased permeability of the alveolar-capillary barrier, and the formation of protein-rich lung edema [36].

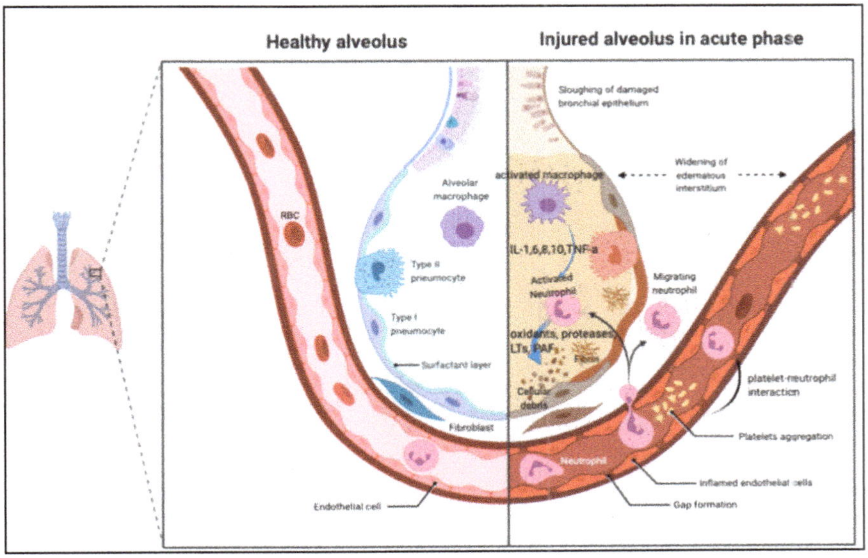

Figure 1. The pathological features of acute respiratory distress syndrome (ARDS) in the acute phase. In the air space, alveolar macrophages secrete cytokines locally to stimulate chemotaxis and activate neutrophils. Neutrophils can release oxidants, proteases, leukotrienes, and other pro-inflammatory molecules, such as platelet-activating factor (PAF). PAF: platelet-activating factor; IL: interleukin; TNF: tumor necrosis factor; LTs: leukotriene.

2. Mechanisms of Platelet in Lung Inflammation

2.1. The Role of Platelet in the ARDS

Platelets are anucleated fragments of bone marrow megakaryocytes of approximately 2–4 μm in diameter, and contain glycogen, mitochondria, and at least three types of granules (dense core granules, lysosomes, and α -granules). Following activation, platelets can secrete the content of the granules, change their shape, and upregulate the expression of adhesion molecules including P-selectin, platelet and endothelial cell adhesion molecule 1 (PECAM-1, also known as CD31), glycoprotein (GP) IIb/IIIa (α IIbβ 3) integrin, fibronectin, and thrombospondin [37]. PECAM1 is a member of the immunoglobulin superfamily of adhesion molecules localized at endothelial cell-cell junctions, and contributes to the maintenance of vascular integrity in resting cells, as well as playing a role in the restoration of vascular integrity following barrier disruption [38]. PECAM1 can be cleaved from endothelial cells by a number of mechanisms, including shear stress, resulting in a secreted, shed form of protein (sPECAM1) that is soluble, and can be released into circulation, exerting proinflammatory effects. The upregulation of PECAM1 and/or reducing sPECAM1 through extracorporeal removal or pharmacologic inhibition might be a novel therapeutic strategy in ARDS [39]. Platelets have an increasingly recognized role in the inflammatory response, leading to the development of ARDS. The possible mechanisms by which platelets contribute to ARDS include the activation of endothelial cells by the release of pro-inflammatory mediators [40–46] and adherence of platelets to lung capillary endothelial cells leading to the activation of attached leukocytes [47], as shown in Figure 2.

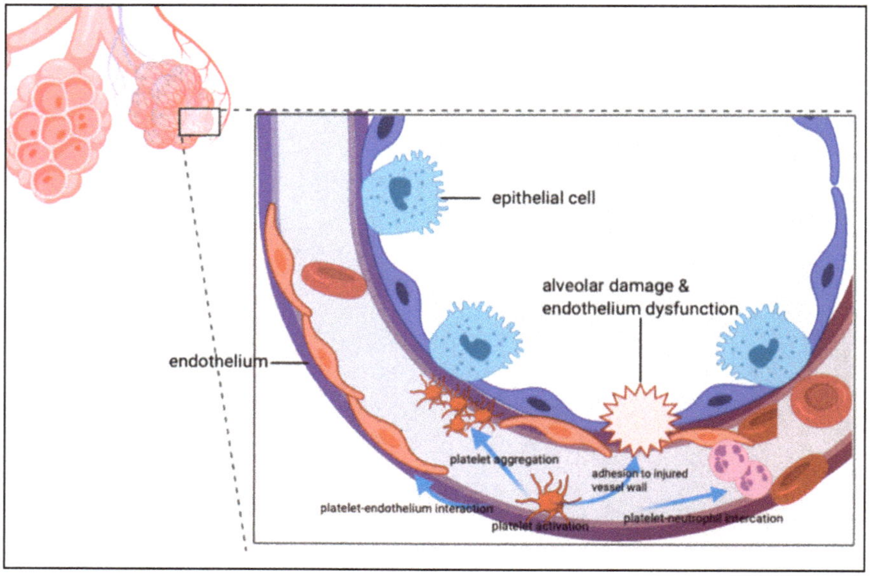

Figure 2. The role of platelets in acute respiratory distress syndrome. Platelets have an increasingly recognized role in the inflammatory response leading to the development of ARDS. The possible mechanisms by which platelets contribute to ARDS include the activation of endothelial cells by the release of pro-inflammatory mediators and adherence of platelets to lung capillary endothelial cells leading to activation of attached leukocytes.

2.2. *Platelet Adhesion to the Injured Vessel Wall*

Not only neutrophils, but also platelets, are shown to adhere to injured capillary endothelium in the acute phase of ARDS. At sites of vascular injury and endothelial denudation, platelets adhere to activated endothelial cells or in the subendothelial matrix [48] directly or indirectly. The direct binding of platelets to extracellular collagen at sites of vascular injury is mediated via several GPs. Platelet surface receptors GP Ia/IIa, GPIV, and GPVI interact directly with collagen, and platelet surface receptors GP Ib/V/IX interact with von Willebrand factor [49]. Binding the GP Ib/IX/V complex to von Willebrand factor initiates the activation of the integrin $\alpha IIb\beta 3$ on platelets, resulting in platelet aggregates via RGD-containing bridging molecules, such as fibrinogen, fibronectin, and thrombospondin [50–52]. In addition, the platelet receptor C-type lectin-like 2 (CLEC-2) has been shown to regulate vascular integrity at sites of acute inflammation [53]. CLEC-2 expressed in platelets is required to limit neutrophil recruitment, which, in turn, limits lung function decline in a mouse model of ARDS. In addition, the expression of the CLEC-2 ligand podoplanin is required in hematopoietic cells to limit neutrophil chemokine expression and, consequently, arterial oxygen saturation decline [54].

2.3. *Platelet-Leukocyte-Endothelium Interactions*

Platelet-neutrophil-endothelium interactions are involved in the lung inflammation of ARDS. As shown in Figure 3, platelet adhesion to the intact endothelium is mediated by at least two different types of adhesion molecules, selectins and integrins. GP IIb/IIIa ($\alpha IIb\beta 3$ integrin) is an important adhesion molecule in platelets that is responsible for mediating platelet aggregation and some platelet-neutrophil-interactions. Injection of platelet-specific monoclonal antibodies against the GP IIb/IIIa receptor in mice causes early signs of acute lung injury with increased cellularity in the lung interstitium and rapid engorgement of alveolar septal vessels [55]. P-selectin, a type I membrane protein, is stored in the α-granules of platelets and Weibel-Palade bodies of endothelial cells, from where it is rapidly expressed on the cell surface by a Ca^{2+}-dependent translocation to the plasma membrane [56]. Upon activation, platelets bind to endothelial cells by expressing P-selectin via GP Ibα and P-selectin glycoprotein ligand-1 (PSGL-1). Following a conformational change, αIIbβ3 integrins establish strong adhesion of platelets by binding to small bridging ligands, such as fibrinogen or vitronectin, which interact with the endothelial adhesion molecules αvβ3 or intercellular adhesion molecule 1 (ICAM-1) [57]. To attract the neutrophils, P-selectin mediates the initial binding ('capturing") of platelets to leukocytes and leukocytes to endothelial cells. Following the adhesion of neutrophils to platelets, neutrophils are activated through PSGL-1 [58], the triggering receptor expressed on myeloid cells (TREM)-1 [59], lipid mediators, and chemokines presented by platelets. In an experimental study, Zhao et al. showed that the blockade of PSGL-1 results in diminished alveolar neutrophil transmigration in lipopolysaccharide (LPS)-induced acute lung injury in mice, indicating that platelets and their interaction with neutrophils are requisite for the development of LPS-induced lung inflammation and injury [60]. TREM-like transcript-1 (TLT-1) is a type-1 immunoglobulin domain receptor that is stored in platelet α-granules and, upon platelet activation, translocate to the surface. TLT-1 uses fibrinogen to govern the transition between inflammation and hemostasis, and facilitates controlled leukocyte transmigration during the progression of ARDS [61]. Collectively, activated platelets play a crucial role in host defense, influencing pulmonary neutrophil recruitment, and contribute to the development of ARDS [40,62,63]. Upon activation, platelets can adhere to other platelets or leukocytes, forming neutrophil platelet aggregates (NPAs) or monocyte-platelet aggregates (MPAs), and to exposed endothelium at sites of inflammation [64]. The presence of circulating leukocyte platelet aggregates (LPAs) is a sensitive indicator of platelet activation, and thrombus formation has been associated with the severity of acute lung injury [65]. Furthermore, Ortiz-Muñoz et al. reported that the dynamic formation of LPAs observed by using lung intravital microscopy sharply increased with acute lung injury [66]. The measurement of LPA in patients with ARDS and other critical illnesses could be a useful biomarker of inflammation, and could be measured serially, to assess therapeutic responses to treatment with pro-resolving lipid mediators.

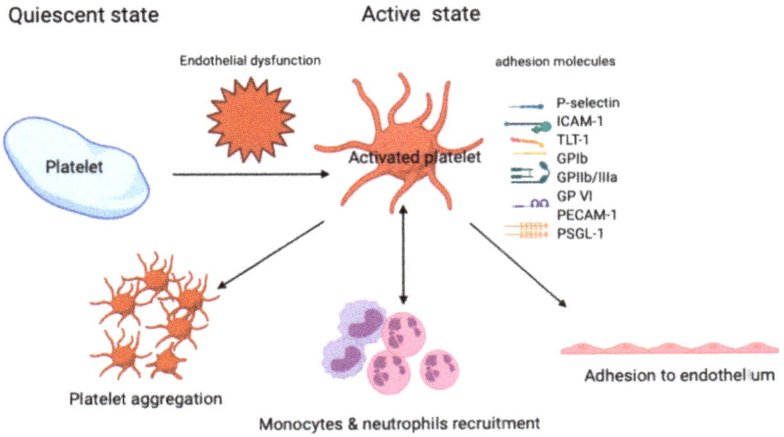

Figure 3. The role of specific adhesion molecules in the platelet-neutrophil interaction, adhesion to endothelium, and platelet aggregation. Triggering receptor expressed on myeloid cells (TREM)-like transcript-1: TLT-1; intercellular adhesion molecule-1: ICAM-1; P-selectin glycoprotein ligand 1: PSGL-1; glycoprotein: GP; Platelet and endothelial cell adhesion molecule-1: PECAM-1.

2.4. Lipid Mediators and Platelet Aggregation

The aggregation of platelets at sites of lung injury to facilitate the recruitment of neutrophils to the injured alveolus is an important mechanism in the development of ARDS [40]. Lipid mediators play a pivotal role in the aggregation of platelets and regulation of inflammation, and arachidonic acid-derived products, such as thromboxane (TX) and leukotrienes (LTs), have been implicated as pro-inflammatory mediators of ARDS [67]. For aggregation, platelets release arachidonic acid through a membrane-bound lipase. Arachidonic acid is converted to TXA2 via a multistep process, which is a powerful mediator of platelet aggregating response. Cyclooxygenase is the key enzyme responsible for the synthesis of prostaglandins (PGs) and TXA2 in platelets. In addition, cyclooxygenase is involved in oxidative stress-induced acute lung injury, suggesting a link between neutrophil-derived oxidative stress and endothelial eicosanoid metabolism [68]. Aspirin has significant antiplatelet properties through the inhibition of cyclooxygenase enzymes that prevent TXA2 production, therefore suppressing platelet aggregation in animal models of acute lung injury [69].

Cytosolic phospholipase A2 (cPLA2) is a key enzyme for the production of inflammatory mediators, such as TXs and LTs, which are generated from arachidonic acid by cyclooxygenase and 5-lipoxygenase, respectively. Nagase et al. reported that the disruption of the gene encoding cPLA2 significantly reduced pulmonary edema, PMN sequestration, and deterioration of the gas exchange in a murine model of LPS-induced acute lung injury [70], indicating that the inhibition of cPLA2-initiated pathways may provide a therapeutic approach to acute lung injury. On the contrary, cPLA2 could act with the reactive oxygen species produced during intestinal ischemia-reperfusion, resulting in the exacerbation of the inflammatory reaction in ARDS [71]. Platelet-activating factor (PAF), a potent phospholipid activator and one of the lipid mediators of platelet aggregation, is also associated with the development of ARDS [72]. The presence of G994T polymorphism in exon 9 of the plasma PAF acetylhydrolase gene has a better survival rate in ARDS [73].

2.5. Neutrophil Extracellular Traps (NETs)

Sepsis syndrome is the primary etiology of ARDS and is associated with a 35–45% incidence of ARDS development [74]. It has been hypothesized that endotoxemia and phagocytosis of bacteria are involved in the pathogenesis of septic syndrome-associated ARDS [75]. Platelets express toll-like receptors (TLRs), including TLR2 and TLR4, that recognize the common bacterial molecules peptidoglycan and LPS, respectively [76]. Activated platelets, particularly in the context of LPS stimulation, trigger the release of extracellular DNA traps (NETs), with proteolytic activity from neutrophils, serving to capture and degrade microbes [76]. These NETs are capable of trapping and killing extracellular pathogens in blood and tissues during infection [77]. However, NETs are not only produced during severe infections, but have also been observed in various inflammatory diseases [78–80]. Caudrillier et al. showed that platelet-induced NETs contribute to lung endothelial injury, and that targeting NET formation with either aspirin or a GP IIb/IIIa inhibitor decreased NET formation and lung injury in the experimental model of transfusion-related acute lung injury (TRALI) [62]. Nitrostyrene derivatives (BNSDs) have been identified as inhibitors of phospholipase and tyrosine kinase, antibacterial agents, and macrophage immune response regulators, and attenuate LPS-mediated acute lung injury via the inhibition of neutrophil-platelet interactions and NET release [81].

3. Antiplatelet Agents in Experimental Studies

3.1. Aspirin

Aspirin is a well-known, irreversible, noncompetitive inhibitor of arachidonic acid cyclooxygenase metabolism and is commonly used in clinical practice. Preclinical studies have shown that aspirin can prevent or treat ARDS by decreasing neutrophil activation and recruitment to the lung, TNF-α expression in pulmonary intravascular macrophages, plasma TX B2 levels, and platelet sequestration in the lungs [62,69,82–85]. Aspirin also reduces the severity of edema and vascular permeability in oxidative stress-induced acute lung injury [68]. Looney et al. showed that treatment with aspirin prevented lung injury and mortality, but blocking P-selectin or CD11b/CD18 pathways did not.

These data suggest a 2-step mechanism of TRALI: priming hematopoietic cells, followed by vascular deposition of activated neutrophils and platelets that then mediate severe lung injury [69]. In addition, Bates et al. showed that delayed postoperative neutrophil apoptosis is significantly preserved in patients taking 300 mg of aspirin on the day before surgery, indicating that aspirin may be able to ameliorate to promote a resolution for persistent inflammation [86].

Another function of aspirin in treating acute lung injury is the acetylation of cyclooxygenase-2 (COX-2) that causes a conformational change, leading to the inhibition of prostanoid synthesis [87]. The acetylation of COX-2 switches catalytic activity to convert arachidonic acid to 15R-hydroxyeicosatetraenoic acid, which can be subsequently converted to 15(R)-epi-lipoxin A4 (15[R]-epi-LXA4), also known as aspirin-triggered lipoxin (ATL) [88]. Lipoxins are endogenous lipid mediators generated during inflammation that can block inflammatory cell recruitment, inhibit cytokine release, and decrease vascular permeability, which collectively are anti-inflammatory properties [89,90]. Ortiz-Muñoz et al. showed that aspirin treatment increased levels of ATL, and treatment with ATL in both lipopolysaccharide and TRALI models protected the lung from acute lung injury [66]. In addition, delayed neutrophil apoptosis is a prominent feature of ARDS [91], which results in prolonging the period of lung injury and hypoxia. Aspirin has previously been shown to preserve neutrophil apoptosis [86], and experimental evidence suggests that ATL restores neutrophil apoptosis and enhances the resolution of alveolar inflammation [92].

Neutrophil recruitment to sites of lung injury may also be modulated through aspirin-triggered anti-inflammatory mediators. In the case of aspirin treatment, aspirin-acetylated COX-2 generates 17R-HDHA, which, following sequential oxygenation by 5-lipoxygenase, results in the production of 17-epi-RvD1, also known as aspirin-triggered RvD1 (AT-RvD1). AT-RvD1 is the 17R epimer of RvD1 (7S, 8R, 17R-trihydroxy-4Z, 9E, 11E, 13Z,15E, 19Z-docosahexaenoic acid), which is more resistant to catalysis than RvD1 [93]. Eickmeier et al. showed that AT-RvD1 inhibited neutrophil-platelet heterotypic interactions by downregulating both P-selectin and its ligand CD24. AT-RvD1 also significantly decreased levels of bronchoalveolar lavage fluid pro-inflammatory cytokines, including IL-1β, IL-6, and TNF-α, and decreased nuclear factor-κB (NF-κB)-phosphorylated p65 nuclear translocation in an acid-initiated lung injury model. This suggests that aspirin therapy might decrease the severity and augment the resolution of ARDS [85]. Tang et al. demonstrated, for the first time, that AT-RvD1– and p-RvD1-treated mice have significantly reduced lung inflammatory responses, including TNF-α, IL-6, keratinocyte cell-derived chemokine, and macrophage inflammatory protein (MIP)-1α and reduced lung injury after immunoglobulin G immune complex deposition, suggesting a new approach to blocking immune complex-induced inflammation [94]. Our study also showed that pretreatment with aspirin reduced NF-κB activation, active oxygen species expression, the number of macrophages, neutrophil infiltration, and lung edema compared with hyperoxia-only treatment in NF-κB-luciferase transgenic mice [95]. Cox et al. showed that AT-RvD1 treatment resulted in reduced oxidative stress, increased glutathione production, and significantly decreased tissue inflammation, indicating that AT-RvD1 is an effective therapy for prolonged hyperoxic exposure in this murine model [96]. A brief summary of the aspirin effect is shown in Figure 4.

3.2. GP IIb/IIIa Antagonists

GP IIb/IIIa receptor inhibitors that mediate platelet-platelet binding through fibrinogen [97] are currently used as a preventive medication for coronary artery disease after percutaneous coronary intervention. Commercially available GP IIb/IIIa receptor inhibitors include abciximab, eptifibatide, and tirofiban.

In a murine model of influenza A virus infections, GP IIb/IIIa antagonist, eptifibatide is shown to protect mice from death caused by influenza viruses, by reducing aggregates of activated platelets [98]. Sharron showed that eptifibatide attenuates platelet granzyme B-mediated apoptosis and results in less severe sepsis and extended survival in a murine model of abdominal sepsis [99], indicating that the GP IIb/IIIa antagonist may be a target for the treatment of sepsis-related ARDS. Caudrillier et al. also showed that another GP IIb/IIIa antagonist, tirofiban, was shown to be effective in the treatment of TRALI by decreasing soluble NET components [62].

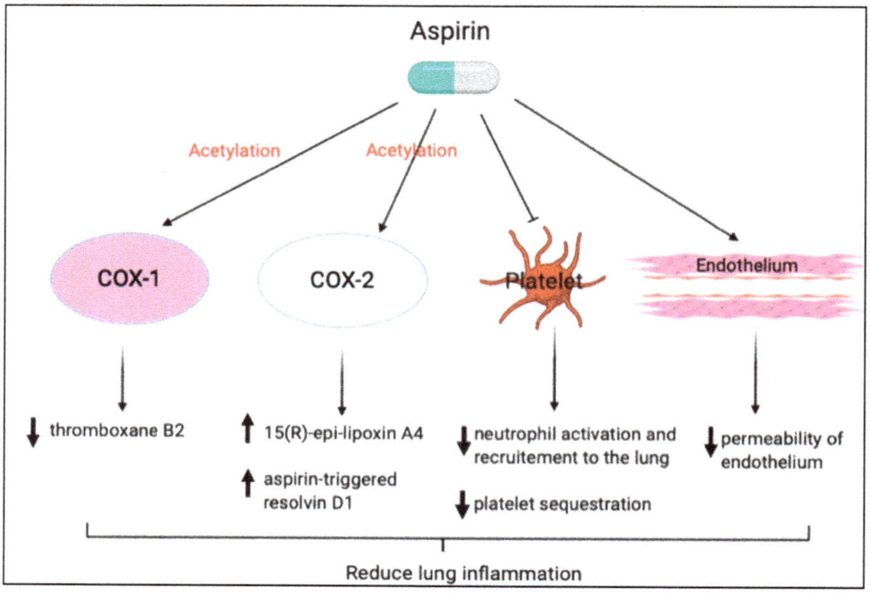

Figure 4. Protective effects of aspirin against lung inflammation. Neutrophil recruitment to the sites of lung injury may also be modulated through aspirin-triggered anti-inflammatory mediators.

3.3. *P2Y12 Inhibitors*

The P2Y12 protein, a chemoreceptor for adenosine diphosphate, is found mainly but not exclusively on the surface of platelets and belongs to the Gi class of a group of G protein-coupled purinergic receptors [100]. Commercially available P2Y12 inhibitors include clopidogrel, prasugrel, and ticagrelor, mainly indicated for cardiovascular diseases. Several studies have shown that clopidogrel not only diminishes the risk of atherothrombotic events, but also reduces the markers of systemic inflammation, including C-reactive protein, soluble CD62P (P-selectin) and CD54, pro-inflammatory cytokines, and platelet-leukocyte conjugates [101]. Harr et al. showed that rats pretreated with clopidogrel were protected from trauma/hemorrhagic shock-related acute lung injury by reducing platelet activation and aggregation, microthrombi formation, and leukocyte recruitment [102]. Le et al. also showed that clopidogrel had a similar effect as the GP IIb/IIIa antagonist, to protect mice from death caused in an experimental model of influenza virus A infection [98]. Tuinman et al. reported that clopidogrel attenuates LPS-induced lung injury in mice, but its effect is inferior to high-dose aspirin [83].

For antiplatelet therapy to treat or prevent ARDS, there are several major differences between animal experiments and human studies. First, the lung injury model of animal experiments cannot fully comply with the process of human acute lung injury. Second, people who develop lung injury usually have comorbidities, which can lead to different outcomes even with the same treatment. Third, the therapeutic dose for animals, once used in humans, may be too high and cause side effects. Fourth, there are too many causes for ARDS in the human body, which results in so-called heterogeneity. For these reasons, it is quite difficult for a single drug to be successful in people with ARDS.

4. Antiplatelet Agents in Clinical Studies

The human study regarding aspirin for treating or preventing ARDS was conducted around 20 years ago. As shown in Table 1, Erlich and colleagues performed a retrospective analysis of 161 patients from Olmsted County, Minnesota, to assess a potential association between prehospital use of antiplatelet agents and the development of ARDS in at-risk patients. Antiplatelet agents included aspirin, clopidogrel, and ticlopidine in their study. They showed that antiplatelet therapy was associated with a reduced incidence of ARDS (12.7% vs 28.0%; OR, 0.37; 95% CI, 0.16–0.84; $p = 0.02$), even after adjusting for confounding variables [103]. Meanwhile, O'Neal et al., from our laboratory, conducted a secondary analysis of a prospective study with 575 patients in the validating acute lung injury markers for diagnosis (VALID) cohort, and showed that concurrent statin and aspirin use, but not aspirin alone, was associated with the reduced risk of ARDS [104]. However, this study was likely underpowered to show an independent association between prehospital aspirin use and the reduced risk of ARDS, given the large proportion of patients who were receiving both prehospital statin and prehospital aspirin therapy. Later, Kor et al., from a group of lung injury prevention study investigators (USCIITG–LIPS), performed a multicenter prospective observational study to evaluate the association between prehospitalization aspirin therapy and incident acute lung injury in a heterogeneous cohort of at-risk medical patients. In total, 3855 at-risk patients were enrolled from 22 hospitals over a 6-month period in the United States and Turkey. Nine hundred seventy-six (25.3%) were receiving aspirin at the time of hospitalization. Two hundred forty (6.2%) patients developed acute lung injury. After adjusting for the propensity to receive aspirin therapy, they found that no statistically significant associations between prehospitalization aspirin therapy and ARDS [105]. However, the overall incidence of ARDS in their study was low (6.2%). To further characterize the possible benefit of prehospital aspirin use in ARDS, we performed a new cross-sectional analysis of the entire prospectively collected VALID cohort, with approximately 1149 critically ill patients (age ≥ 40) enrolled during a 6-year interval. Our data showed that patients with prehospital aspirin had a significantly lower incidence of ARDS (27% vs. 34%, $p = 0.034$). In a multivariable, propensity-adjusted analysis, including age, gender, race, sepsis, and APACHE II, prehospital aspirin use was associated with a decreased risk of ARDS (OR 0.66, 95% CI 0.46–0.94) in the entire cohort, and a subgroup of 725 patients with sepsis (OR 0.60, 95% CI 0.41–0.90) [106]. In a prospective study of 202 patients with ARDS, aspirin therapy, given either before or during the hospital stay, was associated with a reduction in ICU mortality (OR: 0.38, CI: 0.15–0.96, $p = 0.04$) by using multivariate logistic regression analysis [107].

A group of the lung injury prevention study with aspirin (LIPS-A) conducted a multicenter, double-blind, randomized clinical trial, testing whether early administration of aspirin would result in a reduced incidence of ARDS in adult patients at high risk. Approximately 400 participants from 14 hospitals across the United States were enrolled [108]. The results showed that, among at-risk patients presenting to the emergency department, the use of aspirin compared with placebo did not reduce the risk of ARDS at 7 days [109]. However, there were several limitations in this study, including an unexpectedly lower rate of ARDS, a large number of patients who used antiplatelets had been excluded, the time from randomization to first drug administration was longer than anticipated at study onset, and the aspirin dose chosen for this study was too low [109]. Furthermore, most studies did not have a subgroup analysis. ARDS is caused by a variety of etiologies, and we do not know whether aspirin is only beneficial for certain causes. Toner et al. suggested that aspirin can modulate multiple pathogenic mechanisms implicated in the development of sepsis-related ARDS [110]. A bold study that recruited healthy volunteers to receive either 75 or 1200 mg aspirin for 7 days prior to LPS inhalation showed that aspirin reduced pulmonary neutrophilia and tissue-damaging neutrophil proteases (matrix metalloproteinase (MMP)-8/-9), reduced bronchoalveolar lavage concentrations of TNF-α, and reduced systemic and pulmonary TXB2 [45].

Table 1. A summary of recent cohort studies into antiplatelet therapy for ARDS.

Authors	Study Country	Study Design	Patient's Inclusion Criteria	Patient No.	Medications	Dosage (mg)	Medication Given Time Point	Outcome Variables	Results
Erlich el al. [103]	Minnesota, US	Retrospective cohort	at least one major risk factor for ALI & age > 18 years	161	Any kind of antiplatelet medications		at the time of hospital admission	1. development of ALI or ARDS 2. ICU and hospital mortality	Reduced incidence of ALI/ARDS (OR:0.37)
O'Neal Jr et al. [104]	Tennessee, US	Prospective cohort	critically ill patients admitted to the medical or surgical ICU and age >18 years	575	Aspirin combined with statin	81or 365 daily	Prehospital use	1. Development of severe sepsis, ARDS 2. Hospital mortality	Two combined had the lowest rates of severe sepsis, ALI/ARDS and mortality.
Kor et al. [105]	20 hospitals in US & 2 in Turkey	Prospective cohort	non-surgical patients admitted to the hospital with at least one major risk factor for ALI and age >18 years	3855	Aspirin	No mention	at the time of hospital admission	1. development of ALI or ARDS 2. ICU and hospital mortality	No significant effect
Chen et al. [106]	Tennessee, US	Prospective cohort	critically ill patients (age ≥ 40) admitted to the medical or surgical ICU	1149	Aspirin	81 or 365 daily	Prehospital use	1. Development of ARDS 2. Development of sepsis related ARDS	Decreased risk of ARDS (OR: 0.66) in the entire cohort also sepsis (OR: 0.60)
Boyle et al. [107]	United Kingdom	Prospective cohort	patients (>16 years-old) requiring invasive mechanical ventilation admitted to the medical or surgical ICU	202	Aspirin	No mention	both pre-admission and during ICU stay	ICU mortality	Reduction in ICU mortality (OR: 0.38)
Kor et al. [109]	16 US academic hospitals	multicenter, double-blind, RCT	patients at risk for ARDS (Lung Injury Prediction Score ≥4)	7673	Aspirin	325 loading dose followed by 81	within 24 hours of emergency department presentation	1. Development of ARDS by study day 7 2. Hospital length of stay 3. Biomarkers	No significant effect
Hamid et al. [45]	United Kingdom	double-blind, RCT	Healthy volunteers	33	Aspirin	75 or 1200 for 7 days	seven days prior to LPS inhalation	Inflammatory biomarkers	Reduced pulmonary neutrophilia and tissue damaging, reduced BAL concentrations of TNF-α and pulmonary TXB2.

US: United States; RCT: randomized controlled trial; ALI: acute lung injury; ARDS: acute respiratory distress syndrome; BAL: bronchoalveolar lavage; TNF: tumor necrosis factor; TX: thromboxane; OR: odds ratio.

5. Meta-Analysis of Clinical Studies

As shown in Table 2, Panka et al. selected 15 pre-clinical studies and eight clinical studies, and showed that aspirin plays a beneficial role in ARDS prevention and treatment [44]. Yu et al. reviewed six studies and showed aspirin could reduce the rate of ARDS/ALI (OR:0.71) but not the mortality [111]. Jin et al. reviewed seven studies and showed significantly lower odds of ARDS in the prehospital antiplatelet therapy group, compared with subjects with no prehospital antiplatelet therapy (odds ratio: 0.68) [112]. Mohananey et al. included 17 studies, and found that there was a significant reduction in all-cause mortality in patients on antiplatelet therapy, compared to the control (OR: 0.83). Both the incidence of ARDS (OR: 0.67) and the need for mechanical ventilation (OR: 0.74) were lower in the antiplatelet group [113]. On the contrary, Wang et al. analyzed nine eligible studies, and found that antiplatelet therapy did not significantly decrease hospital mortality in high-risk patients, and an association with the incidence of ARDS remains unclear [43].

In summary, it is still unknown whether aspirin can be used to effectively prevent or treat ARDS. This can be attributed to several factors. First, there is considerable heterogeneity in ARDS itself. Several recent research directions are exploring whether different treatments can be given according to different phenotypes of ARDS [114,115]. Therefore, future research should be based on ARDS patients whose phenotype pathology is more aligned with the mechanisms of aspirin. Second, for previous studies, the starting point of aspirin administration, the dose administered, and the duration of administration are all very different. This is also one of the reasons for the inconsistency of the research results. Therefore, whether future research can detect some biomarkers to track their drug response is quite important. Third, even if the above two reasons are resolved, the mechanism of aspirin's action is only a part of the treatment or prevention of ARDS. Perhaps a cocktail therapy, which can combine aspirin with certain medications, would be beneficial for the prevention or treatment of ARDS.

Table 2. Summary of meta-analysis of the effect of aspirin on ARDS.

Authors	Enrolled Types of Studies	Enrolled Study Numbers	Medications	Outcome Variables	Results	Between-Study Heterogeneity	Conclusions
Panka et al. [44]	1 RCT, 7 OS	8	Aspirin	the risk of ARDS	pooled OR was 0.59	Q = 2.44, I^2 = 68%	A beneficial role for Aspirin in ARDS prevention and treatment.
Yu et al. [111]	1 RCT, 5 OS	6	Aspirin	1. the risk of ARDS/ALI 2. mortality.	pooled OR was 0.71	I^2 = 0%, P = 0.419	Aspirin could provide protective effect on the rate of ARDS/ALI, but it could not reduce the mortality.
Jin et al. [112]	7 OS	7	Antiplatelet agents (aspirin 75 to 300 mg daily), (clopidogrel, 75 mg daily), and ticlo- pidine.	1. the risk of ARDS/ALI 2. mortality.	pooled OR was 0.68	I^2 = 34%	Pre-hospital antiplatelet therapy was associated with a reduced rate of ARDS but had no effect on the mortality in the subjects at high risk
Mohanney et al. [113]	17 OS	17	Aspirin and other antiplatelet agents	1. the risk of ARDS/ALI 2. mortality.	pooled OR was 0.67	I^2 = 25%	Antiplatelet therapy had an improved survival, decreased incidence of ARDS
Wang et al. [43]	2 RCT, 7 OS	9	Aspirin and other antiplatelet agents	1. the risk of ARDS/ALI 2. mortality.	pool OR was 0.68 from OS; but no significant difference in RCT	I^2 = 0.0%, p = 0.329 for RCT I^2 = 68.4%, p = 0.004 for OS	Whether antiplatelet therapy is associated with a decreased incidence of ARDS in patients at a high risk of developing the condition remains unclear.

6. Conclusions

In summary, platelets play a crucial role in the pathogenesis of ARDS in a number of experimental studies, and antiplatelet therapy exerts a potential therapeutic benefit for ARDS in clinical studies. The main effects of antiplatelet therapy to reduce the severity of ARDS are possibly based on four directions: (1) reducing platelet adhesion to the injured vessel wall; (2) inhibiting platelet-leukocyte-endothelium interactions; (3) modulating lipid mediator related platelet aggregation, and (4) inhibiting NETs formation. Several observational studies have shown that aspirin is protective against the development of ARDS, and a large multicenter, double-blinded, randomized study showed no beneficial effect of aspirin on the development of ARDS. Future research should be based on ARDS patients whose phenotype pathology is more aligned with the mechanisms of antiplatelet therapy, and specific biomarkers should be developed to track their drug response.

Funding: This research work was funded by the Ministry of Science and Technology, Taiwan and Chiayi Christian Hospital, Chiayi, Taiwan, grant number 104-2314-B-705-005.

Conflicts of Interest: The authors declare no conflict of interest.

References

1. Force, A.D.T.; Ranieri, V.M.; Rubenfeld, G.D.; Thompson, B.T.; Ferguson, N.D.; Caldwell, E.; Fan, E.; Camporota, L.; Slutsky, A.S. Acute respiratory distress syndrome: The Berlin Definition. *JAMA* **2012**, *307*, 2526–2533.
2. Bernard, G.R.; Artigas, A.; Brigham, K.L.; Carlet, J.; Falke, K.; Hudson, L.; Lamy, M.; Legall, J.R.; Morris, A.; Spragg, R. The American-European Consensus Conference on ARDS. Definitions, mechanisms, relevant outcomes, and clinical trial coordination. *Am. J. Respir. Crit. Care Med.* **1994**, *149*, 818–824. [CrossRef] [PubMed]
3. Ware, L.B.; Matthay, M.A. The acute respiratory distress syndrome. *N. Engl. J. Med.* **2000**, *342*, 1334–1349. [CrossRef] [PubMed]
4. Rubenfeld, G.D.; Caldwell, E.; Peabody, E.; Weaver, J.; Martin, D.P.; Neff, M.; Stern, E.J.; Hudson, L.D. Incidence and outcomes of acute lung injury. *N. Engl. J. Med.* **2005**, *353*, 1685–1693. [CrossRef]
5. Chen, W.; Chen, Y.Y.; Tsai, C.F.; Chen, S.C.; Lin, M.S.; Ware, L.B.; Chen, C.M. Incidence and Outcomes of Acute Respiratory Distress Syndrome: A Nationwide Registry-Based Study in Taiwan, 1997 to 2011. *Medicine* **2015**, *94*, e1849. [CrossRef]
6. Acute Respiratory Distress Syndrome Network. Ventilation with lower tidal volumes as compared with traditional tidal volumes for acute lung injury and the acute respiratory distress syndrome. The Acute Respiratory Distress Syndrome Network. *N. Engl. J. Med.* **2000**, *342*, 1301–1308. [CrossRef]
7. Jepsen, S.; Herlevsen, P.; Knudsen, P.; Bud, M.I.; Klausen, N.O. Antioxidant treatment with N-acetylcysteine during adult respiratory distress syndrome: A prospective, randomized, placebo-controlled study. *Crit. Care Med.* **1992**, *20*, 918–923. [CrossRef] [PubMed]
8. Ketoconazole for early treatment of acute lung injury and acute respiratory distress syndrome: A randomized controlled trial. The ARDS Network. *JAMA* **2000**, *283*, 1995–2002.
9. Meade, M.O.; Jacka, M.J.; Cook, D.J.; Dodek, P.; Griffith, L.; Guyatt, G.H.; Canadian Critical Care Trials, G. Survey of interventions for the prevention and treatment of acute respiratory distress syndrome. *Crit. Care Med.* **2004**, *32*, 946–954. [CrossRef]
10. Avecillas, J.F.; Freire, A.X.; Arroliga, A.C. Clinical epidemiology of acute lung injury and acute respiratory distress syndrome: Incidence, diagnosis, and outcomes. *Clin. Chest Med.* **2006**, *27*, 549–557. [CrossRef]
11. Caser, E.B.; Zandonade, E.; Pereira, E.; Gama, A.M.; Barbas, C.S. Impact of distinct definitions of acute lung injury on its incidence and outcomes in Brazilian ICUs: Prospective evaluation of 7,133 patients*. *Crit. Care Med.* **2014**, *42*, 574–582. [CrossRef]
12. Herridge, M.S.; Cheung, A.M.; Tansey, C.M.; Matte-Martyn, A.; Diaz-Granados, N.; Al-Saidi, F.; Cooper, A.B.; Guest, C.B.; Mazer, C.D.; Mehta, S.; et al. One-year outcomes in survivors of the acute respiratory distress syndrome. *N. Engl. J. Med.* **2003**, *348*, 683–693. [CrossRef]
13. Herridge, M.S.; Tansey, C.M.; Matte, A.; Tomlinson, G.; Diaz-Granados, N.; Cooper, A.; Guest, C.B.; Mazer, C.D.; Mehta, S.; Stewart, T.E.; et al. Functional disability 5 years after acute respiratory distress syndrome. *N. Engl. J. Med.* **2011**, *364*, 1293–1304. [CrossRef]
14. Sasannejad, C.; Ely, E.W.; Lahiri, S. Long-term cognitive impairment after acute respiratory distress syndrome: A review of clinical impact and pathophysiological mechanisms. *Crit Care* **2019**, *23*, 352. [CrossRef]
15. Bein, T.; Weber-Carstens, S.; Apfelbacher, C.; Brandstetter, S.; Blecha, S.; Dodoo-Schittko, F.; Brandl, M.; Quintel, M.; Kluge, S.; Putensen, C.; et al. The quality of acute intensive care and the incidence of critical events have an impact on health-related quality of life in survivors of the acute respiratory distress syndrome—A nationwide prospective multicenter observational study. *Ger. Med. Sci.* **2020**, *18*, Doc01. [PubMed]

16. Bachofen, M.; Weibel, E.R. Alterations of the gas exchange apparatus in adult respiratory insufficiency associated with septicemia. *Am. Rev. Respir. Dis.* **1977**, *116*, 589–615. [CrossRef] [PubMed]
17. Matthay, M.A.; Zemans, R.L. The acute respiratory distress syndrome: Pathogenesis and treatment. *Annu. Rev. Pathol.* **2011**, *6*, 147–163. [CrossRef] [PubMed]
18. Huppert, L.A.; Matthay, M.A.; Ware, L.B. Pathogenesis of Acute Respiratory Distress Syndrome. *Semin. Respir. Crit. Care Med.* **2019**, *40*, 31–39. [CrossRef]
19. Kim, T.H.; Hong, S.B.; Lim, C.M.; Koh, Y.; Jang, E.Y.; Huh, J.W. The Role of Exosomes in Bronchoalveloar Lavage from Patients with Acute Respiratory Distress Syndrome. *J. Clin. Med.* **2019**, *8*, 1148. [CrossRef]
20. Pugin, J.; Verghese, G.; Widmer, M.C.; Matthay, M.A. The alveolar space is the site of intense inflammatory and profibrotic reactions in the early phase of acute respiratory distress syndrome. *Crit. Care Med.* **1999**, *27*, 304–312. [CrossRef]
21. Yang, C.Y.; Chen, C.S.; Yiang, G.T.; Cheng, Y.L.; Yong, S.B.; Wu, M.Y.; Li, C.J. New Insights into the Immune Molecular Regulation of the Pathogenesis of Acute Respiratory Distress Syndrome. *Int. J. Mol. Sci.* **2018**, *19*, 588. [CrossRef] [PubMed]
22. Ware, L.B.; Herridge, M. Acute lung injury. *Semin. Respir. Crit. Care Med.* **2013**, *34*, 439–440. [CrossRef]
23. Weiss, S.J. Tissue destruction by neutrophils. *N. Engl. J. Med.* **1989**, *320*, 365–376. [PubMed]
24. Babior, B.M.; Takeuchi, C.; Ruedi, J.; Gutierrez, A.; Wentworth, P., Jr. Investigating antibody-catalyzed ozone generation by human neutrophils. *Proc. Natl. Acad. Sci. USA* **2003**, *100*, 3031–3034. [CrossRef] [PubMed]
25. Stormann, P.; Becker, N.; Vollrath, J.T.; Kohler, K.; Janicova, A.; Wutzler, S.; Hildebrand, F.; Marzi, I.; Relja, B. Early Local Inhibition of Club Cell Protein 16 Following Chest Trauma Reduces Late Sepsis-Induced Acute Lung Injury. *J. Clin. Med.* **2019**, *8*, 896. [CrossRef] [PubMed]
26. Chang, J.C. Acute Respiratory Distress Syndrome as an Organ Phenotype of Vascular Microthrombotic Disease: Based on Hemostatic Theory and Endothelial Molecular Pathogenesis. *Clin. Appl. Thromb. Hemost.* **2019**, *25*, 1076029619887437. [CrossRef] [PubMed]
27. Matthay, M.A.; Wiener-Kronish, J.P. Intact epithelial barrier function is critical for the resolution of alveolar edema in humans. *Am. Rev. Respir. Dis.* **1990**, *142*, 1250–1257. [CrossRef]
28. Perkins, G.D.; Nathani, N.; McAuley, D.F.; Gao, F.; Thickett, D.R. In vitro and in vivo effects of salbutamol on neutrophil function in acute lung injury. *Thorax* **2007**, *62*, 36–42. [CrossRef]
29. Abraham, E. Neutrophils and acute lung injury. *Crit. Care Med.* **2003**, *31*, S195–S199. [CrossRef]
30. Frank, J.A.; Wray, C.M.; McAuley, D.F.; Schwendener, R.; Matthay, M.A. Alveolar macrophages contribute to alveolar barrier dysfunction in ventilator-induced lung injury. *Am. J. Physiol. Lung Cell. Mol. Physiol.* **2006**, *291*, L1191–L1198. [CrossRef]
31. Matthay, M.A.; Zimmerman, G.A.; Esmon, C.; Bhattacharya, J.; Coller, B.; Doerschuk, C.M.; Floros, J.; Gimbrone, M.A., Jr.; Hoffman, E.; Hubmayr, R.D.; et al. Future research directions in acute lung injury: Summary of a National Heart, Lung, and Blood Institute working group. *Am. J. Respir. Crit. Care Med.* **2003**, *167*, 1027–1035. [CrossRef] [PubMed]
32. Matthay, M.A.; Zimmerman, G.A. Acute lung injury and the acute respiratory distress syndrome: Four decades of inquiry into pathogenesis and rational management. *Am. J.Respir. Cell Mol. Biol.* **2005**, *33*, 319–327. [CrossRef] [PubMed]
33. Gadek, J.E. Adverse effects of neutrophils on the lung. *Am. J. Med.* **1992**, *92*, 27S–31S. [CrossRef]
34. Grimminger, F.; Menger, M.; Becker, G.; Seeger, W. Potentiation of leukotriene production following sequestration of neutrophils in isolated lungs: Indirect evidence for intercellular leukotriene A4 transfer. *Blood* **1988**, *72*, 1687–1692. [CrossRef]
35. Fantone, J.C.; Ward, P.A. Role of oxygen-derived free radicals and metabolites in leukocyte-dependent inflammatory reactions. *Am. J. Pathol.* **1982**, *107*, 395–418.
36. Matthay, M.A.; Ware, L.B.; Zimmerman, G.A. The acute respiratory distress syndrome. *J. Clin. Investig.* **2012**, *122*, 2731–2740. [CrossRef]
37. Zarbock, A.; Polanowska-Grabowska, R.K.; Ley, K. Platelet-neutrophil-interactions: Linking hemostasis and inflammation. *Blood Rev.* **2007**, *21*, 99–111. [CrossRef]

38. Privratsky, J.R.; Paddock, C.M.; Florey, O.; Newman, D.K.; Muller, W.A.; Newman, P.J. Relative contribution of PECAM-1 adhesion and signaling to the maintenance of vascular integrity. *J. Cell Sci.* **2011**, *124*, 1477–1485. [CrossRef] [PubMed]
39. Villar, J.; Zhang, H.; Slutsky, A.S. Lung Repair and Regeneration in ARDS: Role of PECAM1 and Wnt Signaling. *Chest* **2019**, *155*, 587–594. [CrossRef]
40. Zarbock, A.; Singbartl, K.; Ley, K. Complete reversal of acid-induced acute lung injury by blocking of platelet-neutrophil aggregation. *J. Clin. Investig.* **2006**, *116*, 3211–3219. [CrossRef]
41. Kiefmann, R.; Heckel, K.; Schenkat, S.; Dorger, M.; Wesierska-Gadek, J.; Goetz, A.E. Platelet-endothelial cell interaction in pulmonary micro-circulation: The role of PARS. *Thromb. Haemost.* **2004**, *91*, 761–770. [CrossRef]
42. Kiefmann, R.; Heckel, K.; Schenkat, S.; Dorger, M.; Goetz, A.E. Role of p-selectin in platelet sequestration in pulmonary capillaries during endotoxemia. *J. Vasc. Res.* **2006**, *43*, 473–481. [CrossRef]
43. Wang, Y.; Zhong, M.; Wang, Z.; Song, J.; Wu, W.; Zhu, D. The preventive effect of antiplatelet therapy in acute respiratory distress syndrome: A meta-analysis. *Crit. Care* **2018**, *22*, 60. [CrossRef]
44. Panka, B.A.; de Grooth, H.J.; Spoelstra-de Man, A.M.; Looney, M.R.; Tuinman, P.R. Prevention or Treatment of Ards With Aspirin: A Review of Preclinical Models and Meta-Analysis of Clinical Studies. *Shock* **2017**, *47*, 13–21. [CrossRef] [PubMed]
45. Hamid, U.; Krasnodembskaya, A.; Fitzgerald, M.; Shyamsundar, M.; Kissenpfennig, A.; Scott, C.; Lefrancais, E.; Looney, M.R.; Verghis, R.; Scott, J.; et al. Aspirin reduces lipopolysaccharide-induced pulmonary inflammation in human models of ARDS. *Thorax* **2017**, *72*, 971–980. [CrossRef] [PubMed]
46. Frantzeskaki, F.; Armaganidis, A.; Orfanos, S.E. Immunothrombosis in Acute Respiratory Distress Syndrome: Cross Talks between Inflammation and Coagulation. *Respiration* **2017**, *93*, 212–225. [CrossRef] [PubMed]
47. Zarbock, A.; Ley, K. The role of platelets in acute lung injury (ALI). *Front. Biosci.* **2009**, *14*, 150–158. [CrossRef] [PubMed]
48. Ruggeri, Z.M. Von Willebrand factor. *Curr. Opin. Hematol.* **2003**, *10*, 142–149. [CrossRef] [PubMed]
49. Ruggeri, Z.M.; Dent, J.A.; Saldivar, E. Contribution of distinct adhesive interactions to platelet aggregation in flowing blood. *Blood* **1999**, *94*, 172–178. [CrossRef]
50. Jurk, K.; Clemetson, K.J.; de Groot, P.G.; Brodde, M.F.; Steiner, M.; Savion, N.; Varon, D.; Sixma, J.J.; Van Aken, H.; Kehrel, B.E. Thrombospondin-1 mediates platelet adhesion at high shear via glycoprotein Ib (GPIb): An alternative/backup mechanism to von Willebrand factor. *FASEB J.* **2003**, *17*, 1490–1492. [CrossRef]
51. Savage, B.; Almus-Jacobs, F.; Ruggeri, Z.M. Specific synergy of multiple substrate-receptor interactions in platelet thrombus formation under flow. *Cell* **1998**, *94*, 657–666. [CrossRef]
52. Kasirer-Friede, A.; Kahn, M.L.; Shattil, S.J. Platelet integrins and immunoreceptors. *Immunol. Rev.* **2007**, *218*, 247–264. [CrossRef]
53. Washington, A.V.; Esponda, O.; Gibson, A. Platelet biology of the rapidly failing lung. *Br. J. Haematol.* **2020**, *188*, 641–651. [CrossRef] [PubMed]
54. Lax, S.; Rayes, J.; Wichaiyo, S.; Haining, E.J.; Lowe, K.; Grygielska, B.; Laloo, R.; Flodby, P.; Borok, Z.; Crandall, E.D.; et al. Platelet CLEC-2 protects against lung injury via effects of its ligand podoplanin on inflammatory alveolar macrophages in the mouse. *Am. J. Physiol. Lung Cell. Mol. Physiol.* **2017**, *313*, L1016–L1029. [CrossRef] [PubMed]
55. Nieswandt, B.; Echtenacher, B.; Wachs, F.P.; Schroder, J.; Gessner, J.E.; Schmidt, R.E.; Grau, G.E.; Mannel, D.N. Acute systemic reaction and lung alterations induced by an antiplatelet integrin gpIIb/IIIa antibody in mice. *Blood* **1999**, *94*, 684–693. [CrossRef]
56. Koedam, J.A.; Cramer, E.M.; Briend, E.; Furie, B.; Furie, B.C.; Wagner, D.D. P-selectin, a granule membrane protein of platelets and endothelial cells, follows the regulated secretory pathway in AtT-20 cells. *J. Cell Biol.* **1992**, *116*, 617–625. [CrossRef]
57. Tabuchi, A.; Kuebler, W.M. Endothelium-platelet interactions in inflammatory lung disease. *Vasc. Pharmacol.* **2008**, *49*, 141–150. [CrossRef]
58. Urzainqui, A.; Serrador, J.M.; Viedma, F.; Yanez-Mo, M.; Rodriguez, A.; Corbi, A.L.; Alonso-Lebrero, J.L.; Luque, A.; Deckert, M.; Vazquez, J.; et al. ITAM-based interaction of ERM proteins with Syk mediates signaling by the leukocyte adhesion receptor PSGL-1. *Immunity* **2002**, *17*, 401–412. [CrossRef]

59. Haselmayer, P.; Grosse-Hovest, L.; von Landenberg, P.; Schild, H.; Radsak, M.P. TREM-1 ligand expression on platelets enhances neutrophil activation. *Blood* **2007**, *110*, 1029–1035. [CrossRef]
60. Zhao, C.; Su, E.M.; Yang, X.; Gao, Z.; Li, L.; Wu, H.; Jiang, Y.; Su, X. Important role of platelets in modulating endotoxin-induced lung inflammation in CFTR-deficient mice. *PLoS ONE* **2013**, *8*, e82683. [CrossRef]
61. Morales-Ortiz, J.; Deal, V.; Reyes, F.; Maldonado-Martinez, G.; Ledesma, N.; Staback, F.; Croft, C.; Pacheco, A.; Ortiz-Zuazaga, H.; Yost, C.C.; et al. Platelet-derived TLT-1 is a prognostic indicator in ALI/ARDS and prevents tissue damage in the lungs in a mouse model. *Blood* **2018**, *132*, 2495–2505. [CrossRef] [PubMed]
62. Caudrillier, A.; Kessenbrock, K.; Gilliss, B.M.; Nguyen, J.X.; Marques, M.B.; Monestier, M.; Toy, P.; Werb, Z.; Looney, M.R. Platelets induce neutrophil extracellular traps in transfusion-related acute lung injury. *J. Clin. Investig.* **2012**, *122*, 2661–2671. [CrossRef] [PubMed]
63. Vieira-de-Abreu, A.; Campbell, R.A.; Weyrich, A.S.; Zimmerman, G.A. Platelets: Versatile effector cells in hemostasis, inflammation, and the immune continuum. *Semin. Immunopathol.* **2012**, *34*, 5–30. [CrossRef] [PubMed]
64. Cerletti, C.; Tamburrelli, C.; Izzi, B.; Gianfagna, F.; de Gaetano, G. Platelet-leukocyte interactions in thrombosis. *Thromb. Res.* **2012**, *129*, 263–266. [CrossRef] [PubMed]
65. Zarbock, A.; Bishop, J.; Muller, H.; Schmolke, M.; Buschmann, K.; Van Aken, H.; Singbartl, K. Chemokine homeostasis vs. chemokine presentation during severe acute lung injury: The other side of the Duffy antigen receptor for chemokines. *Am. J. Physiol. Lung Cell. Mol. Physiol.* **2010**, *298*, L462–L471. [CrossRef]
66. Ortiz-Munoz, G.; Mallavia, B.; Bins, A.; Headley, M.; Krummel, M.F.; Looney, M.R. Aspirin-triggered 15-epi-lipoxin A4 regulates neutrophil-platelet aggregation and attenuates acute lung injury in mice. *Blood* **2014**, *124*, 2625–2634. [CrossRef]
67. Goldman, G.; Welbourn, R.; Kobzik, L.; Valeri, C.R.; Shepro, D.; Hechtman, H.B. Synergism between leukotriene B4 and thromboxane A2 in mediating acid-aspiration injury. *Surgery* **1992**, *111*, 55–61.
68. Wahn, H.; Hammerschmidt, S. Influence of cyclooxygenase and lipoxygenase inhibitors on oxidative stress-induced lung injury. *Crit. Care Med.* **2001**, *29*, 802–807. [CrossRef]
69. Looney, M.R.; Nguyen, J.X.; Hu, Y.; Van Ziffle, J.A.; Lowell, C.A.; Matthay, M.A. Platelet depletion and aspirin treatment protect mice in a two-event model of transfusion-related acute lung injury. *J. Clin. Investig.* **2009**, *119*, 3450–3461. [CrossRef]
70. Nagase, T.; Uozumi, N.; Ishii, S.; Kume, K.; Izumi, T.; Ouchi, Y.; Shimizu, T. Acute lung injury by sepsis and acid aspiration: A key role for cytosolic phospholipase A2. *Nat. Immunol.* **2000**, *1*, 42–46. [CrossRef]
71. Kostopanagiotou, G.; Avgerinos, E.; Costopanagiotou, C.; Arkadopoulos, N.; Andreadou, I.; Diamantopoulou, K.; Lekka, M.; Smyrniotis, V.; Nakos, G. Acute lung injury in a rat model of intestinal ischemia-reperfusion: The potential time depended role of phospholipases A(2). *J. Surg. Res.* **2008**, *147*, 108–116. [CrossRef] [PubMed]
72. Pittet, J.F.; Mackersie, R.C.; Martin, T.R.; Matthay, M.A. Biological markers of acute lung injury: Prognostic and pathogenetic significance. *Am. J. Respir. Crit. Care Med.* **1997**, *155*, 1187–1205. [CrossRef]
73. Lv, W.; Wang, S.; Wang, L.; Wu, Z.; Jiang, Y.; Chen, X.; Gao, R. G994T polymorphism in exon 9 of plasma platelet-activating factor acetylhydrolase gene and lung ultrasound score as prognostic markers in evaluating the outcome of acute respiratory distress syndrome. *Exp. Ther. Med.* **2019**, *17*, 3174–3180. [CrossRef] [PubMed]
74. Hudson, L.D.; Milberg, J.A.; Anardi, D.; Maunder, R.J. Clinical risks for development of the acute respiratory distress syndrome. *Am. J. Respir. Crit. Care Med.* **1995**, *151*, 293–301. [CrossRef] [PubMed]
75. Donnelly, S.C.; Haslett, C. Cellular mechanisms of acute lung injury: Implications for future treatment in the adult respiratory distress syndrome. *Thorax* **1992**, *47*, 260–263. [CrossRef]
76. Semple, J.W.; Italiano, J.E., Jr.; Freedman, J. Platelets and the immune continuum. *Nat. Rev. Immunol.* **2011**, *11*, 264–274. [CrossRef]
77. Brinkmann, V.; Zychlinsky, A. Beneficial suicide: Why neutrophils die to make NETs. *Nat. Rev. Microbiol.* **2007**, *5*, 577–582. [CrossRef]
78. Gupta, A.K.; Hasler, P.; Holzgreve, W.; Gebhardt, S.; Hahn, S. Induction of neutrophil extracellular DNA lattices by placental microparticles and IL-8 and their presence in preeclampsia. *Hum. Immunol.* **2005**, *66*, 1146–1154. [CrossRef]

79. Kessenbrock, K.; Krumbholz, M.; Schonermarck, U.; Back, W.; Gross, W.L.; Werb, Z.; Grone, H.J.; Brinkmann, V.; Jenne, D.E. Netting neutrophils in autoimmune small-vessel vasculitis. *Nat. Med.* **2009**, *15*, 623–625. [CrossRef]
80. Lande, R.; Ganguly, D.; Facchinetti, V.; Frasca, L.; Conrad, C.; Gregorio, J.; Meller, S.; Chamilos, G.; Sebasigari, R.; Riccieri, V.; et al. Neutrophils activate plasmacytoid dendritic cells by releasing self-DNA-peptide complexes in systemic lupus erythematosus. *Sci. Transl. Med.* **2011**, *3*, 73ra19. [CrossRef]
81. Chang, Y.W.; Tseng, C.P.; Lee, C.H.; Hwang, T.L.; Chen, Y.L.; Su, M.T.; Chong, K.Y.; Lan, Y.W.; Wu, C.C.; Chen, K.J.; et al. beta-Nitrostyrene derivatives attenuate LPS-mediated acute lung injury via the inhibition of neutrophil-platelet interactions and NET release. *Am. J. Physiol. Lung Cell. Mol. Physiol.* **2018**, *314*, L654–L669. [CrossRef] [PubMed]
82. Chen, Z.T.; Li, S.L.; Cai, E.Q.; Wu, W.L.; Jin, J.S.; Zhu, B. LPS induces pulmonary intravascular macrophages producing inflammatory mediators via activating NF-kappaB. *J. Cell. Biochem.* **2003**, *89*, 1206–1214. [CrossRef] [PubMed]
83. Tuinman, P.R.; Muller, M.C.; Jongsma, G.; Hegeman, M.A.; Juffermans, N.P. High-dose acetylsalicylic acid is superior to low-dose as well as to clopidogrel in preventing lipopolysaccharide-induced lung injury in mice. *Shock* **2013**, *40*, 334–338. [CrossRef]
84. Kario, K.; Eguchi, K.; Hoshide, S.; Hoshide, Y.; Umeda, Y.; Mitsuhashi, T.; Shimada, K. U-curve relationship between orthostatic blood pressure change and silent cerebrovascular disease in elderly hypertensives: Orthostatic hypertension as a new cardiovascular risk factor. *J. Am. Coll. Cardiol.* **2002**, *40*, 133–141. [CrossRef]
85. Eickmeier, O.; Seki, H.; Haworth, O.; Hilberath, J.N.; Gao, F.; Uddin, M.; Croze, R.H.; Carlo, T.; Pfeffer, M.A.; Levy, B.D. Aspirin-triggered resolvin D1 reduces mucosal inflammation and promotes resolution in a murine model of acute lung injury. *Mucosal Immunol.* **2013**, *6*, 256–266. [CrossRef]
86. Bates, J.J.; Watson, R.W.; Glynn, C.M.; O'Neill, A.J.; Fitzpatrick, J.M.; Buggy, D.J. Aspirin preserves neutrophil apoptosis after cardiopulmonary bypass. *Shock* **2004**, *21*, 495–499. [CrossRef] [PubMed]
87. Claria, J.; Serhan, C.N. Aspirin triggers previously undescribed bioactive eicosanoids by human endothelial cell-leukocyte interactions. *Proc. Natl. Acad. Sci. USA* **1995**, *92*, 9475–9479. [CrossRef] [PubMed]
88. Serhan, C.N. Lipoxins and aspirin-triggered 15-epi-lipoxins are the first lipid mediators of endogenous anti-inflammation and resolution. *Prostaglandins Leukot. Essent. Fat. Acids* **2005**, *73*, 141–162. [CrossRef] [PubMed]
89. Levy, B.D.; Clish, C.B.; Schmidt, B.; Gronert, K.; Serhan, C.N. Lipid mediator class switching during acute inflammation: Signals in resolution. *Nat. Immunol.* **2001**, *2*, 612–619. [CrossRef] [PubMed]
90. Serhan, C.N. Resolution phase of inflammation: Novel endogenous anti-inflammatory and proresolving lipid mediators and pathways. *Annu. Rev. Immunol.* **2007**, *25*, 101–137. [CrossRef] [PubMed]
91. Matute-Bello, G.; Liles, W.C.; Radella, F., 2nd; Steinberg, K.P.; Ruzinski, J.T.; Jonas, M.; Chi, E.Y.; Hudson, L.D.; Martin, T.R. Neutrophil apoptosis in the acute respiratory distress syndrome. *Am. J. Respir. Crit. Care Med.* **1997**, *156*, 1969–1977. [CrossRef] [PubMed]
92. El Kebir, D.; Jozsef, L.; Pan, W.; Wang, L.; Petasis, N.A.; Serhan, C.N.; Filep, J.G. 15-epi-lipoxin A4 inhibits myeloperoxidase signaling and enhances resolution of acute lung injury. *Am. J. Respir. Crit. Care Med.* **2009**, *180*, 311–319. [CrossRef] [PubMed]
93. Sun, Y.P.; Oh, S.F.; Uddin, J.; Yang, R.; Gotlinger, K.; Campbell, E.; Colgan, S.P.; Petasis, N.A.; Serhan, C.N. Resolvin D1 and its aspirin-triggered 17R epimer. Stereochemical assignments, anti-inflammatory properties, and enzymatic inactivation. *J. Biol. Chem.* **2007**, *282*, 9323–9334. [CrossRef]
94. Tang, H.; Liu, Y.; Yan, C.; Petasis, N.A.; Serhan, C.N.; Gao, H. Protective actions of aspirin-triggered (17R) resolvin D1 and its analogue, 17R-hydroxy-19-para-fluorophenoxy-resolvin D1 methyl ester, in C5a-dependent IgG immune complex-induced inflammation and lung injury. *J. Immunol.* **2014**, *193*, 3769–3778. [CrossRef] [PubMed]
95. Chen, C.M.; Tung, Y.T.; Wei, C.H.; Lee, P.Y.; Chen, W. Anti-Inflammatory and Reactive Oxygen Species Suppression through Aspirin Pretreatment to Treat Hyperoxia-Induced Acute Lung Injury in NF-kappaB-Luciferase Inducible Transgenic Mice. *Antioxidants* **2020**, *9*, 429. [CrossRef]
96. Cox, R., Jr.; Phillips, O.; Fukumoto, J.; Fukumoto, I.; Tamarapu Parthasarathy, P.; Arias, S.; Cho, Y.; Lockey, R.F.; Kolliputi, N. Aspirin-Triggered Resolvin D1 Treatment Enhances Resolution of Hyperoxic Acute Lung Injury. *Am. J. Respir. Cell Mol. Biol.* **2015**, *53*, 422–435. [CrossRef] [PubMed]

97. Schmitt-Sody, M.; Metz, P.; Gottschalk, O.; Zysk, S.; Birkenmaier, C.; Goebl, M.; von Schulze Pellengahr, C.; Veihelmann, A.; Jansson, V. Selective inhibition of platelets by the GPIIb/IIIa receptor antagonist Tirofiban reduces leukocyte-endothelial cell interaction in murine antigen-induced arthritis. *Inflamm. Res.* **2007**, *56*, 414–420. [CrossRef]
98. Le, V.B.; Schneider, J.G.; Boergeling, Y.; Berri, F.; Ducatez, M.; Guerin, J.L.; Adrian, I.; Errazuriz-Cerda, E.; Frasquilho, S.; Antunes, L.; et al. Platelet activation and aggregation promote lung inflammation and influenza virus pathogenesis. *Am. J. Respir. Crit. Care Med.* **2015**, *191*, 804–819. [CrossRef]
99. Sharron, M.; Hoptay, C.E.; Wiles, A.A.; Garvin, L.M.; Geha, M.; Benton, A.S.; Nagaraju, K.; Freishtat, R.J. Platelets induce apoptosis during sepsis in a contact-dependent manner that is inhibited by GPIIb/IIIa blockade. *PLoS ONE* **2012**, *7*, e41549. [CrossRef]
100. Dorsam, R.T.; Kunapuli, S.P. Central role of the P2Y12 receptor in platelet activation. *J. Clin. Investig.* **2004**, *113*, 340–345. [CrossRef]
101. Muhlestein, J.B. Effect of antiplatelet therapy on inflammatory markers in atherothrombotic patients. *Thromb. Haemost.* **2010**, *103*, 71–82. [CrossRef] [PubMed]
102. Harr, J.N.; Moore, E.E.; Wohlauer, M.V.; Fragoso, M.; Gamboni, F.; Liang, X.; Banerjee, A.; Silliman, C.C. Activated platelets in heparinized shed blood: The "second hit" of acute lung injury in trauma/hemorrhagic shock models. *Shock* **2011**, *36*, 595–603. [CrossRef] [PubMed]
103. Erlich, J.M.; Talmor, D.S.; Cartin-Ceba, R.; Gajic, O.; Kor, D.J. Prehospitalization antiplatelet therapy is associated with a reduced incidence of acute lung injury: A population-based cohort study. *Chest* **2011**, *139*, 289–295. [CrossRef] [PubMed]
104. O'Neal, H.R., Jr.; Koyama, T.; Koehler, E.A.; Siew, E.; Curtis, B.R.; Fremont, R.D.; May, A.K.; Bernard, G.R.; Ware, L.B. Prehospital statin and aspirin use and the prevalence of severe sepsis and acute lung injury/acute respiratory distress syndrome. *Crit. Care Med.* **2011**, *39*, 1343–1350. [CrossRef]
105. Kor, D.J.; Erlich, J.; Gong, M.N.; Malinchoc, M.; Carter, R.E.; Gajic, O.; Talmor, D.S.; Illness, U.S.C.; Injury Trials Group: Lung Injury Prevention Study Investigators. Association of prehospitalization aspirin therapy and acute lung injury: Results of a multicenter international observational study of at-risk patients. *Crit. Care Med.* **2011**, *39*, 2393–2400. [CrossRef]
106. Chen, W.; Janz, D.R.; Bastarache, J.A.; May, A.K.; O'Neal, H.R., Jr.; Bernard, G.R.; Ware, L.B. Prehospital aspirin use is associated with reduced risk of acute respiratory distress syndrome in critically ill patients: A propensity-adjusted analysis. *Crit. Care Med.* **2015**, *43*, 801–807. [CrossRef]
107. Boyle, A.J.; Di Gangi, S.; Hamid, U.I.; Mottram, L.J.; McNamee, L.; White, G.; Cross, L.J.; McNamee, J.J.; O'Kane, C.M.; McAuley, D.F. Aspirin therapy in patients with acute respiratory distress syndrome (ARDS) is associated with reduced intensive care unit mortality: A prospective analysis. *Crit. Care* **2015**, *19*, 109. [CrossRef] [PubMed]
108. Kor, D.J.; Talmor, D.S.; Banner-Goodspeed, V.M.; Carter, R.E.; Hinds, R.; Park, P.K.; Gajic, O.; Gong, M.N.; Illness, U.S.C.; Injury Trials Group: Lung Injury Prevention with Aspirin Study Group. Lung Injury Prevention with Aspirin (LIPS-A): A protocol for a multicentre randomised clinical trial in medical patients at high risk of acute lung injury. *BMJ Open* **2012**, *2*. [CrossRef] [PubMed]
109. Kor, D.J.; Carter, R.E.; Park, P.K.; Festic, E.; Banner-Goodspeed, V.M.; Hinds, R.; Talmor, D.; Gajic, O.; Ware, L.B.; Gong, M.N.; et al. Effect of Aspirin on Development of ARDS in At-Risk Patients Presenting to the Emergency Department: The LIPS-A Randomized Clinical Trial. *JAMA* **2016**, *315*, 2406–2414. [CrossRef] [PubMed]
110. Toner, P.; McAuley, D.F.; Shyamsundar, M. Aspirin as a potential treatment in sepsis or acute respiratory distress syndrome. *Crit. Care* **2015**, *19*, 374. [CrossRef]
111. Yu, H.; Ni, Y.N.; Liang, Z.A.; Liang, B.M.; Wang, Y. The effect of aspirin in preventing the acute respiratory distress syndrome/acute lung injury: A meta-analysis. *Am. J. Emerg. Med.* **2018**, *36*, 1486–1491. [CrossRef]
112. Jin, W.; Chuang, C.C.; Jin, H.; Ye, J.; Kandaswamy, E.; Wang, L.; Zuo, L. Effects of Pre-Hospital Antiplatelet Therapy on the Incidence of ARDS. *Respir. Care* **2020**, *65*, 1039–1045. [CrossRef] [PubMed]
113. Mohananey, D.; Sethi, J.; Villablanca, P.A.; Ali, M.S.; Kumar, R.; Baruah, A.; Bhatia, N.; Agrawal, S.; Hussain, Z.; Shamoun, F.E.; et al. Effect of antiplatelet therapy on mortality and acute lung injury in critically ill patients: A systematic review and meta-analysis. *Ann. Card. Anaesth.* **2016**, *19*, 626–637. [PubMed]

114. Sinha, P.; Churpek, M.M.; Calfee, C.S. Machine Learning Classifier Models Can Identify ARDS Phenotypes Using Readily Available Clinical Data. *Am. J. Respir. Crit. Care Med.* **2020**, *201*, A1014. [CrossRef]
115. Sinha, P.; Delucchi, K.L.; McAuley, D.F.; O'Kane, C.M.; Matthay, M.A.; Calfee, C.S. Development and validation of parsimonious algorithms to classify acute respiratory distress syndrome phenotypes: A secondary analysis of randomised controlled trials. *Lancet Respir. Med.* **2020**, *8*, 247–257. [CrossRef]

biomedicines

MDPI

Review

Targeting Redox Imbalance as an Approach for Diabetic Kidney Disease

Keiichiro Matoba [1,*], Yusuke Takeda [1], Yosuke Nagai [1], Tamotsu Yokota [1], Kazunori Utsunomiya [2] and Rimei Nishimura [1]

1 Division of Diabetes, Metabolism, and Endocrinology, Department of Internal Medicine, The Jikei University School of Medicine, Tokyo 105-8461, Japan; ms05-takeda@jikei.ac.jp (Y.T.); y.nagai@jikei.ac.jp (Y.N.); yokotat@jikei.ac.jp (T.Y.); rimei@jikei.ac.jp (R.N.)

2 Center for Preventive Medicine, The Jikei University School of Medicine, Tokyo 105-8461, Japan; kazu-utsunomiya@jikei.ac.jp

* Correspondence: matoba@jikei.ac.jp

Received: 1 February 2020; Accepted: 20 February 2020; Published: 22 February 2020

Abstract: Diabetic kidney disease (DKD) is a worldwide public health problem. It is the leading cause of end-stage renal disease and is associated with increased mortality from cardiovascular complications. The tight interactions between redox imbalance and the development of DKD are becoming increasingly evident. Numerous cascades, including the polyol and hexosamine pathways have been implicated in the oxidative stress of diabetes patients. However, the precise molecular mechanism by which oxidative stress affects the progression of DKD remains to be elucidated. Given the limited therapeutic options for DKD, it is essential to understand how oxidants and antioxidants are controlled in diabetes and how oxidative stress impacts the progression of renal damage. This review aims to provide an overview of the current status of knowledge regarding the pathological roles of oxidative stress in DKD. Finally, we summarize recent therapeutic approaches to preventing DKD with a focus on the anti-oxidative effects of newly developed anti-hyperglycemic agents.

Keywords: diabetic kidney disease; oxidative stress; redox imbalance

---

1. Introduction

The current diabetes pandemic has emerged as a global health burden. Despite accumulating evidence supporting the prevention of obesity and related metabolic disorders, the number of diabetic patients is rapidly increasing, particularly in middle- and low-income countries [1]. According to the estimates of the International Diabetes Federation, diabetes affects 425 million people globally, and the number is expected to increase to more than 600 million in 2045 [2].

It is a major concern that diabetes is associated with the development of micro and macrovascular complications. Diabetic kidney disease (DKD) is the leading cause of end-stage renal disease and is therefore a critical issue for healthcare systems [3–5]. The reason for the diabetes pandemic can be explained, at least in part, by the aging of the population and the increase in obese subjects. DKD is characterized by functional and structural abnormalities in the glomeruli, including glomerular hyperfiltration, mesangial expansion, the thickening of the glomerular basement membrane, and podocyte loss. These changes ultimately result in the glomerulosclerosis associated with albuminuria and a decline in the glomerular filtration rate (GFR). Numerous studies have assessed the link between albuminuria and the cardiovascular risk in patients with DKD and have demonstrated that albuminuria is not only a hallmark of DKD, but also an independent risk factor for cardiovascular death. The detrimental interaction between diabetic renal injury and coronary heart disease is termed reno-cardiac syndrome [6]. Indeed, in the UK Prospective Diabetes Study (UKPDS), annual cardiovascular mortality rates were found to increase to 3%, 4.6%, and 19.2% with the progression to microalbuminuria, macroalbuminuria, and renal failure, respectively [7]. Importantly, cardiovascular events were the most common cause of death in all stages of DKD. It is therefore essential to establish effective therapeutic strategies against DKD. To this end, a detailed understanding of the molecular basis that drives DKD is required.

Emerging evidence suggests that DKD is associated with multiple metabolic disorders (e.g., hyperglycemia, hypertension, and dyslipidemia), hemodynamic changes, activation of the renin-angiotensin system (RAS), and inflammation [8]. While there is no doubt that multifactorial intervention for these abnormalities is necessary for the prevention of DKD acceleration [9,10], the current standards of care do not eliminate the risk of DKD. Given the limited therapeutic options for inhibiting DKD, there has been an ongoing effort to elucidate the biological mechanisms responsible for renal injury and to develop novel drugs.

There is a growing appreciation of the roles of oxidative cellular injury caused by free radicals in the process of diabetic vascular complications. Oxidative stress is defined as an imbalance between the formation of highly reactive molecules and the antioxidant mechanism. Reactive oxygen species (ROS) are chemicals, such as superoxide anion (O_2-), hydroxyl radical (OH), and hydrogen peroxide (H_2O_2), which are generated in cells. Nicotinamide adenine dinucleotide phosphate (NADPH) oxidase is the most important source of superoxide anion and is upregulated in the kidney in diabetes [11]. Consistent with this data, superoxide is increased in the diabetic kidneys and in renal cells incubated under high glucose conditions. Moreover, excess free fatty acids, mainly derived from the obese state, induce the generation of ROS through oxidative phosphorylation in mitochondria. Another possible reason for the oxidative stress in diabetes is decreased antioxidants. As a result, excess ROS can damage DNA, protein, and lipids, making them nonfunctional. These findings highlight the importance of oxidative stress in the mechanisms that facilitate renal injury in the context of diabetes. We herein review the roles of oxidative stress in diabetic renal damage and finally describe medicines that have the potential to inhibit the renal ROS production in patients with DKD.

2. Oxidative Stress in Diabetes and DKD

Elevated ROS is considered to be a causal link between high glucose conditions and DKD progression. The various possible sources for the overproduction of ROS in diabetes include (Figure 1): (1) Activation of the polyol pathway leading to the accumulation of sorbitol and fructose, NADPH redox imbalances, and changes in signal transduction; (2) The increased flux of the hexosamine pathway; (3) Increased protein kinase C (PKC) activity and subsequent cascades of stress; (4) The non-enzymatic glycation of proteins generating advanced glycation end-products (AGEs); and (5) Activation of the small GTPase Rho and its target, Rho-kinase (ROCK).

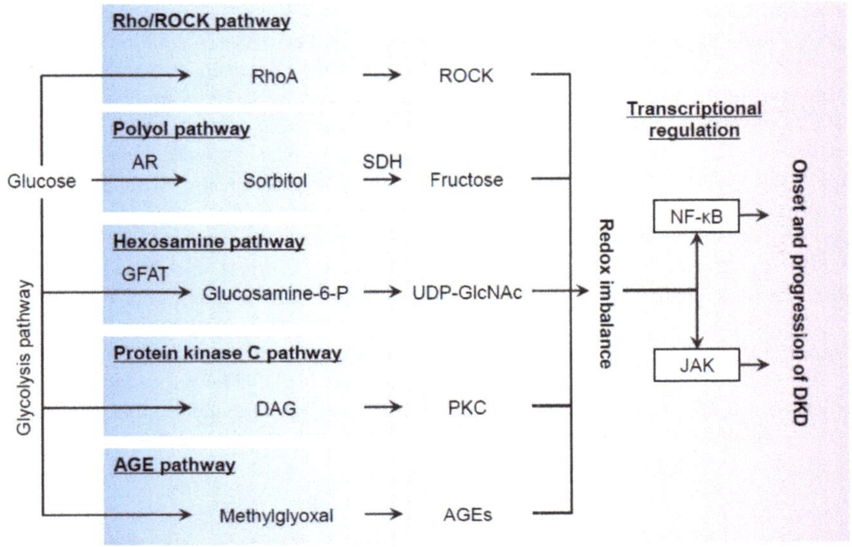

Figure 1. In the setting of diabetes, excess glucose activates several pathways including the polyol pathway, hexosamine pathway, as well as signals that lead to activation of Rho-kinase (ROCK), PKC and generation of AGEs. All of these activation results in oxidant/antioxidant imbalance that proceeds to DKD. AR, aldose reductase; SDH, sorbitol dehydrogenase; GFAT, glutamine:fructose-6-phosphate aminotransferase; glucosamine-6-P, glucosamine-6-phosphate; UDP-GlcNAc, uridine diphosphate-N-acetyl glucosamine; DAG, diacylglycerol; PKC, protein kinase C; AGEs, advanced glycation end-products.

2.1. The Polyol Pathway

Among the various pathways, the polyol pathway plays an important role in the development of DKD. It has been suggested that the polyol pathway generates not only osmotic stress, but also hyperglycemic oxidative stress in renal tissue. Under homeostatic conditions, cellular glucose is predominantly oxidized into glucose-6-phosphate and enters the glycolytic pathway to generate energy in the form of ATP. In states such as diabetes, however, the flux of glucose through the polyol pathway is increased.

In the polyol pathway, glucose is converted to sorbitol by aldose reductase (AR), the first and rate-limiting enzyme of this pathway, with the aid of its cofactor NADPH. AR has been detected in a number of tissues, including tissue of the liver, skeletal muscle, heart, eyes, neuron, and kidney. It has been extensively studied for a potential role in diabetic vascular complications including DKD [12]. In physiological settings, AR breaks down the toxic aldehyde products produced by lipid peroxidation, such as 4-hydroxyl-nonenal (HNE) and its glutathione conjugates (GSH-NHE) into inactive alcohols. Whereas the catalytic action of AR to mediate glucose reduction is negligible under euglycemic conditions, this enzyme is activated in diabetes. Not only in diabetic rodents, but the activity of AR is also increased in renal glomeruli in people with diabetes [13]. Supporting these findings, the accumulation of sorbitol has been demonstrated in glomerular mesangial cells incubated under high glucose conditions [14], which can induce cellular osmotic stress and damage diabetic glomeruli [15]. The fact that AR inhibitor treatment can prevent the development of DKD highlights the significance of the polyol pathway in the biology of DKD. For example, epalrestat, an inhibitor of AR, can attenuate albuminuria, podocyte foot process fusion, and interstitial fibrosis in type 2 diabetic db/db mice [16]. Moreover, AR-deficient mice are resistant to the progression of diabetic kidney injury [17]. In these mice, glomerular hypertrophy, extracellular matrix accumulation, and the overproduction of collagen

4 were inhibited in comparison to wild type mice. The increase in urinary albumin excretion was also prevented in the AR-null mice. In contrast to this experimental evidence, AR inhibitors only have a partial effect in preventing DKD in patients [18]. The incongruity between animal and human data may be due to the short length of clinical trials and variable potency of AR inhibitors.

As the second step in the polyol pathway, sorbitol is oxidized to fructose by sorbitol dehydrogenase (SDH), with its co-factor nicotinamide adenine dinucleotide (NAD). As such, the increased polyol flux leads to an increase in the NADH/NAD ratio. Since NAD is an important factor in many enzyme-catalyzed reactions, other metabolic pathways are also affected. The sirtuin signaling pathway is a major pathway affected by the reduction of NAD. Mammalian sirtuin is a NAD-dependent protein deacetylase with various functions in energy homeostasis, cell survival, and DNA repair [19]. As a consequence, decreased NAD levels eventually lead to the over-acetylation of proteins. Thus, supplementation with NAD precursors or analogues can serve as an effective therapeutic intervention for recovering sirtuin activity and preventing diseases, including diabetes and DKD [20,21]. Moreover, an NADH/NAD redox imbalance can reduce the availability of NADPH for regenerating antioxidant GSH. Importantly, NADH is used as a substrate for NADH oxidase to generate superoxide anions and this occurs in diabetes. Moreover, excess NADH also inhibits glycolysis and the subsequent Krebs cycle, which provides more glucose in the polyol pathway.

2.2. The Hexosamine Pathway

It is now clear that the increased flux of fructose-6-phosphate (fructose-6-P) into the hexosamine pathway also contributes to oxidative stress in the context of diabetes. Under normoglycemic conditions, most of the glucose is metabolized through the glycolysis pathway, and only 2–5% enters the hexosamine pathway and a small amount of fructose-6-P is produced [22]. However, under hyperglycemic conditions, excess fructose-6-P is derived from this pathway to provide a substrate for glutamine:fructose-6-phosphate aminotransferase (GFAT), the rate limiting enzyme of the hexosamine pathway. GFAT mediates the conversion of fructose-6-P to glucosamine-6-phosphate (glucosamine-6-P), and the consequent uridine diphosphate-N-acetyl glucosamine (UDP-GlcNAc).

UDP-GlcNAc is used for the production of glycosyl chains of proteins and lipids. Specific cytoplasmic and nuclear proteins are modified post-translationally by UDP-GlcNAc, and over-modification leads to pathologic changes in the gene expression. For example, transcriptional factors, such as specificity protein 1 (SP1), are modulated by UDP-GlcNAc [23] which leads to the induction of transforming growth factor β1 (TGF-β1) and plasminogen activator inhibitor-1 (PAI-1). Both of these factors contribute to the accumulation of extracellular matrix and diabetic glomerular sclerosis [24]. Consistent with these data, it has been reported that the inhibition of GFAT attenuates the hyperglycemia-induced increases of TGF-β1 in mesangial cells [25]. UDP-GlcNAc also stimulates the production of ROS and pro-apoptotic caspase-3 activity, which contribute to mesangial cell damage [26].

Importantly, the overexpression of GFAT results in the elevation of nuclear factor κB (NF-κB) promotor activity in mesangial cells [27], and excess UDP-GlcNAc provokes oxidative renal cell damage by upregulating the expression of tumor necrosis factor α (TNF-α). Given the well-established link between inflammation and oxidative stress [28], it is reasonable to suggest that the excess glucose flux through the hexosamine pathway leads to redox imbalance, at least in part, via the inflammatory response. Taken together, the activated hexosamine pathway is a piece of one machinery that diabetes leads to oxidative renal damage. Although recent investigations have expanded our knowledge regarding the molecular mechanisms of the hexosamine pathway, its pathological role in patients remains to be established.

2.3. The PKC Pathway

In the setting of diabetes, the increased flux of dihydroxyacetone phosphate (DHAP) to glycerol-3-phosphate leads to the generation of diacylglycerol (DAG), a physiological activator of PKC. PKC phosphorylates subunits of NADPH oxidase, which has been recognized to contribute to the production of ROS. The denouement of elevated PKC signaling is the activation of MAPK signaling and inducible nitric oxide synthase, culminating in structural and functional derangements. Indeed, the PKC-mediated oxidant production elicits endothelial dysfunction and apoptosis. By blocking PKC, the metabolic signaling cascade is interrupted and the production of ROS is reduced. Inhibiting the formation of DAG is one of the options for regulating the PKC signaling pathway.

PKC consists of a family of at least 12 members. PKC-α, PKC-β, PKC-δ, PKC-ε, and PKC-ζ are detected in the glomeruli [29]. PKC plays a pivotal role in renal dysfunction under diabetic conditions. It has been demonstrated that PKC isoforms are activated in diabetic glomeruli and mesangial cells cultured in high glucose media, which contribute to mesangial expansion as well as thickening of the glomerular basement membrane. The importance of PKC-β in DKD has been demonstrated in a loss-of-function study in mice. The amelioration of histological abnormalities and TGF-β1 induction was achieved in PKC-β knockout mice [30]. The urinary excretion of 8-hydroxydeoxyguanosine (8-OHdG) and isoprostane—parameters of oxidative stress—in PKC-β-deficient diabetic mice were reduced in comparison to wild-type mice. Mechanistically, the activity of NADPH oxidase and the mRNA expression levels of p47phox, Nox2, and Nox4 were attenuated in these mice. These findings, coupled with the work of others, have led to the increasing appreciation that PKC-β is an essential determinant of the ROS production.

2.4. The AGE-RAGE Pathway

Another important pathway whereby glucose can activate oxidative stress is AGE signaling. AGEs are generated exogenously and endogenously through non-enzymatic reactions of amino acids, proteins, glucose, and metabolites (e.g., glycolaldehyde, glyceraldehyde, glyoxal, methylglyoxal, 3-deoxyglucosone, and fructose) [31]. The receptor for AGE (RAGE) is a multi-ligand cell surface receptor that can be induced under diabetic conditions. The AGE-RAGE system is one of the major pathways involved in the onset and progression of diabetic vascular complications, including neuropathy, retinopathy, and nephropathy. The flux of glucose through the polyol pathway would increase the formation of toxic AGE compounds, ultimately leading to the production of free radicals, and a decrease in nitric oxide and taurine. Therefore, there is crosstalk between AR-dependent and -independent mechanisms of oxidative stress, which makes it difficult to understand the relative contributions of each. AGEs are known to accumulate intracellularly, which stimulates various signaling pathways, including the inflammatory response. Accumulated AGEs specifically stimulate the production of inflammatory cytokines and adhesion molecules via regulation of transcriptional factor NF-κB, as well as the PKC pathway. The proposed mechanisms by which AGEs interfere with these functions include the disruption of molecular confirmation and the reduction of the degradation capacity by its deposition or activation of RAGE.

In renal mesangial cells, type 4 collagen is upregulated by exposure to AGEs. However, this induction was prevented by the anti-RAGE ribozyme, suggesting that the AGE-mediated induction of the expression of type 4 collagen is dependent on RAGE. It has indeed been reported that diabetic mice that overexpress human RAGE in vascular cells exhibited kidney enlargement, glomerular hypertrophy with mesangial expansion and increased urinary albumin excretion [32]. Moreover, these phenotypes were prevented by the administration of an AGE inhibitor, indicating that the AGE-RAGE signal is an effective target for overcoming DKD. Other studies have evaluated the effects of the specific inhibition of RAGE with DNA aptamer and demonstrated that RAGE-aptamer attenuates the development of experimental DKD by inhibiting oxidative stress [33,34].

2.5. ROCK Signaling

The small GTP-binding protein Rho and its downstream target Rho-associated coiled-coil containing protein kinase (Rho-kinase, ROCK) are implicated in a variety of cellular processes, including cell proliferation, contraction, and migration. ROCK signaling is activated by glucose, cytokines, and ROS [35–37]. Initial insights linking ROCK to diabetic vascular complications were gleaned from our studies identifying ROCK as a critical molecule of the pathological changes of the microvasculature and large blood vessels. For instance, the inhibition of ROCK results in the attenuation of albuminuria, glomerular hypertrophy, and macrophage infiltration in mouse models of diabetes [24,38]. Furthermore, the beneficial effects of ROCK inhibition are observed in the diabetic retina and neuron. Yokota et al. showed that enhanced expression of retinal vascular endothelial growth factor (VEGF) was attenuated by the treatment with ROCK inhibitor in streptozotocin-induced diabetic rat [39]. ROCK blockade also restores normal motor nerve conduction velocity in diabetic rats by mediating proper localization of adhesion-related molecules in myelinating Schwann cells [40]. Another study in endothelial cells demonstrated that ROCK acts as a key player in vascular inflammation [41].

ROCK has two isoforms (ROCK1 and ROCK2) that share 65% sequence homology, but have different activation machinery. Genetic deletion models of ROCK1 and ROCK2 revealed distinctive roles in the regulation of cellular function. For instance, ROCK1 knockout modes demonstrate impaired closure of eyelid and umbilical ring [42], whereas ROCK2 deletion leads to intrauterine growth retardation [43]. Takeda et al. showed the strong contribution of endothelial ROCK2 to the induction of adhesion molecules and chemokines via NF-κB activation [37]. In addition, Nagai et al. reported ROCK2-mediated fibrotic reactions in mesangial cells [36]. Taken together, these findings raise the possibility that ROCK isoform-specific therapeutic approach may be effective for the prevention of diabetic vascular complications.

We provided evidence implicating ROCK as an essential regulator of the redox balance and the progression of DKD [44]. In the streptozotocin-induced diabetic rat, renal Nox4 (a catalytic subunit of NADPH oxidase) and urinary 8-OHdG were increased, suggesting oxidative stress in the diabetic kidney. Of note, ROCK inhibitor attenuated the renal Nox4 expression and the urinary increase of 8-OHdG. Moreover, ROCK regulates the mesangial production of inflammatory cytokines through the mechanism of NF-κB [45]. Whereas some experiments have identified the direct regulation of ROCK in either IκBα degradation or p65 phosphorylation, a mechanism through which ROCK is involved in the nuclear import of p65, without affecting either IκBα degradation or the phosphorylation of p65, has also been documented [38]. Collectively, these findings suggest a direct or inflammation-mediated effect of ROCK on oxidative stress in the diabetic kidney.

3. ROS-Mediated Stress Signaling in DKD

As described above, ROS is produced under diabetic conditions. In addition to its direct effects on cellular protein and DNA, ROS activates several signaling cascades that are implicated in the histological and functional changes in DKD.

3.1. NF-κB and AP-1

Experimental work over the past decade has revealed the mechanistic basis of the interplay between inflammation and oxidative stress. The inflammatory signal is mainly orchestrated by transcriptional factor NF-κB, which consists of a heterodimer of the Rel family proteins: p65 and p50. Under physiological conditions, NF-κB is sequestered in the cytoplasm by IκB family proteins, the best characterized of which is IκBα. The phosphorylation of IκBα results in its ubiquitination and subsequent proteasomal degradation, which results in the exposure of its nuclear localization signal. The following recognition of NF-κB by karyopherin β directs it to the nuclear pore complex, thus allowing for entry into the nucleus. The coactivator p300 generates a complex with p65/p50 dimer to stabilize the chromatin structure for efficient transcription.

Increased renal NF-κB levels are detected in the kidneys of diabetic experimental models, which activate glomerular and tubular cells to induce renal injury [35,45]. Downstream targets of NF-κB include adhesion molecules and pro-inflammatory cytokines (e.g., interleukin 6, TNF-α), which all drive oxidative stress and the development of DKD. In addition to the role as downstream events of NF-κB activation, ROS activates NF-κB signaling [46]. For instance, H_2O_2 stimulates NF-κB to produce an array of inflammatory mediators. In turn, these activate the further production of ROS. Activating protein 1 (AP-1) is another major redox-sensitive transcriptional factor. ROS activates c-Fos and c-Jun, both of which are components of AP-1. Similar to NF-κB, glucose and oxidative stress activate AP-1-mediated inflammatory signaling, which will contribute to the formation of the vicious inflammation-oxidative stress cycle. Further clinical trial and mechanistic investigations are required in order to validate the role of AP-1 in the pathogenesis of DKD.

3.2. *JAK-STAT*

Janus kinase/signal transducer and activator of transcription (JAK-STAT) is activated by extracellular ligands, such as cytokines, chemokines, and growth factors to induce a number of cellular responses. ROS has also been shown to activate the JAK-STAT pathway under excessive glucose levels and is associated with glomerular expansion [47]. For example, H_2O_2 stimulates the activity of JAK family members, JAK2 and tyrosine kinase 2 (TYK2) [48].

The fundamental role of the JAK-STAT signal is originally established in lymphoid cells. However, this signal also has definitive roles in renal cells (i.e., glomerular mesangial cells, podocytes, and tubular epithelial cells) [49]. The overexpression of podocyte JAK2 results in the worsening of renal injury in mouse models of DKD [50]. As a bridge to clinical translation, the activation of JAK-STAT signaling is observed in the kidney of DKD patients. A transcriptomic investigation performed in glomerular samples obtained from subjects with DKD has shown that all downstream targets of JAK-STAT were highly expressed in the glomeruli of patients in comparison to healthy subjects. Notably, the degree of gene induction of the JAK-STAT pathway was tightly and inversely correlated with the decline in GFR. Moreover, Baricitinib, an inhibitor of the JAK family of protein tyrosine kinases that selectively inhibits JAK1 and JAK2, attenuates albuminuria in diabetic patients. As such, inhibiting oxidative stress may have the potential to block JAK-STAT signaling and the progression of DKD.

3.3. *Nrf2-Keap1*

The antioxidant defense mechanism (e.g., superoxide dismutase, glutathione reductase, glutathione peroxidase, and GSH) is essential for scavenging of ROS. However, this system is impaired in diabetes [51]. The defense response is mainly regulated by nuclear factor erythroid 2-related factor 2 (Nrf2), which governs the expression of antioxidants and detoxification enzymes. The cytosolic inhibitor Kelch-like ECH-associated protein 1 (Keap1) acts as a "sensor" for cellular oxidative stress. Keap1 is proposed to mediate Nrf2 activity via its capacity to inhibit Nrf2 nuclear translocation.

The upregulation of Nrf2-Keap1-dependent antioxidants attenuates renal oxidative overload. Notably, activation of Nrf2 improves histological findings in the glomerulus of streptozotocin-induced diabetic mice by attenuating oxidative stress, the expression of TGF-β1, and the production of extracellular matrix [52]. In addition, Nrf2 inhibits glucose-induced mesangial hypertrophy. Although the Nrf2 activator known as bardoxolone has been demonstrated to be reno-protective in patients with DKD, significant increase of heart failure was reported in the bardoxolone–treated group [53–55]. A clinical trial excluding high-risk patients is ongoing in Japan [56]. Moreover, bardoxolone is currently being studied in patients with Alport syndrome enrolled in the United States, Europe, Japan, and Australia. The potential to prevent or delay kidney function decline will be evaluated in these studies.

4. Targeting Oxidative Stress for the Prevention of DKD

Therapeutic options for the management of DKD are currently limited to systemic intervention for diabetes-related metabolic changes (i.e., hyperglycemia, hypertension, and dyslipidemia). Given the importance of oxidative stress for many of the pathological aspects of kidney injury, the redox imbalance could be a potential therapeutic target for the prevention of renal failure in diabetic patients. Several studies have shown that the inhibition of oxidative stress can prevent metabolic dysfunction, fibrotic signals, and proteinuria. Agents that are already in use in clinical practice such as statins, metformin, and thiazolidinediones have been demonstrated to suppress oxidative stress by inhibiting NADPH oxidase [57,58]. In addition to these drugs, recent clinical trials have established compelling evidence of beneficial cardiorenal outcomes of sodium glucose co-transporter 2 (SGLT2) inhibitors and glucagon-like peptide-1 (GLP-1) receptor agonists, beyond their glucose-lowering effect. The regulation of oxidative stress is one of the assumed mechanisms of the beneficial effects of these agents.

4.1. SGLT2 Inhibitors

SGLT2 inhibitors are a novel class of anti-hyperglycemic agents that are being used increasingly frequently for the management of diabetes. This drug blocks SGLT2 at the renal proximal tubule, leading to the limitation of glucose reabsorption of filtered glucose, which in turn results in glycosuria and blood glucose reduction. This effect is independent of the action of insulin. In addition to its glucose-lowering action, SGLT2 inhibitors induce natriuresis, thereby causing a reduction of blood pressure, improvement of glomerular hyperfiltration and albuminuria, at least in part, by activating tubuloglomerular feedback [59].

The Food and Drug Administration mandate the assessment of the cardiovascular safety of all novel hypoglycemic agents prior to seeking approval. The secondary outcome analyses in these trials have demonstrated the potential of SGLT2 inhibitors to reduce the risks of DKD and end-stage renal disease. Empagliflozin has been shown to improve renal composite outcomes (i.e., doubling of creatinine, renal replacement therapy, or renal death) in patients with type 2 diabetes [60]. Similar results were reported in trials with canagliflozin. The Canagliflozin and Renal Endpoints in Diabetes with Established Nephropathy Clinical Evaluation (CREDENCE) trial was conducted to investigate the efficacy and safety of canagliflozin for attenuating clinically important cardiorenal outcomes in patients with DKD [61]. Importantly, the CREDENCE trial was restricted to patients who were already taking the maximum tolerated dose of an angiotensin-converting enzyme inhibitor or angiotensin receptor blocker. A significant reduction was observed in the relative risk of the renal composite outcomes in subjects treated with canagliflozin. In addition to the renal benefits, the rates of cardiovascular death, myocardial infarction, or stroke and hospitalization for heart failure were lower in the canagliflozin group. Remarkably, there was no increase in the rates of amputation or bone fracture. Based on these large clinical trials, SGLT2 inhibitors are recommended for high-risk DKD patients with an estimated GFR of >30 mL/min/1.73 m^2 or urinary albumin excretion >30 mg/g creatinine (particularly >300 mg/g creatinine), to reduce the risk of DKD progression [3,62].

Decreased GSH levels and elevated oxidized glutathione (GSSG) levels are detected in the renal cortex of type 2 diabetic mice. Tanaka et al. showed that ipragliflozin treatment ameliorated albuminuria, glomerular expansion with the improvement of this redox imbalance [63]. The administration of empagliflozin also attenuated renal fibrosis, inflammation, as well as elevation of 8-OHdG in streptozotocin-induced diabetic mice [64]. Furthermore, the glucose-induced ROS generation was suppressed by siRNA against SGLT2 in tubular cells [65].

The basic mechanism to explain the effects on oxidative stress may involve anti-inflammatory actions of SGLT2 inhibitors [59]. Diabetic patients treated with canagliflozin showed lower plasma levels of TNF receptor and interleukin 6 in comparison to glimepiride group [66]. Animal studies also suggested anti-inflammatory actions of SGLT2 inhibitors. For example, empagliflozin significantly reduced mRNA levels of inflammatory mediators, such as monocyte chemoattractant protein 1 and interleukin 6 [67]. Additionally, SGLT2 inhibitors have been shown to modulate energy metabolism by inducing energy loss, fat utilization, and the browning of white adipose tissue [68]. Therefore, the beneficial effects of SGLT2 inhibitors on renal oxidative stress are partly mediated by weight loss, the improvement of insulin resistance, and the reduction of adipose tissue inflammation.

4.2. GLP-1 Receptor Agonists

GLP-1 is a gut-derived hormone secreted from intestinal L-cells upon meal ingestion that was originally found to mediate glucose handling by regulating the pancreatic islet cell activity, food intake, and gastrointestinal function. In addition to pancreatic β cells, the GLP-1 receptor is detected in renal tubular cells and the kidney vessels. Activation of GLP-1 receptor stimulates adenylate cyclase to drive the production of cAMP and protein kinase A (PKA) activation, primary effectors of GLP-1-mediated insulin secretion. Findings from small clinical studies as well as large cardiovascular safety trials with GLP-1 receptor agonists suggest its renoprotective effects, mainly in patients with macroalbuminuria [69–71]. However, no change was observed in renal hard endpoints, possibly due to low the incidence of renal death. It is reasonable to suggest that the beneficial actions of GLP-1 receptor agonists are partly through effects on body weight and associated risk factors for DKD. Similarly to SGLT2 inhibitors, natriuresis is induced by the GLP-1-mediated inhibition of the sodium-hydrogen exchanger 3, which is located at the brush border of the renal proximal tubule. In addition, GLP-1 receptor agonists improve dyslipidemia by reducing the production and secretion of intestinal chylomicrons. However, given the finding that beneficial effects of GLP-1 receptor agonists on albuminuria were observed even after adjustment for HbA1c and other traditional metabolic abnormalities, it is plausible that direct actions contributed to their effects on albuminuria.

Studies have shown that cAMP and PKA signaling are linked to the anti-oxidative response. GLP-1-mediated cAMP elevation demonstrates anti-oxidative effects by inhibiting AGE-RAGE signaling [72]. Therefore, it is likely that GLP-1 receptor agonists are protective against renal oxidative stress, independently of blood glucose levels. Indeed, disruption of the GLP-1 receptor in mice resulted in the progression of DKD with the elevation of renal NADPH and superoxide. Conversely, liraglutide suppressed these inductions through the actions on cAMP and PKA activity [73]. Of note, these improvements have been observed without major alterations in glucose metabolism, further supporting the hypothesis of direct renal effects of GLP-1 receptor agonists.

5. Conclusions and Future Perspectives

Given the high mortality of DKD and increased healthcare costs, kidney protection is a critical issue in the management of diabetes. There is now satisfactory evidence to illustrate the causal link between oxidative stress and the progression of DKD. When considered alongside the fact that it is still difficult to diagnose at an early stage due to a lack of reliable biomarkers, serum or urinary oxidative stress markers may be useful for making a diagnosis of DKD, especially with the combination of urinary albumin levels. Whether redox imbalance is either a trigger or consequence of DKD progression is still debated. However, it is conceivable that it is both. Experimental studies using gene deletion models of specific enzymes or kinases have greatly expanded our understanding of oxidative stress. In addition to traditional antioxidants such as vitamin C and E, clinical and experimental data support the possibility that novel classes of anti-hyperglycemic agents have beneficial effects on oxidative stress and the renal outcome. In particular, SGLT2 inhibitors and GLP-1 receptor agonists are potential pharmaceuticals that could reduce renal oxidative stress through direct or indirect actions. A robust understanding of the mechanism underlying these agents' renal benefits will be required to facilitate the establishment of novel therapeutic strategies against DKD.

Author Contributions: K.M. wrote the manuscript. Y.T., Y.N., T.Y., K.U., and R.N. helped edit the manuscript and revised the manuscript for important intellectual content. All authors have read and agreed to the published version of the manuscript.

Funding: This work was supported by a Grant-in-Aid for Scientific Research from Japan Society for the Promotion of Science (to Keiichiro Matoba and Rimei Nishimura), the MSD Life Science Foundation (to Keiichiro Matoba), and the Takeda Science Foundation (to Keiichiro Matoba), along with the Suzuken Memorial Foundation (to Keiichiro Matoba).

Conflicts of Interest: Keiichiro Matoba has received research support from Sanofi KK, Tanabe Pharma, and Takeda Pharmaceutical. Kazunori Utsunomiya has received research support from Terumo, Novo Nordisk Pharma, Taisho Pharmaceutical, Böehringer Ingelheim, Kyowa Hakko Kirin, Sumitomo Dainippon Pharma, and Ono Pharmaceutical as well as speaker honoraria from Tanabe Pharma, Sanofi KK, Sumitomo Dainippon Pharma, Eli Lilly, and Böehringer Ingelheim. Rimei Nishimura has received speaker honoraria from Astellas Pharma, Nippon Boehringer Ingelheim, Eli Lilly Japan KK, Kissei Pharmaceutical, Medtronic Japan, MSD, Novartis Pharma KK, Novo Nordisk Pharma, Sanofi KK, and Takeda Pharmaceutical and contract research fees for collaborative research with the Japan Diabetes Foundation.

References

1. Gaps in Access to Diabetes Medicines and Supplies Continue to Dominate. International Diabetes Federation. Available online: https://www.idf.org/e-library/diabetes-voice/archive/125-july-2017-improving-access-to-diabetes-care.html?layout=article&aid=347 (accessed on 22 February 2020).
2. Huang, Y.; Karuranga, S.; Malanda, B.; Williams, D. Call for data contribution to the IDF Diabetes Atlas 9th Edition 2019. *Diabetes Res. Clin. Pract.* **2018**, *140*, 351–352. [CrossRef]
3. American Diabetes Association 11. Microvascular Complications and Foot Care: Standards of Medical Care in Diabetes-2020. *Diabetes Care* **2020**, *43*, S135–S151. [CrossRef] [PubMed]
4. Saran, R.; Robinson, B.; Abbott, K.C.; Agodoa, L.Y.; Bhave, N.; Bragg-Gresham, J.; Balkrishnan, R.; Dietrich, X.; Eckard, A.; Eggers, P.W.; et al. US Renal Data System 2017 Annual Data Report: Epidemiology of Kidney Disease in the United States. *Am. J. Kidney Dis.* **2018**, *71*, A7. [CrossRef] [PubMed]
5. Fox, C.S.; Matsushita, K.; Woodward, M.; Bilo, H.J.G.; Chalmers, J.; Heerspink, H.J.L.; Lee, B.J.; Perkins, R.M.; Rossing, P.; Sairenchi, T.; et al. Associations of kidney disease measures with mortality and end-stage renal disease in individuals with and without diabetes: a meta-analysis. *Lancet* **2012**, *380*, 1662–1673. [CrossRef]
6. Kingma, J.; Simard, D.; Rouleau, J. Renocardiac syndromes: physiopathology and treatment stratagems. *Can. J. Kidney Health Dis.* **2015**, *2*, 41. [CrossRef]
7. Adler, A.I.; Stevens, R.J.; Manley, S.E.; Bilous, R.W.; Cull, C.A.; Holman, R.R. UKPDS Group Development and progression of nephropathy in type 2 diabetes: The United Kingdom Prospective Diabetes Study (UKPDS 64). *Kidney Int.* **2003**, *63*, 225–232. [CrossRef]
8. Kawanami, D.; Matoba, K.; Utsunomiya, K. Signaling pathways in diabetic nephropathy. *Histol. Histopathol.* **2016**, *31*, 1059–1067.
9. Gæde, P.H.; Lund-Andersen, H.; Parving, H.-H.; Pedersen, O. Effect of a Multifactorial Intervention on Mortality in Type 2 Diabetes. *N. Engl. J. Med.* **2008**, *358*, 580–591.
10. Ueki, K.; Sasako, T.; Okazaki, Y.; Kato, M.; Okahata, S.; Katsuyama, H.; Haraguchi, M.; Morita, A.; Ohashi, K.; Hara, K.; et al. Effect of an intensified multifactorial intervention on cardiovascular outcomes and mortality in type 2 diabetes (J-DOIT3): an open-label, randomised controlled trial. *Lancet Diabetes Endocrinol.* **2017**, *5*, 951–964. [CrossRef]
11. Wan, C.; Su, H.; Zhang, C. Role of NADPH Oxidase in Metabolic Disease-Related Renal Injury: An Update. *Oxidative Med. Cell. Longev.* **2016**, *2016*, 1–8. [CrossRef]
12. Tang, W.H.; Martin, K.A.; Hwa, J. Aldose Reductase, Oxidative Stress, and Diabetic Mellitus. *Front. Pharmacol.* **2012**, *3*, 87. [CrossRef] [PubMed]
13. Kasajima, H.; Yamagishi, S.-I.; Sugai, S.; Yagihashi, N.; Yagihashi, S. Enhanced in situ expression of aldose reductase in peripheral nerve and renal glomeruli in diabetic patients. *Virchows Archiv* **2001**, *439*, 46–54. [CrossRef] [PubMed]
14. Haneda, M.; Kikkawa, R.; Arimura, T.; Ebata, K.; Togawa, M.; Maeda, S.; Sawada, T.; Horide, N.; Shigeta, Y. Glucose inhibits myo-inositol uptake and reduces myo-inositol content in cultured rat glomerular mesangial cells. *Metabolism* **1990**, *39*, 40–45. [CrossRef]
15. Hotta, N. New concepts and insights on pathogenesis and treatment of diabetic complications: polyol pathway and its inhibition. *Nagoya J. Med. Sci.* **1997**, *60*, 89–100. [PubMed]

16. He, J.; Gao, H.-X.; Yang, N.; Zhu, X.-D.; Sun, R.-B.; Xie, Y.; Zeng, C.-H.; Zhang, J.; Wang, J.-K.; Ding, F.; et al. The aldose reductase inhibitor epalrestat exerts nephritic protection on diabetic nephropathy in db/db mice through metabolic modulation. *Acta Pharmacol. Sin.* **2018**, *40*, 86–97. [CrossRef] [PubMed]
17. Liu, H.; Luo, Y.; Zhang, T.; Zhang, Y.; Wu, Q.; Yuan, L.; Chung, S.S.M.; Oates, P.J.; Yang, J.Y. Genetic deficiency of aldose reductase counteracts the development of diabetic nephropathy in C57BL/6 mice. *Diabetologia* **2011**, *54*, 1242–1251. [CrossRef]
18. Dunlop, M.E. Aldose reductase and the role of the polyol pathway in diabetic nephropathy. *Kidney Int.* **2000**, *58*, S3–S12. [CrossRef]
19. Singh, C.K.; Chhabra, G.; Ndiaye, M.A.; Garcia-Peterson, L.M.; Mack, N.J.; Ahmad, N. The Role of Sirtuins in Antioxidant and Redox Signaling. *Antioxid. Redox Signal.* **2018**, *28*, 643–661. [CrossRef]
20. Turkmen, K.; Karagoz, A.; Kucuk, A. Sirtuins as novel players in the pathogenesis of diabetes mellitus. *World J. Diabetes* **2014**, *5*, 894–900. [CrossRef]
21. Güçlü, A.; Erdur, F.; Turkmen, K. The Emerging Role of Sirtuin 1 in Cellular Metabolism, Diabetes Mellitus, Diabetic Kidney Disease and Hypertension. *Exp. Clin. Endocrinol. Diabetes* **2015**, *124*, 131–139.
22. Schleicher, E.D.; Weigert, C. Role of the hexosamine biosynthetic pathway in diabetic nephropathy. *Kidney Int.* **2000**, *58*, S13–S18. [CrossRef] [PubMed]
23. Jokela, T.A.; Makkonen, K.M.; Oikari, S.; Kärnä, R.; Koli, E.; Hart, G.W.; Tammi, R.H.; Carlberg, C.; Tammi, M.I. Cellular Content of UDP-N-acetylhexosamines Controls Hyaluronan Synthase 2 Expression and Correlates with O-Linked N-Acetylglucosamine Modification of Transcription Factors YY1 and SP1*. *J. Biol. Chem.* **2011**, *286*, 33632–33640. [CrossRef] [PubMed]
24. Matoba, K.; Kawanami, D.; Okada, R.; Tsukamoto, M.; Kinoshita, J.; Ito, T.; Ishizawa, S.; Kanazawa, Y.; Yokota, T.; Murai, N.; et al. Rho-kinase inhibition prevents the progression of diabetic nephropathy by downregulating hypoxia-inducible factor 1α. *Kidney Int.* **2013**, *84*, 545–554. [CrossRef]
25. Kolm-Litty, V.; Sauer, U.; Nerlich, A.G.; Lehmann, R.; Schleicher, E.D. High glucose-induced transforming growth factor beta1 production is mediated by the hexosamine pathway in porcine glomerular mesangial cells. *J. Clin. Investig.* **1998**, *101*, 160–169. [CrossRef] [PubMed]
26. Singh, L.P.; Cheng, D.W.; Kowluru, R.; Levi, E.; Jiang, Y. Hexosamine induction of oxidative stress, hypertrophy and laminin expression in renal mesangial cells: effect of the anti-oxidant α-lipoic acid. *Cell Biochem. Funct.* **2007**, *25*, 537–550. [CrossRef]
27. James, L.R.; Tang, D.; Ingram, A.; Ly, H.; Thai, K.; Cai, L.; Scholey, J.W. Flux through the hexosamine pathway is a determinant of nuclear factor kappaB- dependent promoter activation. *Diabetes* **2002**, *51*, 1146–1156. [CrossRef]
28. Suryavanshi, S.V.; Kulkarni, Y.A. NF-kappabeta: A potential target in the management of vascular complications of diabetes. *Front. Pharmacol.* **2017**, *8*, 798. [CrossRef]
29. Huwiler, A.; Schulze-Lohoff, E.; Fabbro, D.; Pfeilschifter, J. Immunocharacterization of protein kinase C isoenzymes in rat kidney glomeruli, and cultured glomerular epithelial and mesangial cells. *Exp. Nephrol.* **1993**, *1*, 19–25.
30. Ohshiro, Y.; Ma, R.C.; Yasuda, Y.; Hiraoka-Yamamoto, J.; Clermont, A.C.; Isshiki, K.; Yagi, K.; Arikawa, E.; Kern, T.S.; King, G.L. Reduction of diabetes-induced oxidative stress, fibrotic cytokine expression, and renal dysfunction in protein kinase C beta-null mice. *Diabetes* **2006**, *55*, 3112–3120. [CrossRef]
31. Akamine, T.; Takaku, S.; Suzuki, M.; Niimi, N.; Yako, H.; Matoba, K.; Kawanami, D.; Utsunomiya, K.; Nishimura, R.; Sango, K. Glycolaldehyde induces sensory neuron death through activation of the c-Jun N-terminal kinase and p-38 MAP kinase pathways. *Histochem. Cell Biol.* **2019**, 1–9. [CrossRef]
32. Yamamoto, Y.; Kato, I.; Doi, T.; Yonekura, H.; Ohashi, S.; Takeuchi, M.; Watanabe, T.; Yamagishi, S.; Sakurai, S.; Takasawa, S.; et al. Development and prevention of advanced diabetic nephropathy in RAGE-overexpressing mice. *J. Clin. Investig.* **2001**, *108*, 261–268. [CrossRef] [PubMed]
33. Matsui, T.; Higashimoto, Y.; Nishino, Y.; Nakamura, N.; Fukami, K.; Yamagishi, S.-I. RAGE-Aptamer Blocks the Development and Progression of Experimental Diabetic Nephropathy. *Diabetes* **2017**, *66*, 1683–1695. [CrossRef] [PubMed]
34. Sanajou, D.; Ghorbanihaghjo, A.; Argani, H.; Aslani, S. AGE-RAGE axis blockade in diabetic nephropathy: Current status and future directions. *Eur. J. Pharmacol.* **2018**, *833*, 158–164. [CrossRef] [PubMed]
35. Matoba, K.; Kawanami, D.; Nagai, Y.; Takeda, Y.; Akamine, T.; Ishizawa, S.; Kanazawa, Y.; Yokota, T.; Utsunomiya, K. Rho-Kinase Blockade Attenuates Podocyte Apoptosis by Inhibiting the Notch Signaling Pathway in Diabetic Nephropathy. *Int. J. Mol. Sci.* **2017**, *18*, 1795. [CrossRef] [PubMed]

36. Nagai, Y.; Kawanami, D.; Matoba, K.; Takeda, Y.; Utsunomiya, K. 505-P: ROCK2 Regulates TGF-Beta-Induced Expression of CTGF and Profibrotic Genes via NF-kappa B and Cytoskeleton Dynamics in the Mesangial Cells. *Diabetes* **2019**, *68*, 505. [CrossRef]
37. Takeda, Y.; Matoba, K.; Kawanami, D.; Nagai, Y.; Akamine, T.; Ishizawa, S.; Kanazawa, Y.; Yokota, T.; Utsunomiya, K. ROCK2 Regulates Monocyte Migration and Cell to Cell Adhesion in Vascular Endothelial Cells. *Int. J. Mol. Sci.* **2019**, *20*, 1331. [CrossRef]
38. Matoba, K.; Kawanami, D.; Tsukamoto, M.; Kinoshita, J.; Ito, T.; Ishizawa, S.; Kanazawa, Y.; Yokota, T.; Murai, N.; Matsufuji, S.; et al. Rho-kinase regulation of TNF-alpha-induced nuclear translocation of NF-kappaB RelA/p65 and M-CSF expression via p38 MAPK in mesangial cells. *Am. J. Physiol. Ren. Physiol.* **2014**, *307*, F571–F580. [CrossRef]
39. Yokota, T.; Utsunomiya, K.; Taniguchi, K.; Gojo, A.; Kurata, H.; Tajima, N. Involvement of the Rho/Rho Kinase Signaling Pathway in Platelet-Derived Growth Factor BB-induced Vascular Endothelial Growth Factor Expression in Diabetic Rat Retina. *Jpn. J. Ophthalmol.* **2007**, *51*, 424–430. [CrossRef]
40. Kanazawa, Y.; Takahashi-Fujigasaki, J.; Ishizawa, S.; Takabayashi, N.; Ishibashi, K.; Matoba, K.; Kawanami, D.; Yokota, T.; Tajima, N.; Utsunomiya, K. The Rho-kinase inhibitor fasudil restores normal motor nerve conduction velocity in diabetic rats by assuring the proper localization of adhesion-related molecules in myelinating Schwann cells. *Exp. Neurol.* **2013**, *247*, 438–446. [CrossRef]
41. Kawanami, D.; Matoba, K.; Okada, R.; Tsukamoto, M.; Kinoshita, J.; Ishizawa, S.; Kanazawa, Y.; Yokota, T.; Utsunomiya, K. Fasudil inhibits ER stress-induced VCAM-1 expression by modulating unfolded protein response in endothelial cells. *Biochem. Biophys. Res. Commun.* **2013**, *435*, 171–175. [CrossRef]
42. Shimizu, Y.; Thumkeo, D.; Keel, J.; Ishizaki, T.; Oshima, H.; Oshima, M.; Noda, Y.; Matsumura, F.; Taketo, M.M.; Narumiya, S. ROCK-I regulates closure of the eyelids and ventral body wall by inducing assembly of actomyosin bundles. *J. Cell Biol.* **2005**, *168*, 941–953. [CrossRef] [PubMed]
43. Thumkeo, D.; Keel, J.; Ishizaki, T.; Hirose, M.; Nonomura, K.; Oshima, H.; Oshima, M.; Taketo, M.M.; Narumiya, S. Targeted Disruption of the Mouse Rho-Associated Kinase 2 Gene Results in Intrauterine Growth Retardation and Fetal Death. *Mol. Cell. Biol.* **2003**, *23*, 5043–5055. [CrossRef] [PubMed]
44. Gojo, A.; Utsunomiya, K.; Taniguchi, K.; Yokota, T.; Ishizawa, S.; Kanazawa, Y.; Kurata, H.; Tajima, N. The Rho-kinase inhibitor, fasudil, attenuates diabetic nephropathy in streptozotocin-induced diabetic rats. *Eur. J. Pharmacol.* **2007**, *568*, 242–247. [CrossRef] [PubMed]
45. Matoba, K.; Takeda, Y.; Nagai, Y.; Kawanami, D.; Utsunomiya, K.; Nishimura, R. Unraveling the Role of Inflammation in the Pathogenesis of Diabetic Kidney Disease. *Int. J. Mol. Sci.* **2019**, *20*, 3393. [CrossRef] [PubMed]
46. Toth-Manikowski, S.; Atta, M.G. Diabetic Kidney Disease: Pathophysiology and Therapeutic Targets. *J. Diabetes Res.* **2015**, *2015*, 1–16. [CrossRef] [PubMed]
47. Gloire, G.; Legrand-Poels, S.; Piette, J. NF-κB activation by reactive oxygen species: Fifteen years later. *Biochem. Pharmacol.* **2006**, *72*, 1493–1505. [CrossRef] [PubMed]
48. Simon, A.R.; Rai, U.; Fanburg, B.L.; Cochran, B. Activation of the JAK-STAT pathway by reactive oxygen species. *Am. J. Physiol. Content* **1998**, *275*, C1640–C1652. [CrossRef]
49. Tuttle, K.R.; Brosius, F.C., 3rd; Adler, S.G.; Kretzler, M.; Mehta, R.L.; Tumlin, J.A.; Tanaka, Y.; Haneda, M.; Liu, J.; Silk, M.E.; et al. JAK1/JAK2 inhibition by baricitinib in diabetic kidney disease: results from a Phase 2 randomized controlled clinical trial. *Nephrol. Dial. Transplant.* **2018**, *33*, 1950–1959. [CrossRef]
50. Zhang, H.; Nair, V.; Saha, J.; Atkins, K.B.; Hodgin, J.B.; Saunders, T.L.; Myers, M.G.; Werner, T.; Kretzler, M.; Brosius, F.C. Podocyte-specific JAK2 overexpression worsens diabetic kidney disease in mice. *Kidney Int.* **2017**, *92*, 909–921. [CrossRef]
51. David, J.A.; Rifkin, W.J.; Rabbani, P.S.; Ceradini, D.J. The Nrf2/Keap1/ARE pathway and oxidative stress as a therapeutic target in type II diabetes mellitus. *J. Diabetes Res.* **2017**, *2017*, 4826724.
52. Zheng, H.; Whitman, S.A.; Wu, W.; Wondrak, G.T.; Wong, P.K.; Fang, D.; Zhang, D.D. Therapeutic Potential of Nrf2 Activators in Streptozotocin-Induced Diabetic Nephropathy. *Diabetes* **2011**, *60*, 3055–3066. [CrossRef] [PubMed]
53. Pergola, P.E.; Raskin, P.; Toto, R.D.; Meyer, C.J.; Huff, J.W.; Grossman, E.B.; Krauth, M.; Ruiz, S.; Audhya, P.; Christ-Schmidt, H.; et al. Bardoxolone Methyl and Kidney Function in CKD with Type 2 Diabetes. *N. Engl. J. Med.* **2011**, *365*, 327–336. [CrossRef] [PubMed]

54. De Zeeuw, D.; Akizawa, T.; Audhya, P.; Bakris, G.L.; Chin, M.; Christ-Schmidt, H.; Goldsberry, A.; Houser, M.; Krauth, M.; Heerspink, H.J.L.; et al. Bardoxolone methyl in type 2 diabetes and stage 4 chronic kidney disease. *N. Engl. J. Med.* **2013**, *369*, 2492–2503. [CrossRef]
55. Chin, M.P.; Bakris, G.L.; Block, G.A.; Chertow, G.M.; Goldsberry, A.; Inker, L.A.; Heerspink, H.J.; O'Grady, M.; Pergola, P.E.; Wanner, C.; et al. Bardoxolone Methyl Improves Kidney Function in Patients with Chronic Kidney Disease Stage 4 and Type 2 Diabetes: Post-Hoc Analyses from Bardoxolone Methyl Evaluation in Patients with Chronic Kidney Disease and Type 2 Diabetes Study. *Am. J. Nephrol.* **2018**, *47*, 40–47. [CrossRef] [PubMed]
56. Hirakawa, Y.; Tanaka, T.; Nangaku, M. Mechanisms of metabolic memory and renal hypoxia as a therapeutic target in diabetic kidney disease. *J. Diabetes Investig.* **2017**, *8*, 261–271. [CrossRef] [PubMed]
57. Bruder-Nascimento, T.; Callera, G.E.; Montezano, A.C.; De Chantemele, E.J.B.; Tostes, R.C.; Touyz, R.M. Atorvastatin inhibits pro-inflammatory actions of aldosterone in vascular smooth muscle cells by reducing oxidative stress. *Life Sci.* **2019**, *221*, 29–34. [CrossRef] [PubMed]
58. An, H.; Wei, R.; Ke, J.; Yang, J.; Liu, Y.; Wang, X.; Wang, G.; Hong, T. Metformin attenuates fluctuating glucose-induced endothelial dysfunction through enhancing GTPCH1-mediated eNOS recoupling and inhibiting NADPH oxidase. *J. Diabetes Complicat.* **2016**, *30*, 1017–1024. [CrossRef]
59. Kawanami, D.; Matoba, K.; Takeda, Y.; Nagai, Y.; Akamine, T.; Yokota, T.; Sango, K.; Utsunomiya, K. SGLT2 Inhibitors as a Therapeutic Option for Diabetic Nephropathy. *Int. J. Mol. Sci.* **2017**, *18*, 1083. [CrossRef]
60. Wanner, C.; Inzucchi, S.E.; Lachin, J.M.; Fitchett, D.; Von Eynatten, M.; Mattheus, M.; Johansen, O.E.; Woerle, H.J.; Broedl, U.C.; Zinman, B. Empagliflozin and Progression of Kidney Disease in Type 2 Diabetes. *N. Engl. J. Med.* **2016**, *375*, 323–334. [CrossRef]
61. Perkovic, V.; Jardine, M.J.; Neal, B.; Bompoint, S.; Heerspink, H.J.; Charytan, D.M.; Edwards, R.; Agarwal, R.; Bakris, G.; Bull, S.; et al. Canagliflozin and Renal Outcomes in Type 2 Diabetes and Nephropathy. *N. Engl. J. Med.* **2019**, *380*, 2295–2306. [CrossRef]
62. Buse, J.B.; Wexler, D.J.; Tsapas, A.; Rossing, P.; Mingrone, G.; Mathieu, C.; D'Alessio, D.A.; Davies, M. 2019 update to: Management of hyperglycaemia in type 2 diabetes, 2018. A consensus report by the American Diabetes Association (ADA) and the European Association for the Study of Diabetes (EASD). *Diabetologia* **2020**, *63*, 221–228. [CrossRef]
63. Tanaka, S.; Sugiura, Y.; Saito, H.; Sugahara, M.; Higashijima, Y.; Yamaguchi, J.; Inagi, R.; Suematsu, M.; Nangaku, M.; Tanaka, T. Sodium–glucose cotransporter 2 inhibition normalizes glucose metabolism and suppresses oxidative stress in the kidneys of diabetic mice. *Kidney Int.* **2018**, *94*, 912–925. [CrossRef]
64. Ojima, A.; Matsui, T.; Nishino, Y.; Nakamura, N.; Yamagishi, S. Empagliflozin, an Inhibitor of Sodium-Glucose Cotransporter 2 Exerts Anti-Inflammatory and Antifibrotic Effects on Experimental Diabetic Nephropathy Partly by Suppressing AGEs-Receptor Axis. *Horm. Metab. Res.* **2015**, *47*, 686–692. [CrossRef]
65. Maeda, S.; Matsui, T.; Takeuchi, M.; Yamagishi, S.-I. Sodium-glucose cotransporter 2-mediated oxidative stress augments advanced glycation end products-induced tubular cell apoptosis. *Diabetes/Metab. Res. Rev.* **2013**, *29*, 406–412. [CrossRef]
66. Heerspink, H.J.L.; Perco, P.; Mulder, S.; Leierer, J.; Hansen, M.K.; Heinzel, A.; Mayer, G. Canagliflozin reduces inflammation and fibrosis biomarkers: a potential mechanism of action for beneficial effects of SGLT2 inhibitors in diabetic kidney disease. *Diabetologia* **2019**, *62*, 1154–1166. [CrossRef]
67. Vallon, V.; Gerasimova, M.; Rose, M.A.; Masuda, T.; Satriano, J.; Mayoux, E.; Koepsell, H.; Thomson, S.C.; Rieg, T. SGLT2 inhibitor empagliflozin reduces renal growth and albuminuria in proportion to hyperglycemia and prevents glomerular hyperfiltration in diabetic Akita mice. *Am. J. Physiol. Physiol.* **2013**, *306*, F194–F204. [CrossRef]
68. Xu, L.; Nagata, N.; Nagashimada, M.; Zhuge, F.; Ni, Y.; Chen, G.; Mayoux, E.; Kaneko, S.; Ota, T. SGLT2 Inhibition by Empagliflozin Promotes Fat Utilization and Browning and Attenuates Inflammation and Insulin Resistance by Polarizing M2 Macrophages in Diet-induced Obese Mice. *EBioMedicine* **2017**, *20*, 137–149. [CrossRef]
69. Kawanami, D.; Matoba, K.; Sango, K.; Utsunomiya, K. Incretin-Based Therapies for Diabetic Complications: Basic Mechanisms and Clinical Evidence. *Int. J. Mol. Sci.* **2016**, *17*, 1223. [CrossRef]
70. Greco, E.V.; Russo, G.T.; Giandalia, A.; Viazzi, F.; Pontremoli, R.; De Cosmo, S. GLP-1 Receptor Agonists and Kidney Protection. *Medicina* **2019**, *55*, 233. [CrossRef]

71. Marso, S.P.; Bain, S.; Consoli, A.; Eliaschewitz, F.G.; Jódar, E.; Leiter, L.; Lingvay, I.; Rosenstock, J.; Seufert, J.; Warren, M.L.; et al. Semaglutide and Cardiovascular Outcomes in Patients with Type 2 Diabetes. *N. Engl. J. Med.* **2016**, *375*, 1834–1844. [CrossRef]
72. Sourris, K.C.; Yao, H.; Jerums, G.; Cooper, M.E.; Ekinci, E.I.; Coughlan, M.T. Can targeting the incretin pathway dampen RAGE-mediated events in diabetic nephropathy? *Curr. Drug Targets* **2016**, *17*, 1252–1264. [CrossRef]
73. Fujita, H.; Morii, T.; Fujishima, H.; Sato, T.; Shimizu, T.; Hosoba, M.; Tsukiyama, K.; Narita, T.; Takahashi, T.; Drucker, D.J.; et al. The protective roles of GLP-1R signaling in diabetic nephropathy: possible mechanism and therapeutic potential. *Kidney Int.* **2014**, *85*, 579–589. [CrossRef]

MDPI
St. Alban-Anlage 66
4052 Basel
Switzerland
Tel. +41 61 683 77 34
Fax +41 61 302 89 18
www.mdpi.com

Biomedicines Editorial Office
E-mail: biomedicines@mdpi.com
www.mdpi.com/journal/biomedicines

MDPI

www.ingramcontent.com/pod-product-compliance
Lightning Source LLC
LaVergne TN
LVHW070047120526
838202LV00101B/1505
* 9 7 8 3 0 3 6 5 6 0 2 3 6 *